THE WHOLE INTERNIST CATALOG

A COMPENDIUM OF CLUES TO DIAGNOSIS AND MANAGEMENT

ARLAN J. GOTTLIEB, M.D.
KENNETH W. ZAMKOFF, M.D.
MICHAEL S. JASTREMSKI, M.D.
ANTHONY SCALZO, M.D.
KENNETH J. IMBODEN, M.D.

All of the University of New York
Upstate Medical Center and
Veterans Administration Medical Center
Syracuse, New York

1980

W.B. SAUNDERS COMPANY

PHILADELPHIA   LONDON   TORONTO

W. B. Saunders Company: West Washington Square
Philadelphia, PA 19105

1 St. Anne's Road
Eastbourne, East Sussex BN 21 3UN, England

1 Goldthorne Avenue
Toronto, Ontario M8Z 5T9, Canada

Library of Congress Cataloging in Publication Data

Gottlieb, Arlan J
  The whole internist catalog.

  1. Internal medicine. I. Title.
RC46.G57   616   79-66034
ISBN 0-7216-4179-2

The Whole Internist Catalog   ISBN 0-7216-4179-2

Last digit is the print number: 9   8   7   6   5   4   3   2   1

To those who seek better ways to care for the sick

If you wish to suggest an article for the 2nd Volume (a helpful hint, practical advice, or whatever), please cut out this page and send it to the first-named author with the information and your name and address. Credit will be given to you if the item is used.

> To: Arlan J. Gottlieb, M.D.
> Division of Hematology
> State University of New York
> Upstate Medical Center
> 750 East Adams Street
> Syracuse, New York 13210

I wish to suggest the following article for the 2nd Volume of THE WHOLE INTERNIST CATALOG:

(Name) _____

_____

_____

PREFACE

There are many excellent, comprehensive formal textbooks of internal medicine and its subspecialties. This volume has not been written to replace any of them, nor is it meant to be a comprehensive manual of procedures, therapeutics, or laboratory medicine. We have tried to present answers to some common, practical problems. In addition, we have sought to provide information that, once discovered, has always seemed hard to find a second time.

The contents are drawn from many sources including textbooks, journals, magazines, and opinion. In the process of translating these materials we hope we have neither oversimplified them nor been too editorial. It is our belief that medicine should be practiced with both a concern for the patient and a zest for learning. The content and style of the book attempts to convey this enthusiasm to the reader.

We believe this book would be most useful if the readers would spend some time familiarizing themselves with its contents; it will then be ready when needed. The references provided are not meant to be complete, but represent a "starter set" for a literature review.

We stopped because we were tired — not because we were through. There's much more to be said, and enough material has been collected for a second volume. We would appreciate hearing from you concerning what you would like to see included in a second volume as well as your thoughts on this one.

Our thanks to our colleagues at the Upstate Medical Center for their contributions.

ARLAN J. GOTTLIEB
KENNETH W. ZAMKOFF
MICHAEL S. JASTREMSKI
ANTHONY J. SCALZO
KENNETH J. IMBODEN

ACKNOWLEDG-MENTS

As the adult develops from the child, *The Whole Internist Catalog* grew from *The Whole Pediatrician Catalog* by McMillan, Nieburg, and Oski. We are most grateful to Frank Oski, M.D., for his help in initiating this project as well as his encouragement and suggestions throughout the course of the work. Our thanks to the medical house staff and students whose curiosity made it necessary to find these answers and to Jack Hanley, Dave McCraw, and Joanne Shore of Saunders for their help.

The highly entertaining book by Wilfred Funk, *Word Origins and Their Romantic Stories* (published in 1978 by Bell Publishing Company, New York), served as the source of the majority of the word derivations.

An extensive listing of medical aphorisms, including many of those employed in this volume, has been compiled by Robert Matz, M.D., and published in the *Journal of the American Medical Association.*

The Word Processing Center of The Department of Medicine, Upstate Medical Center, under the direction of Ms. Margaret Snyder, provided invaluable assistance with the drafts and redrafts of manuscript as did Miss Margaret King, Stephanie Laskey, Evelyn Phillips, and Janet Rayo.

Finally, our special thanks to Paul Kronenberg, M.D., for his participation at the time of pubescence.

There is no heavier burden than a great potential.

LINUS VAN PELT (PEANUTS)

CONTENTS

1
APPROACH TO THE PATIENT

THE CHIEF COMPLAINTS

It would be wise for the medical community to heed the example set by commercial organizations and review the complaints most frequently voiced by patients. A survey of such complaints was recently compiled from responses of 300 patients who voted "Always," "Sometimes," or "Never" in describing the frequency of a complaint. The ten most common complaints are as follows:

1. Doctors are more interested in disease than in health. (Most votes: "Always")
2. Doctors fail to keep appointment times. (Most votes: "Always")
3. Office staff members give patients little or no respect. (Most votes: "Always")
4. Doctors act like God. (Most votes: "Always")
5. Doctors and staff give no privacy. (Most votes: "Sometimes")
6. Fees are not explained on statements. (Most votes: "Sometimes")
7. Doctors abuse investigatory techniques. (Most votes: "Sometimes")
8. Office hours inadequate. (Most votes: "Sometimes")
9. Medical problems are not adequately explained. (Most votes: "Sometimes")
10. Inadequate waiting room facilities. (Most votes: "Never")

Reference: Physician's Management, February 1978, p. 39.

ASCLEPIUS–THE FIRST DOCTOR

Asclepius was the son of Apollo and Coronis. Just prior to her delivery, Coronis decided to marry a fellow mortal. In a jealous rage, Apollo put Coronis and her husband to death. Apollo rescued the yet unborn Asclepius from the mother's funeral pyre and remanded the child to the care of the centaur Chiron. From Chiron, Asclepius learned the science and art of medicine and became world renowned as a healer. He was armed by the blood of the Gorgons (given to him by Athene) and a magical plant cure (learned from a serpent). When the dead were brought to life by Asclepius' healing powers, Hades complained. Zeus agreed that the lot of mortals was to follow their destiny and that

Patient's Rule *(concerning his symptoms):*
It's not a matter of life or death — it's much more important than that.

Asclepius was guilty of defiling the order of nature. Accordingly, Asclepius was struck dead with a thunderbolt. An outraged Apollo revenged his son's death by exterminating the Cyclops who had forged the thunderbolt.

Asclepius had two sons, both of whom took part in the Trojan War as physicians. His daughters, Iaso, Panacea, Aegle, and Hygieia were also closely associated with the healing cult. Asclepius was sometimes portrayed as a serpent god, but more often as a friendly, compassionate, learned man. He ultimately was enshrined among the stars. His daughter, Hygieia, became the goddess of health and, with Panacea, Asclepius, and Apollo, is remembered in the Hippocratic Oath.

WHAT THE MIND DOES NOT KNOW THE NOSE WILL NOT SMELL

Occasionally a particular disease or ingestion of a toxic substance is suggested by the odor of a patient's body or breath.

ODOR	PRODUCT OR DISEASE STATE
Acetone	Diabetes mellitus
Acrid (pear-like)	Paraldehyde
Alcohol (fruit-like)	Alcohol
Ammonia (urine)	Uremia, cholera
Bitter almonds	Cyanide
Cottage cheese	Tophaceous gout
Cinnamon	Pulmonary tuberculosis
Disinfectants	Phenol, creosote
Feces (putrid)	Anerobic infections
Foul armpits	Paratyphoid fever
Garlic	Malathion, parathion, arsenic, phosphorus, tellurium
Halitosis	Acute illness, poor dental hygiene, sinusitis, gastric malignancy
Honey	Pemphigus vulgaris
Mice	Diphtheria
Musty fish (raw liver)	Hepatic failure
Pungent, aromatic	Ethchlorvynol (Placidyl)
Rotten eggs	Hydrogen sulfide, mercaptans
Shoe polish	Nitrobenzene
Sweet	Pseudomonas
Sweet acetone (russet apples)	Lacquer, alcohol, ketoacidosis, chloroform
Stale tobacco	Nicotine
Violets	Turpentine
Wet leaves	Pulmonary tuberculosis
Wintergreen	Methyl salicylate

> *Mentor* — Means a wise and sage teacher. Mentor was the friend to whom Ulysses (Odysseus) entrusted care of his hearth and home prior to leaving on his trip. Zeus chose to assume Mentor's form to counsel Telemachus, Ulysses' son, when things went badly for *chez* Ulysses and faithful Penelope.

PERFORATE NASAL SEPTUM

1. Cocaine abuse
2. Nasal spray abuse
3. Wegener's granulomatosis and lethal midline granuloma
4. Vasculitis
5. Leprosy
6. Tuberculosis
7. Syphilis
8. Nasal surgery
9. Prolonged nasogastric intubation
10. Self-mutilation

CLUBBING

It is hard to decide whether a midsystolic click or clubbing of the fingers is the most debated physical finding. One suspects it may be the latter.

Clubbing was described by Hippocrates more than 2300 years ago, yet its pathogenesis remains a mystery.

Pathologic clubbing (secondary to an underlying illness or disease) should be distinguished from hereditary thickening of the distal phalanges (with curved nails frequently seen in blacks) and from pachydermoperiostosis, in which idiopathic clubbing is present from the first decade.

The earliest signs of clubbing are (1) loss of the normal 15-degree angle between the dorsal surface of the phalanx and the nail's proximal portion and (2) increased convexity of the nailbeds in cross-sectional and sagittal planes. Then, with proliferation of underlying tissue, the nail base softens, and the nail will rock with pressure. In addition to the loosening of the nail, eponychia and paronychia may be found. The patient may complain of accelerated nail growth, hangnails, warmth, and/or sweating of the digits.

As clubbing advances, the distal interphalangeal joints may show hyperextensibility. Fingers may take on a banjo or drumstick appearance.

The spectrum of involvement is wide, from only one phalanx being affected to all the fingers and toes. There may also be concomitant periostitis and new bone formation of the distal long bones (hypertrophic osteoarthropathy), gynecomastia, leonine facies, and involvement of clavicles and ribs.

A common misconception is that clubbing is associated with chronic obstructive pulmonary disease. It is true that a patient with severe chronic bronchitis (blue-bloater) may have clubbing, but if someone with pure emphysema (pink-puffer) develops clubbing, they should be evaluated for one of the diseases listed here.

Etiology of Clubbing

PRIMARY INTRATHORACIC NEOPLASMS

Bronchogenic carcinoma*
Tumors of the pleura
Mediastinal Hodgkin's disease*

INFECTIONS

Lung abscess
Bronchiectasis
Empyema
Subacute bacterial endocarditis*
Intestinal tuberculosis
Amebic or bacillary dysentery
Cavitary pulmonary tuberculosis*

OTHER

Pneumoconiosis*
Cyanotic heart disease
Primary cholangiolitic cirrhosis*
Toxic, biliary, and portal cirrhosis
Hepatic amyloidosis
Ulcerative colitis
Regional enteritis
Sprue
Idiopathic steatorrhea
Colonic polyposis
Hyperparathyroidism
Following thyroidectomy for Graves' disease
Metastatic lesion to lung (rare)
Neoplasms of the small intestine
Carcinoma of the colon
Desquamative interstitial pneumonitis*

UNILATERAL CLUBBING

Aneurysms of the aorta, subclavian, or innominate artery
Brachial arteriovenous fistulae
Apical lung cancer
Axillary tumors

UNIDIGITAL CLUBBING

Injury to the median nerve
Tophaceous gout
Sarcoidosis

*More frequently associated with hypertrophic osteoarthropathy.

THE SPLEEN: SPLENOMEGALY VERSUS SCANOMEGALY

The normal spleen weighs approximately 80 to 200 grams in the adult male and 70 to 180 grams in the adult female. It is a posterior structure in its normal condition, rotating anteriorly as it enlarges. An enlarged spleen may not be palpable in patients with an obese abdomen, in those who are unable to cooperate fully with the examiner, and in subjects with a deep chest. If the spleen is not felt with the patient supine, the physician should seek it with the patient in the right lateral decubitus position. Only then should it be considered nonpalpable.

Textbooks disagree as to the degree of enlargement necessary before the spleen can be palpated. It has been stated that 50 per cent of spleens enlarged to scan are palpable and that 20 per cent of spleens weighing more than 900 grams are not palpable. Obviously, not all spleens, and certainly not all examiners, are created equal. The most frequent errors in splenic palpation involve incomplete relaxation of the abdominal musculature of the patient and of the musculature of the palpating hand. A light touch is preferred.

If the spleen is not palpable, or if imaging is desired, x-ray, abdominal ultrasonography, and scanning with colloidal preparations of various radionuclides are readily available. A recent publication by Aito[1] compared these modalities and concluded the following:

1. X-ray and nuclear medicine scanning give a definite result concerning splenic size in 87 per cent and 100 per cent of cases, respectively. Splenic size could not be determined in 21 per cent of the ultrasound studies.

2. All spleens weighing more than 300 grams (estimated weight) were palpable. The average weight of a palpable spleen in his series was 285 grams.

3. The following general criteria were given for splenic enlargement:

X-ray. The spleen is not enlarged if it is not seen by this method, if it is less than 5 cm in width, or if it is less than 85 per cent of the size of the (normal) kidney. The spleen is enlarged if it is more than 6 cm wide, if it is more than 13.6 cm long, or if the length × width is more than 75 sq cm.

Colloid Scanning. The spleen is enlarged if the lateral scan area is more than 80 sq cm or if the length is greater than 14 cm.

The problem concerning the assessment of splenomegaly (palpable spleen) versus "scanomegaly" (nonpalpable spleen, spleen enlarged to x-ray or scanning procedure) can be vexing. Obviously, our diagnostic clues to disease have been built on centuries of experience with the physical examination, while scanning procedures have been with us for only a relatively short period of time. The spleen contains 25 per cent of the lymphoid mass of the body and may enlarge as a response to infection or inflammation. In such cases, splenomegaly may have the same significance as an elevated sedimentation rate.

It is our feeling that splenic scanning is overused. If a spleen is definitely felt on physical examination, there is little reason to confirm this with a liver-spleen scan. Extreme caution should be exercised when the liver-spleen scan is used in the evaluation of patients with suspected malignancy. Patchy isotope uptake, and even focal defects, may prove to be due to causes other than malignancy. Finally, we are unsure of the cost-benefit ratio of knowing that the spleen is enlarged to scan in a myriad of conditions. Unless it is done to assess prognosis or response to treatment, such scanning procedures may result in "hospital bill–omegaly" rather than the addition of important information to the patient's data base.

References: Aito, H.: Ann. Clin. Res., 6 (Suppl. 15):1, 1974; Silverman, S., DeNardo, G. L., Glatstein, E., and Lipton, M. J.: Am. J. Med., 52:362, 1972.

Thanks to Steve Landaw, M.D., Ph.D., for this contribution.

S-P-L-E-E-N

Some acronyms are too good to pass up. How about the mechanisms of splenic enlargement?

1. Sequestration
   a. Loss of red cell deformability (i.e., hereditary spherocytosis)
   b. Antibody coating of red cells
2. Proliferation
   a. Secondary to chronic immunologic stimulation (i.e., infectious mononucleosis, cytomegalovirus, SBE, chronic malaria)
3. Lipid — (Gaucher's, Niemann Pick)
4. Engorgement
   a. Portal hypertension
   b. Splenic trauma
   c. Sequestration crisis of some hemoglobinopathies and thalassemia
5. Endowment
   a. Congenital splenomegaly (i.e., hemangiomas, hydromas)
6. iNvasion
   a. Lymphoma and leukemia
   b. Granulomatous disease

In the adult, few conditions give you *really* big spleens. By big we mean down below the left and maybe the right iliac crest.

Remembering this list may help you to the diagnosis quickly:

1. Chronic granulocytic leukemia and myelofibrosis. Rare in polycythemia vera unless there is considerable fibrosis.
2. Lymphoma — usually the less aggressive histologies
3. Hairy cell leukemia (malignant-reticuloendotheliosis)
4. Sarcoidosis (rare)
5. Gaucher's disease
6. Kala-Azar
7. Chronic malaria

...and that's pretty much it.

References: Boles, E. T., Jr., Baxter, C. F., and Newton, W. A., Jr.: Clin. Pediatr., 2:161, 1963; McMillan, J., Nieburg, P., and Oski, F. A.: The Whole Pediatrician Catalogue. Philadelphia, W. B. Saunders Company, 1977, p. 21.

SOME SOUNDS OF THE BODY

Noises generated within the patient's body may be valuable diagnostic aids. Bruits, hums, murmurs, breath sounds, and bowel sounds are typical examples of body sounds that are heard by the physician with the aid of a stethoscope but are usually inaudible to the patient. On the other hand, there are body noises that are heard by the patient, but rarely by the physician.

HEAD NOISES

A patient who complains of rhythmic rushing or beating in their head may have a moderate-sized cerebral aneurysm, especially when the internal carotid is involved. More commonly this throbbing is the result of hypertension, atherosclerosis, or anemia. The beating or rushing is synchronous with the heart.

Complaints of a crisp, clear "tick-tick-tick" in the ear, a clicking nostril, or a clicking or snapping sound in the throat may lead the physician to entertain a diagnosis of auditory hallucinations! In reality, the cause is a spasmotic contraction of intratympanic, palatine, and eustachian tube muscles. This type of muscular behavior can be observed directly in cases of fatigue, nervousness, or tension, which cause twitching of the muscles of the eyelid. All conditions can be treated with rest, reassurance, and mild sedation.

LAUGHING AS A DISEASE

The therapeutic effect of laughter is well known. Sydenham said, "The arrival of a good clown exercises a more beneficial influence upon the health of a town than of 20 asses laden with drugs."

We rarely think of laughter as a disease. Powerful laughter may do injury, breaking ribs or leading to choking and aspiration. The novelist Anthony Trollope is one of the few people recorded as dying from a fit of laughter. Trousseau first described laughter as a manifestation of an obscure variety of *epilepsy*. Involuntary or inappropriate laughter may occur in various organic diseases of the central nervous system, such as *multiple sclerosis*. Wood, Svien, and Daly have reported an interesting example of involuntary laughter associated with a *neurinoma of the fifth nerve*. The laughing stopped after surgical removal of the offending lesion. In examples of involuntary laughter, the apparent response of mirth may be as puzzling to the victim as it is to the bystander. Involuntary laughter is distinct from the emotional incontinence of grotesque laughter sometimes found in patients with *tumors of the frontal lobe*. Subjectively, they are greatly amused and believe that things are very funny. The wide variation in provoking lesions suggests that there is no small focal laughter center.

Kuru, the strange "laughing disease" found among the Fore tribes of New Guinea, is associated with organic degeneration of the central nervous system. Though the disease appears confined to certain tribes in certain districts, it is not clear whether hereditary factors or environmental ones are primarily responsible. Laughing, however, is only part of the very complex neurological disorder; sudden death is another. Present evidence suggests that it is a long-delayed response to a chronic infection.

Rankin and Philip have described an epidemic of laughing and crying that disorganized community life for six months in an African tribe in Tanganyika (now Tanzania). It began in a mission school for girls, which was forced to close down when more than half the pupils became affected. Most of those involved were adolescent girls and younger boys. It seemed to spread by example. Laughing and crying lasted for some minutes or a few hours, then things would quiet down, only to recur later. Restlessness and occasional vomiting were noted. Physical examination revealed nothing abnormal, except for the hyperkinetic state and exaggerated tendon jerks. After one or two weeks, the disorder abated. Certain paranoid fears and evidence of hysteric reactions were reported. No example was found among the better educated or more experienced members of the community, regardless of age.

Reference: Bean, William B.: Rare Diseases and Lesions: Their Contributions to Clinical Medicine. Springfield, Ill., Charles C Thomas, Publisher, 1967, pp. 100–101.

SINGULTUS

The hiccough, or singultus, is a common human affliction that is usually of little consequence. On occasion the singultus can be a "multitus" and lead to embarrassment, discomfort, incapacitation, and even death! There have been many treatments suggested for simple hiccoughs, including fright and swallowing sugar.

For sustained hiccoughs the following may be tried:

1. Thorazine, 25 to 50 mg orally every 4 to 6 hours
2. Quinidine, 200 mg orally every 4 to 6 hours
3. Electrical "overstimulation" of the phrenic nerve
4. Sectioning the phrenic nerve
5. "Benny's treatment" (highly successful):
   a. 100 per cent O_2 for 5 minutes
   b. Using an eyedropper, instill 1 ml of spirits of ammonia in the posterior nasopharynx, and have the patient immediately *sniff* and *swallow* the ammonia.
   c. 100 per cent O_2 for 5 to 10 minutes.

Benny's treatment is extremely irritating, but it is successful because of the chemical overstimulation of the phrenic nerve. The ammonia causes sinus tachycardia and therefore should be used with caution, if at all, in cardiac patients. Thorazine or quinidine should be tried first.

Some Causes of Hiccough

IRRITATION OF THE PHRENIC NERVE
 Idiopathic
 Contiguous infection/inflammation
 Tumors involving the nerve

CYCLICAL DIAPHRAGMATIC SPASM *(After laughing, crying, or coughing)*

SUPRADIAPHRAGMATIC IRRITATION
 Pneumonitis
 Effusion/empyema
 Inferior myocardial infarction
 Pericarditis

INFRADIAPHRAGMATIC IRRITATION
 Gastric ulcer
 Cholecystitis
 Inflammatory bowel disease
 Ruptured viscus
 Subphrenic or lesser sac abscess
 Perinephric abscess

THE MOST COMMON
 Excess alcohol
 Excessive smoking
 Eating large boluses of food with inadequate liquid
 Air swallowing
 "Nerves"

IT'S A GAS

Scientific inquiry into flatus and its effects on man has occurred only recently. We now at last have a better understanding of the properties of intestinal gas.

The normal intestinal tract contains between 30 to 200 ml of gas. The major components are N_2, CO_2, CH_4, and H_2. Swallowed air accounts for the majority of the nitrogen. Hydrogen, methane, and carbon dioxide result from luminal bacterial production. It is interesting to note that patients with functional bowel complaints had slower transport times of artificially instilled gas. Moreover, they experienced discomfort with an amount of gas that produced no symptoms in normal subjects.

Besides recommending to symptomatic patients proper eating and drinking habits to avoid aerophagia, there is little the physician can do to alleviate their ills. To fill this obvious gap in our therapeutics, the following list gives in order of their flatulence potential ten commonly ingested beans to be avoided by the distressed patient.

1. Soybeans
2. Pink beans
3. Black beans
4. Pinto beans
5. California small white beans
6. Great northern beans
7. Lima beans (baby)
8. Garbanzos
9. Lima beans (large)
10. Blackeyes

References: Wallechinsky, D., Wallace, I., and Wallace, A.: The Book of Lists. New York, William Morrow & Co., Inc., 1977, p. 386; Levitt, M. D.: New Engl. J. Med., 284:*1394*, 1971; Lasser, R. B. Bond, J. H., and Levitt, M. D.: New Engl. J. Med., *293*:524, 1975.

Z-Z-Z-Z-Z-Z

Forty-five per cent of normal subjects occasionally snore, while another 25 per cent admit to habitual snoring. Snoring is more common in older, obese men, although it is an affliction borne by people of all ages and both sexes. It appears that the only significant medical sequela to heavy snoring (besides insomnia in one's sleeping partner[s]) is a greater frequency of hypoventilation during sleep. Whether hypoventilation during sleep in heavy snorers predisposes to the sleep apnea syndrome is yet to be determined.

Reference: Zwillich, C.: Arch. Intern. Med., *139*:24, 1979.

NIGHTMARES

Dream analysis is a widely used psychiatric tool, but did you know that recurrent nightmares may be the major manifestation of a variety of serious medical conditions? The following is a list of conditions that may be associated with recurrent nightmares. If you know of others, please drop us a line.

Hypoglycemia
Hyperthyroidism
Hypoxia
Sick sinus syndrome (bradyarrhythmias)
Digitalis toxicity
Pinworms
Steroid excess (endogenous or exogenous)
Cerebritis
Drug withdrawal
Reserpine

MALINGERING

Some of the most bizarre syndromes may be observed in patients who are malingering. Patients "in the know" medically should be particularly suspect. In a recent review of 32 patients with factitious fever, 16 patients had a medical or paramedical background. Included were nurses, a graduate student in bacteriology, an ex–medical student, lab techs, a Navy corpsman, and a pharmacist. The rest of the group included 12 students and 4 patients with occupations bearing no relationship to medicine. Thermometer manipulation and self-induced infections were recurrent themes. The increased use of electronic thermometers with their short cords and a witness attached will do away with many of these recurrent fevers of unknown origin.

Syndromes of self-mutilation produced by injection or auto-scarification are varied, and their etiology is often obscured by the ingratiating nature of the patient and the lack of apparent secondary gain. Keep your guard up when pathologic findings fail to follow physiologic guidelines. Be very, very careful and very, very sure before raising the possibility of malingering to a patient.

The inventiveness of the malingering doctor, nurse, or layman with a medical background may be such that an apparent physiologic disease process is produced. Medical cognoscenti are particularly suspect for the use of agents producing recognizable and plausible physiologic aberrations. The use of vitamin K antagonists or heparin to produce a bleeding diathesis is a case in point. The prolonged coagulation studies correct when the patient's plasma is mixed in equal quantities with normal plasma in the case of surreptitious ingestion of vitamin K antagonists. The same studies fail to correct and show a "circulating anticoagulant" when heparin is being used.

Hypoglycemia is another recurrent theme. Use of a radioimmunoassay employing an antibody to the "C-peptide" portion of the native insulin molecule will help establish the diagnosis of exogenous hyperinsulinism or insulinoma in the non-malingerer. The "C-peptide" assay will also be elevated when hypoglycemia is produced by oral hypoglycemic agents of the sulfonylurea class, since these agents stimulate the release of insulin into the portal circulation. Tolbutamide, chloropropamide, and acetohexamide in particular may produce prolonged hypoglycemia. Chloropropamide has a half-life of 36 hours and is excreted by the kidneys, leading to a markedly prolonged hypoglycemia action in the patient with renal disease.

CHARACTERISTICS OF MUNCHAUSEN'S SYNDROME

1. Feigned severe illness of a dramatic and emergency nature.
2. Dramatic, but plausible, history (often part truth and part fabrication).
3. Willingness to undergo physical investigation and treatment, including operative intervention.
4. Evidence of many previous hospital procedures (surgical scars).
5. Aggressive and unruly behavior ("evasive and truculent").
6. Background of many hospitalizations and extensive travel (usually concealed).
7. Departure from hospital against medical advice.
8. Absence of any readily discernible ulterior motive.

References: Audan, R. P., Fauci, A. S., Dale, D. C., et al.: Ann. Intern. Med., *90*:230, 1979; Pallis, C. A., and Barnji, A. N.: Br. Med. J., *1*:973, 1979.

URINE TEMPERATURE: A CLUE TO EARLY DIAGNOSIS OF FACTITIOUS FEVER

The urine temperature is within 1 to 1.5°C of the oral temperature taken simultaneously.

Reference: Murray, H. W., Tuazon, C. U., Guerrero, I. C., et al.: New Engl. J. Med., *296*:23, 1977.

> *Every psychoneurotic ultimately dies of organic disease.*

HYPOCHONDRIASIS

Nondisease may well be the most common illness that the primary care physician treats. Estimates of the number of "worried well" in outpatient populations have ranged from 20 to 60 per cent. Many physicians are ill equipped both by inclination and by training to manage these people appropriately.

Hypochondriasis can be defined as an inappropriate or excessive concern with one's physical or mental health. It can occur with or without definable organic abnormalities and may be an entity in itself or a symptom of another problem. The four functional classes of hypochondriasis suggested by Idzorek provide a nice framework for the primary physician to use in structuring an approach to this problem.

First, hypochondriasis can be a symptom of an acute situational stress reaction in people who are neither neurotic nor psychotic. The reassurance of a careful physical examination, coupled with an opportunity for the patient to verbalize his personal problems to an understanding, empathetic physician, is usually all that is necessary to treat these people successfully. It is important to recognize and appropriately manage this problem early in its course before a chronic pattern of somatic complaints develops.

Inappropriate and excessive somatic concerns often accompany primary depression. Treatment of this form of hypochondriasis should be directed toward the primary process and not at the somatic symptom. Standard programs of psychotherapy and antidepressants should be used. Psychiatric consultation may be indicated in the management of some of these patients.

Third, hypochondriasis can be a symptom of psychosis. The sudden onset of peculiar or bizarre symptoms, especially in young adults, should alert the physician to the possibility of a developing psychotic reaction. Again, treatment should be directed at the underlying psychosis and not at the hypochondriacal symptoms. These patients will often need specific psychiatric treatment.

Finally, there is a group that Idzorek calls "true hypochondriacs." They have no underlying mental illness but do have chronic, excessive, and inappropriate concern about somatic complaints. They tend to bother their physicians frequently, to "doctor-shop," and to have large numbers of diagnostic evaluations and surgical procedures. At one end of the spectrum are the patients with a single specific chronic somatic complaint but no accompanying functional loss. At the other are patients whose somatic complaints prevent them from functioning in society and seem to be their only reasons for existence. These true hypochondriacs are challenging and frustrating patients to care for; however, the following active supportive program can be used to manage the patient so that contacts are less frequent and occur at times more convenient to the physician.

1. The physician should attempt to show interest and concern towards the patient at the initial evaluation — this will make the patient feel more comfortable and increase his feeling of security.

2. The physician should attempt to "listen" to the patient and then do a good physical examination — this will result in very positive feelings by the patient towards the physician, which will tend to establish good rapport for the duration of the relationship.

3. Once it is recognized that the patient is a true hypochondriac (whether mild or severe in intensity), the physician should then let the

patient discuss his symptoms as much as he wishes during the time limit of the appointment.

4. The physician should not challenge symptoms or indicate to the patient that his problems are psychogenic.

5. Any medical explanation should be simple.

6. The physician should do only the minimum examinations and tests that need to be done for the *physician* to feel certain about the patient's physical condition, as these various activities tend to arouse the hypochondriac's somatic concerns even greater.

7. Arrange specific appointments in the future for the patient — this is very important as it will not only increase the patient's feelings of security but make him more likely to wait until the next session to discuss any "new problems." In future appointments, the above mentioned guidelines should be continued, with the emphasis on letting the patient discuss his somatic concerns as much as he wishes in the time limit of the appointment.

8. If the patient calls at night or on weekends, the physician should simply remind the patient that he (the physician) is well acquainted with the patient's physical condition and that further evaluation can wait until the next scheduled appointment.

The goal of this program is management, not cure; remember that to be well may be terrifying to the true hypochondriac.

Reference: Idzorek, S.: Resident and Staff Physician, December 1977, p. 95. Parts reprinted with the permission of the author and publisher.

ON ADMISSION TO THE HOSPITAL -WRITING THE ADMITTING ORDERS

When a patient is admitted to the hospital, an organized set of instructions to the nursing staff will help to assure efficient patient management. By adopting a standard routine for writing admission orders, the number of omissions that can compromise the care and evaluation of the patient will be reduced. The following is a suggested sequence for writing the admission orders.

SEQUENCE	COMMENT
Designate the floor to which patient is admitted	e.g., Admit to the Coronary Care Unit...
Age and sex of the patient	e.g., this 50 y.o. male (or female) ...
Admitting diagnosis	e.g., with a diagnosis of acute myocardial infarction

SEQUENCE	COMMENT
Condition of the patient	e.g., good, fair, poor, critical (in _____ condition)
Vital signs	State the frequency and any special measurements desired (e.g., supine and standing blood pressure and pulse). Place limits on the vital signs, which, if exceeded, require a physician to be notified.
Allergy	List any allergies. State no known allergies if this is the case.
Diet	Be specific in the type of diet the patient needs. Are *calorie counts* required? Is *fluid restriction* required?
Activities	Is the patient to remain in bed? Can the patient use toilet facilities or does he require a bedside commode? Can the patient ambulate as tolerated?
Nursing procedures	e.g., How often is the patient to be *weighed?* (Every patient's weight on admission *must* be recorded.) Is the patient to have *intake* and *output* recorded? Is the patient to have *fractional urines* for glucose determinations? Are stools to be examined for occult blood? Does the patient need *special care* of some sort (eye care, pulmonary toilet, skin care, dressing changes, ostomy care, Foley catheter care, etc.)? Are *isolation precautions* required?
Medications	List the medications to be given and when and how.
Intravenous orders	List the IV orders. Drugs that are to be administered intravenously can be listed under IV orders.
Diagnostic studies	All laboratory and x-ray studies to be done initially are placed here.

Date and sign the orders. Write the orders so they can be easily read and understood.

The problem with calling in a consultant is that you may feel obligated to take his advice.

> *Consultation* — Comes from the Latin *consultare,* meaning to "deliberate or counsel," but with a definite implication of a joint activity, because of the prefix *con,* meaning "with" or, better, "together." (Joseph D. Sapria)

THE DOCTOR'S BAG

The following is a suggested list of equipment and drugs that might be considered the basic tools of the trade for a physician who must deal with medical situations away from an equipped facility. The standard black bag will not hold all the equipment suggested. However, a large fishing tackle box will hold everything except the cylinders of oxygen, and the compartments facilitate organization and localization of the contents.

Contents of the Doctor's Bag

1. One 1000 ml Ringer's lactate solution
2. One 250 ml 5% glucose in water solution
3. One ampule of 50 ml 50% glucose*
4. 2 ml, 5 ml, 20 ml syringes
5. 14 gauge 2½ inch, 18 gauge 2½ inch, 20 gauge 2½ inch intravenous catheters and 20 gauge 1½ inch needles, 22 gauge 1½ inch needles, 25 gauge 1 inch needles
6. 19 gauge and 21 gauge butterfly needles
7. Intravenous tubing
8. Tourniquet
9. Alcohol sponges
10. Stethoscope
11. Sphygmomanometer
12. Ophthalmoscope-otoscope
13. Endotrachael tube — cuffed — small, medium, and large

14. Plastic laryngoscope with light
15. Nasogastric tube and Toomey syringe
16. Suture kit
17. Needle holder
18. Tissue forceps
19. Scissors
20. Three mosquito hemostats
21. Tongue depressors
22. Neurologic hammer
23. Prescription pad and triplicate narcotic form
24. E cylinder of oxygen with flow valve and face masks
25. Adhesive tape
26. Oral airways
27. Ace bandages
28. Eye patches
29. Gauze
30. Sterile gloves
31. Steristrips
32. ambu bag
33. Esophageal obturator airway

Drugs in the Doctor's Bag

1. Atropine sulfate 0.4 mg/ml — 20 mg vial*
2. Chlorpromazine (Thorazine) 25 mg/ml — 2 ml ampules
3. Diazepam (Valium) 10 mg/2 ml ampules
4. Diazoxide (Hyperstat) 15 mg/ml — 20 ml ampules
5. Digoxin (Lanoxin) 0.25 mg/ml — 2 ml ampules
6. Diphenhydramine (Benadryl) 50 mg/ml — 10 ml vial
7. Epinephrine (Adrenalin) 1/1000 solution — 1 ml ampules; 1/10,000 solution — 10 ml syringe*
8. Furosemide (Lasix) 10 mg/ml — 2 ml ampules
9. Hydrocortisone sodium succinate (Solu-Cortef) 250 mg vials
10. Levarterenol (Levophed) 0.2% solution — 2 and 4 ml ampules
11. Lidocaine hydrochloride (Xylocaine) 20 mg/ml — 50 ml vials* (for intravenous use); lidocaine hydrochloride (Xylocaine) 1% solution — 20 ml vials (for local anesthesia)
12. Morphine sulfate 15 mg/ml — 1 ml ampules*
13. Meperidine hydrochloride (Demerol) 50 mg/ml — 2 ml ampules
14. Nitroglycerin — sublingual 0.4 mg tablets
15. Prochlorperazine maleate (Compazine) suppositories
16. Sodium phenobarbital 130 mg/ml
17. Theophylline ethylenediamine (Aminophylline) 250 mg/ml 10 ml ampules
18. Naloxone hydrochloride (Narcan) 0.4 mg/ml — 1 ml ampules

19. Edrophonium chloride (Tensilon) 10 mg/ml — 10 ml vials
20. Sodium bicarbonate 44.6 mEq/ampule — 50 ml ampule
21. Activated charcoal U.S.P.
22. Calcium chloride 100 mg/ml — 10 ml syringes*
23. Vials isotonic sodium chloride (for dilutions)

---

*Also available in unit dose syringes.

Reference: Burket, G. E.: Rational Drug Therapy, *10*:1, 1976; Mayne, B. R.: Sports Medicine, September 1975, p. 67.

PRESCRIPTION CHECKLIST

The Right Drug

1. Have you considered the indications carefully?
2. Have you reviewed the possible side effects?
3. Is there a potential for drug interaction in the patient?
4. Are the benefit/risk and benefit/cost ratios favorable for this particular patient?

The Right Information

5. Does the patient understand why the drug is being given?
6. Does the patient understand the potential side effects and know which of these, if any, might require expeditious action?
7. Does the patient understand how, when, and for how long to take the drug? Are you sure?
8. Are there any specific "do's and don'ts" (e.g., alcohol) the patient should be aware of while taking the medication?

The Right Script

9. Is the prescription accurate?
10. Does it conform to what you told the patient?
11. Is it legible?
12. Have you provided for enough of the drug to complete the contemplated therapy? Have you limited the quantity dispensed if you are employing the drug in a therapeutic trial?
13. Did you sign your prescription?

1

14. Is your BNDD number necessary?

15. Did you use the right form (i.e., triplicate narcotic form, Medicaid)?

> *Apothecary* — From the ancient Greek *apothoke,* which meant "storehouse." It wasn't until the seventeenth century in London that the Apothecaries Company separated from the Grocers' Guild after agreeing to sell only drugs. And now...

And

16. Can the patient get the medication?
17. Can the patient afford the medication?
18. Have you told the patient whether to refrigerate the medication?

Prescription Alphabet Soup

Here are some traditional abbreviations that are understood if they can be read.

D — day	B — twice	Sig. — label (*signa*)
W — week	T — thrice	P.R.N. — as necessary (*pro re nata*)
Q — each	Q — four	M.D.D. — maximum daily dose
H — hours	I — times	
	O — every other	

caps — capsules	a — before (*ante*)
tabs — tablets	p — post, dinner (*post, prandium*)
oz — ounces	s — sleep (*somni*)
teasp — teaspoon (5 ml)	Disp. — dispense
tbsp — tablespoon (15 ml)	M — mix
	c — food (*cibus*)

Prejudices

1. We have everything labeled.
2. We never use QD for daily, since it can be confused with QID and QOD
3. We use generic names when possible.
4. We limit the dispensed quantity of certain drugs to avoid abuse or unsupervised self-administration.

TERMINATING THE PHYSICIAN-PATIENT RELATIONSHIP

Current residency training programs — especially in family practice, medicine and pediatrics — often require that the resident be responsible for the ongoing primary care of a group of patients for the entire duration of the training. These physician-patient relationships will need to be terminated as the resident finishes the training program. The doctor-patient relationship itself has an important therapeutic effect, and there is potential for serious adverse effects on the patients (and, to a lesser extent, on the physician) when termination of this relationship is unsatisfactory. Patients may develop new or worsening symptoms, stop keeping their appointments or taking their medication, begin making additional emergency calls and visits, or become angry at the departing physician or the new physician.

The following measures have been suggested as a means to terminate the physician-patient relationship with minimal mutual trauma.

1. Inform the patient early. Plan on discussing termination several times before it actually occurs.
2. When you tell the patient, give him time to express his feelings. Don't wait until the end of the visit as you are walking out the door.
3. Do not take negative responses as a personal insult. Explore the origins of the feelings in a compassionate and understanding manner.
4. Make certain that the patient has heard your plans to leave. Reinforce it at the next visit.
5. Explain to the patient why you are leaving, but don't "over-explain."
6. Ask the patient his preference for subsequent medical care.
7. If the patient begins breaking appointments, call him up and find out why.
8. After the patient has had sufficient opportunity to adjust to the loss, identify and, if possible, introduce the patient to his new physician.

Reference: Freidin, R. B., and Lazerson, A. M.: J.A.M.A., *241*:819, 1979.

PATIENT'S BILL OF RIGHTS

1. The patient has the right to considerate and respectful care.

2. The patient has the right to obtain from his physician complete current information concerning his diagnosis, treatment, and prognosis in terms the patient can be reasonably expected to understand.

3. The patient has the right to receive from his physician information necessary to give informed consent prior to the start of any procedure and/or treatment.

4. The patient has the right to refuse treatment to the extent permitted by law and to be informed of the medical consequences of his action.

5. The patient has the right to every consideration of his privacy concerning his own medical program.

6. The patient has the right to expect that all communications and records pertaining to his care should be treated as confidential.

7. The patient has the right to expect that within its capacity, the hospital must make reasonable response to the request of a patient for services.

8. The patient has the right to obtain information as to any relationship of his hospital to other health care and educational institutions insofar as his care is concerned.

9. The patient has the right to be advised if the hospital proposes to engage in or perform human experimentation affecting his care or treatment.

10. The patient has the right to expect reasonable continuity of care.

11. The patient has the right to examine and receive an explanation of his bill regardless of source of payment.

12. The patient has the right to know what hospital rules and regulations apply to his conduct as a patient.

Reference: National policy statement of the American Hospital Association.

Loeb's Laws of Medicine:
A. *If what you're doing is working, keep doing it.*
B. *If what you're doing is not working, stop doing it.*
C. *If you don't know what to do, don't do anything.*
D. *Above all, never let a surgeon get your patient.*

PATIENT'S BILL OF RIGHTS

2
CRITICAL CARE

"Life is short, and the art long; opportunity is fleeting; experiment perilous, and judgment difficult"

Corpus Hippocraticum

DEFINITION OF CRITICAL CARE MEDICINE (CCM) AND CCM PHYSICAN SPECIALISTS

The discipline of critical care medicine (CCM) has evolved over the last few decades in conjunction with the development of techniques and technology for acute and long-term life support of patients with multiple organ system derangement. CCM is concerned with all aspects of the management of patients with immediate life-threatening conditions. CCM is a multidisciplinary endeavor that crosses traditional departmental and specialty lines, since the problems encountered in the critically ill patient encompass various aspects of many different specialties.

The CCM physician is a subspecialist whose knowledge is, of necessity, broad, involving all aspects of the management of the critically ill patient, and whose base of operation is the intensive care unit (ICU). This physician has completed training in a primary specialty and in the CCM aspects of many disciplines, enabling him to integrate the efforts of various specialists on the patient care team in the ICU, utilize recognized techniques for vital support, teach other physicians, nurses, and health professionals the practice of intensive care, foster research, and perform administrative functions in the ICU.

Thus, CCM is a unique discipline, based in the intensive care unit, with its primary concern being the total care of the patient with a critical illness.

"It is the function of the ICU director to maintain all the patient's systems in an equal state of failure and all his medical consultants equally unhappy."

C. Bryan-Brown, M.D.

ALPHABET SOUP

You can expect to encounter a variety of cardiovascular symbols and formulae in the intensive care unit since invasive hemodynamic monitoring is so commonly performed now. The table on the following pages should help you understand this area of medical jargon.

When using these parameters in patient management, remember:

1. Analysis of numbers alone is meaningless. They must be correlated with your clinical examination.

2. No one parameter is adequate in all patients at all times. You need to examine the interrelationships among the various factors to get the whole picture.

3. Trends are more useful than isolated values.

4. Think "optimal" rather than "normal." Normal values are generally determined on a normal, healthy population. Critically ill patients are far from normal and healthy and may, in fact, do best at levels of cardiovascular performance that are quite deviant from the "normal range."

Reference: Desoutels, D. A., et al.: Respiratory Care, *23*:43, 1978. Table reproduced (with modifications) with the permission of author and publisher.

Shoemaker's Dictum
It is unwise to monitor patients to achieve normal values because that will erase compensations that have survival value. The proper objective of monitoring is to achieve survival.

PARAMETER	ABBREVIATION	FORMULA	UNITS	MEANING/USE
Mean arterial pressure	$\overline{\text{MAP}}$	$DP\ \dfrac{SP^*-DP^*}{3}$	Torr	Useful endpoint for titrating vasoactive agents. Used to calculate systemic vascular resistance.
Central venous pressure	CVP	Directly measured	Torr cm H_2O	Used as index of volume status and right ventricular preload.
Pulmonary artery occlusion pressure ("wedge pressure")	PAo	Directly measured	Torr	Index of volume status and left ventricular preload. More reliable than CVP.
Mean pulmonary artery pressure	$\overline{\text{PAP}}$	$DP + \dfrac{SP^{**}-DP^{**}}{3}$	Torr	Used to calculate pulmonary vascular resistance.
Cardiac output	C.O.	Directly measured	Liters/min	Prime measurement of hemodynamic function.
Cardiac index	CI	$\dfrac{\text{C.O.}}{\text{Body surface area}}$	Liters/min/sq meter	
Stroke volume	SV	C.O./Pulse	ml	Provides some information about cardiac performance.
Systemic vascular resistance	SVR	$\dfrac{\overline{\text{MAP}}-\text{CVP}}{\text{C.O.}} \times 80$	dynes/cm/sec^{-5}	Measure of resistance of arterial tree. Useful in differential diagnosis of various shock states.

2

Parameter	Abbreviation	Formula	Units	Description
Pulmonary vascular resistance	PVR	$\dfrac{\overline{PAP}-PAo}{C.O.} \times 80$	dynes/cm/sec^{-5}	Measure of resistance of pulmonary vascular bed. Elevated in pulmonary embolism, COAD, acute respiratory failure.
Left ventricular stroke work	LVSW	SV($\overline{MAP}$–PA) 0.0136	gram/meter	Measure of left ventricular performance.
Right ventricular stroke work	RVSW	SV($\overline{PAP}$–CVP) 0.0136	gram/meter	Measure of right ventricular performance.
Arterio-venous oxygen difference	C(a-$\bar{v}$)O$_2$	Directly measured from arterial and mixed venous blood gases	ml/100 ml	Index of adequacy of tissue oxygenation.
Oxygen transport	O$_2$ Trans. (O$_2$ Del)	C.O. $\times$ CaO$_2$ CaO$_2$ = arterial oxygen content	ml/min	Amount of oxygen delivered to the tissues.
Oxygen consumption	O$_2$ Cons.	C.O. $\times$ C(a-$\bar{v}$)O$_2$	ml/min	Amount of oxygen extracted by the tissues.
Oxygen utilization coefficient	O$_2$ Util. Coef.	$\dfrac{O_2 \text{ Cons.}}{O_2 \text{ Trans.}}$	–	Index of efficiency of oxygen utilization.
Index	I	$\dfrac{\text{Parameter}}{\text{Body surface area}}$	–	Eliminates body size as variable and thus aids in interpreting values of various measurements.

*SP, DP—systolic, diastolic pressure (systemic)
**SP, DP—systolic, diastolic pressure (pulmonary artery)

BEDSIDE PULMONARY ARTERY CATHETERIZATION

Balloon flotation catheterization of the pulmonary artery at the patient's bedside is now a routine and invaluable procedure in critical care medicine. This procedure allows the physician to measure right- and left-sided cardiac pressures, cardiac output (by thermodilution), and mixed venous blood gases. Placement of a Swan-Ganz catheter is indicated in any situation in which accurate assessment of the circulatory system and prompt recognition of critical alteration in cardiovascular dynamics are necessary. To quote Dr. Swan, "The indication for the use of a flotation catheter is any situation in which a physician would consider placing a central venous pressure line for the purposes of cardiovascular monitoring." With experience, the placement of these catheters is as easy as the placement of a central venous pressure line. The cardiovascular data obtained are both more accurate and more complete than those obtained by CVP monitoring.

Balloon flotation catheters are inserted percutaneously or by cut-down via the basilic, internal jugular, subclavian, or femoral vein. The following check list will help you prepare for insertion:

Crash cart handy
Calibrate transducer and level with patient (make sure you use the venous and not the arterial scale)
Test balloon and record volume
Test thermistor
Flush PA (distal) line
Flush CVP (proximal) line
Check fit of:
    Guide wire through needle
    Introducer over guide wire
    Catheter through introducer

The catheterization is then performed. Pressure monitoring is used to follow the course of the catheter through the various cardiac chambers as shown in Figure 2–1.

HEMODYNAMIC ASPECTS OF
BALLOON CATHETER INSERTIONS
INTO THE PULMONARY ARTERY

FIG. 2–1.

(A) Right atrium, (B) right ventricle, (C) pulmonary artery, (D) pulmonary artery occlusion pressure ("wedge"), (E) desired catheter behavior for long-term monitoring.

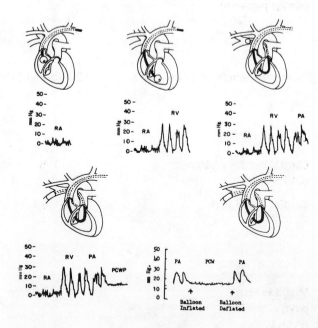

The first table on the following page summarizes the parameters that can be measured with the thermodilution Swan-Ganz catheter. You can use the individual parameters and their interrelationships to diagnose and manipulate the patient's cardiorespiratory status.

Most of the problems with using these catheters are technical. The second table summarizes the more common problems, their causes, and solutions.

PARAMETER	NORMAL VALUE	SIGNIFICANCE
Pulmonary artery occlusion pressure (PAo) (wedge pressure)	6–12 mm Hg	Measure of left ventricular preload (except in mitral stenosis and high levels of PEEP). Decreased = Hypovolemia. Increased = Hypervolemia and/or left ventricular dysfunction.
Pulmonary artery pressure (PAP)	20-25/8–12 mm Hg	Gradient between PA diastolic and PAo increases with increased pulmonary vascular resistance (e.g., pulmonary embolism, acute respiratory failure).
Central venous pressure (CVP)	1–5 mm Hg	Measure of right ventricular preload.
Cardiac index (CI)	3.5–4.0 L/min/sq m	Prime indicator of hemodynamic function. Manipulations of other parameters directed at improving cardiac function.
Mixed venous oxygen tension (PvO$_2$)	40 torr	Index of tissue oxygenation. Decrease = inadequate oxygen delivery to the tissues. Increase = deranged tissue oxygen utilization (e.g., sepsis, cyanide intoxication).

PROBLEM	CAUSES	SOLUTION
Damped tracing	Obstruction in line (clot, air bubble, kinked catheter)	Remove obstruction
No PAo tracing	Balloon rupture Equipment failure	Change catheter Check transducer and oscilloscope
	Faulty catheter position	Reposition
Persistent PAo tracing (Note: Do not inflate balloon with catheter in PAo position.)	Balloon left inflated Distal position	Deflate balloon Reposition
Right ventricular tracing	Faulty position	Reposition
Erratic, spiking wave form	Catheter fling	Introduce small air bubble into transducer
Blood backing up	Break in system (open stopcock, loose dome, cracked line)	Fix break

MORTICIAN'S APPROACH TO FEMORAL VENIPUNCTURE

2

The securing of an intravenous infusion life line is an integral part of advanced cardiac life support. Peripheral venipuncture is often technically quite difficult during a cardiac arrest because of vascular collapse, which necessitates central venous catheterization. The femoral vein should be the site of choice for central venipuncture during a cardiac arrest because cannulation of the femoral vein does not interfere with continuing ventilation and chest compression.

The procedure is performed in the following manner: After the skin has been cleansed, the femoral vein is located two finger breadths below the inguinal ligament, medial to the femoral artery. Usually an 8 or 12 inch through-the-needle catheter set is used. The puncture is made with the needle attached to a 5 or 10 ml syringe, with the needle at a 45° angle with the skin. Suction on the syringe is maintained as the needle is advanced until blood appears in the syringe, indicating that the vein has been entered. The needle is then advanced another millimeter or so to insure that the entire bevel of the needle is in the vein. The catheter is inserted, the needle removed, and the IV solution administered.

The main problem with this technique is localization of the femoral artery landmark in patients with weak or absent arterial pulses. Embalmers are commonly faced with this problem, since none of their clients has a palpable pulse. Here is their foolproof technique for locating the position of the femoral artery in pulseless patients:

1. Place the thumb on the anterior-superior iliac spine.

2. Place the fifth finger of the same hand in the midpoint of the pubic symphysis.

3. Fold the middle finger of the same hand downward. The femoral artery lies immediately below the downward-folded finger.

4. The femoral vein is then entered by inserting the needle medial to the downward-folded finger.

> *The River Lethe* — Flows at the boundaries of Hades. Those drinking the waters forgot their pasts. Thence come "lethargic" — soporific, apathetic, forgetful — and "Alethia."

HEAT STROKE-EMERGENCY THERAPY

Heat stroke is a life-threatening medical emergency. Without accurate diagnosis and appropriate therapy, death or serious disability will almost certainly occur. Heat stroke is characterized by anhydrosis, a change in mental status, and a rectal temperature greater than 40°C (104°F). Although there have been a few reports of heat stroke cases in which the patient continued sweating, usually a patient will have hot, dry skin. The skin is usually red, but if shock has supervened, it may be ashen gray. Central nervous system dysfunction may be manifested as seizures, confusion, delirium, disorientation, or combative psychotic behavior. There may be opisthotonos, Babinski's toe sign, and focal neurological signs. Coma may occur.

Heat stroke carries a mortality rate of 10 to 80 per cent in various reported studies. The mortality rate approaches 100 per cent in untreated patients. Survival depends on aggressive treatment to bring about rapid cooling.

Many deaths occur because of failure to recognize the syndrome of heat stroke. It must be clearly understood, however, that even if the diagnosis of heat stroke is in doubt when the patient is first examined in an emergency facility, the very fact that the patient's temperature is 40°C or higher demands effective and rapid cooling. Such a grossly nonphysiologic temperature will surely cause morbidity and mortality unless treated aggressively, no matter what the underlying cause.

Emergency Therapy for Heat Stroke

— Vital signs. Quick physical exam. Available history.
— Establish and maintain an airway: For tachypnea, use high-flow O_2 mask. For gasping or agonal respirations, use endotracheal tube with 80 to 100 per cent oxygen.
— CVP line. Normal saline, no more than 200 ml an hour to start (many patients with heat stroke are *not* dehydrated). No potassium chloride until the potassium level has been determined and an adequate urine flow is established.
— Electrocardiogram.
— Foley catheter with urine culture.
— Guaiac of rectal contents.
— Draw bloods: Arterial blood gases from the radial artery. (If disseminated intravascular coagulation occurs, a femoral puncture could be the site for future bleeding). Blood gases should be corrected for body temperature. CBC, clotting functions, platelet count, electrolytes, BUN, creatinine, glucose, calcium, SGOT.
— Immerse the patient in a tub filled with ice water. Massage the body vigorously. If shivering occurs give 50 mg Thorazine intramuscularly. If no tub is available, pack the axilla and groin with ice, cover the patient with sheets drenched in ice water and alco-

2

hol, and douse the patient frequently with ice water. Promote evaporation by using fans or air-conditioning. Iced gastric lavages may be helpful. Ice water enemas are time-consuming and relatively ineffective.
— Temperature may be monitored by nasopharyngeal thermometer or in-dwelling electronic rectal thermometer.
— Remove the patient from cooling when the temperature approaches 38°C (100°F).
— After effective cooling repeat the laboratory analyses. Include uric acid levels, amylase, liver function tests, magnesium, and CPK. Blood cultures should be obtained.

There is no sound reason to use steroid therapy. Dextran should not be used, as it interferes with clotting. Digitalis should be used with caution, since hypokalemia and respiratory alkalosis may be present. There is no rationale for prophylactic antibiotic therapy. The maintenance of a brisk urine flow is of prime importance, since rhabdomyolysis and concomitant acute renal failure are common in heat stroke.

RUN FOR YOUR LIFE

For the past two years Blue Cross–Blue Shield of Central New York has sponsored a 10 km race called "Run For Your Life." The run is dedicated to physical fitness and takes place in late spring. On both occasions the day was hot, humid, and windless. We know of eight cases of resultant heat stroke that required hospital admission.

COOKED GOOSE

When a patient has a rectal temperature of 40°C or higher, he must be cooled as rapidly as possible no matter what the cause. The need for immediate therapy notwithstanding, investigation for the underlying cause should also be initiated without delay. None of the disease states listed below should be overlooked, as every one of them has a serious mortality rate.

Heat stroke
Hypothalamic dysfunction
Meningitis
Delirium tremens
Midbrain hemorrhage
Falciparum malaria
Rocky Mountain fever

Typhus
Sepsis (e.g., meningococcemia, staphylococcemia)
Influenza
Reaction to drugs or anesthetic agents (malignant hyperthermia)
Hypernephroma

TEMPERATURE CONVERSION AND CORRECTION FACTORS FOR ARTERIAL BLOOD GASES

Extremes of body temperature that are sometimes encountered in the critically ill patient can cause significant variance between the actual arterial blood gas values and those that are obtained in the laboratory at room temperature. The accompanying table can be used to make these temperature corrections for arterial blood gases if your laboratory does not routinely do this. For example, reported blood gases of pH 7.30, $PaCO_2$ 50 torr, and PaO_2 100 torr in a patient with a body temperature of 33°C are actually pH 7.36, $PaCO_2$ 41.2, and PaO_2 71.2.

	↑ 1°C*†	↓ 1°C*†
pH	↓ .015	↑ .015
PCO_2 (mm Hg)	↑ 4.4%	↓ 4.4%
PO_2 (mm Hg)	↑ 7.2%	↓ 7.2%

*Change with reference to 37°C.
†Per cent change of the value measured at standard 37°C.

Reference: Reuler, J. B.: Ann. Intern. Med. *89*:519, 1978. Table reprinted with the permission of the author and publisher.

HYPOTHERMIA

The *appropriate management* of hypothermia can turn a clinically dead patient into a normal person within hours. Alcoholics, the elderly, and newborns are the high risk populations for this disorder; but the recent popularity of outdoor winter sports has increased its incidence in the young and otherwise healthy. The correct diagnosis must precede appropriate management. Consider hypothermia when presented with any comatose hypotensive patient. Remember that extreme environmental conditions are not necessary to produce hypothermia (we treated a case on May 13, when the ambient temperature was in the 50's). The characteristic "J" (Osborn) wave (Figure 2–2) in the EKG may be the clinical clue that makes the diagnosis.

2

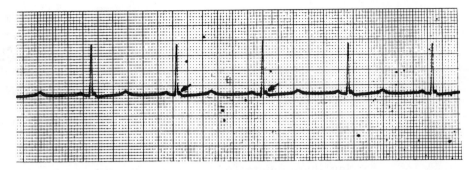

FIG. 2-2

The characteristic "J" wave seen in the EKG of this hypothermic patient is marked with arrows. As described by Osborn, the wave is a "camel humped" deflection. It is usually seen as a slowly inscribed deflection at the QRS-ST junction or J point. J waves may also be seen in CNS disease and in some normal individuals.

There are some physiologic effects of hypothermia that have an important bearing on management.

PHYSIOLOGIC EFFECT	MANAGEMENT IMPLICATION
1. Decreased oxygen requirement	1. Protective — preserves neurologic function in spite of depressed perfusion
2. Increased myocardial irritability	2. High risk of V-fib when temperature is below 28–30°C
3. Respiratory depression and bronchorrhea	3. Secondary pulmonary complications (e.g., aspiration pneumonia)
4. Alteration in arterial blood gases	4. Adjust to ambient body temperature
5. Acidosis — respiratory and metabolic (lactic)	5. Correct, but be careful with the $NaHCO_3$ to avoid alkalosis during rewarming
6. Depressed hepatic function	6. Prolonged drug effect
7. Increased urine flow	7. Hypovolemia
8. Extracellular fluid shifts	8. Hypovolemia
9. Hyperglycemia when cold, followed by hypoglycemia with rewarming	9. Don't give insulin
10. Pancreatic injury	10. Secondary pancreatitis
11. Neurologic depression	11. May be completely reversible — "Nobody is dead until they are warm and dead"

The therapy for hypothermia consists of general supportive measures combined with specific rewarming techniques. The *do's* and *don't's* of general supportive care are: ·

Do

1. Handle the patient carefully and gently to avoid precipitation of ventricular fibrillation.
2. Accurately record and monitor core temperature with a recording thermometer with a low temperature range (the operating room usually has one).
3. Admit patient to ICU if core temperature is less than 33°C.
4. Continuously monitor the EKG.
5. Oxygenate, ventilate, and maintain tracheal toilet.
6. Replace volume — warm the fluids with a blood warmer.
7. Correct the arterial blood gases for body temperature.
8. Carefully give sodium bicarbonate for metabolic acidosis.
9. Give thyroxine and corticosteroids if myxedema is suspected.

Don't

1. Don't move or manipulate the patient unless absolutely necessary.
2. Don't insert any intracardiac catheters.
3. Don't give most drugs — they have little effect when the patient is cold, and may produce toxicity with rewarming.
4. Don't treat hyperglycemia unless it is extreme; there is a risk of hypoglycemia with rewarming.

Areas of frostbite should be locally and rapidly rewarmed by means of water baths at 40–43.6°C. Patients with frostbite should receive tetanus prophylaxis.

Rewarming should be instituted simultaneously with the general support measures. The following table lists the rewarming methods that have been described. External rewarming alone may cause further heat loss from peripheral vasodilitation and paradoxical core cooling that, in turn, predisposes to ventricular arrhythmias. Patients with a core temperature less than 32°C probably do best with a combination of core rewarming and passive external rewarming. The method of core rewarming chosen should be based on available resources and the clinical setting.

TYPE OF REWARMING	METHODS
Passive rewarming	1. Removal from environmental exposure 2. Insulating material (e.g., blankets)
Active external rewarming	1. Immersion in heated water 2. Electric blankets 3. Heated objects (e.g., water bottle)
Active core rewarming	1. Intragastric balloon 2. Colonic irrigation 3. Mediastinal irrigation via thoractomy 4. Hemodialysis 5. Peritoneal dialysis 6. Extracorporeal blood rewarming 7. Inhalation rewarming

Should ventricular fibrillation occur, cardiopulmonary resuscitation should be instituted and continued until the patient has been rewarmed, since the protective effect of hypothermia on the brain makes complete neurologic recovery possible even after prolonged periods of cardiac arrest. Remember, "no one is dead until they are warm and dead."

Reference: Reuler, J. B., Ann. Intern. Med., *89*:519, 1978. Table on rewarming methods reprinted with permission of the author and publisher.

HOW COLD IS IT?

High winds and low temperatures can lead to frostbite on exposed skin. Children, alcoholics, and senior citizens are especially vulnerable to cold weather. The table (Fig. 2–3) below can be used to predict the danger from exposure posed by varying environmental conditions.

CHILL FACTOR

Wind in m.p.h.	Local Temperature in Degrees Fahrenheit										
	32	23	14	5	-4	-13	-22	-31	-40	-49	-58
	Equivalent Temperature (Wind Plus Local Temperature)										
Calm	32	23	14	5	-4	-13	-22	-31	-40	-49	-58
5	29	20	10	1	-9	-18	-28	-37	-47	-56	-65
10	18	7	-4	-15	-26	-37	-48	-59	-70	-81	-92
15	13	-1	-13	-25	-37	-49	-61	-73	-88	-97	-109
20	7	-6	-19	-32	-44	-57	-70	-83	-98	-109	-121
25	3	-10	-24	-37	-50	-64	-77	-90	-104	-117	-130
30	1	-13	-27	-41	-54	-68	-82	-97	-109	-123	-137
35	-1	-15	-29	-43	-57	-71	-85	-99	-113	-127	-142
40	-3	-17	-31	-45	-59	-74	-87	-102	-116	-131	-145
45	-3	-18	-32	-46	-61	-75	-89	-104	-118	-132	-147
50	-4	-18	-33	-47	-62	-76	-91	-105	-120	-134	-148
	little danger for those properly clothed ⟶		considerable danger ⟶		extreme danger ⟶						

FIG. 2–3

Differential environmental risk from chill factor. The chill factor is computed by relating the wind velocity to the local temperature. Zones of varying risk are demarcated by heavy black lines.

Reference: Emergency Victim Care. Instructional Materials Laboratory, Ohio State University, 1973.

SNAKE BITE

There are a large number of poisonous snakes whose venoms can cause a diverse range of clinical syndromes. Local effects include severe pain, swelling, ecchymosis, and lymphadenopathy, which may progress to necrosis and gangrene of the extremity, requiring amputation. Systemic effects may include pulmonary failure, circulatory collapse, convulsions, bulbar paralysis, renal failure, and disseminated intravascular coagulation.

Important: Many first aid books recommend that the offending snake be killed and brought along for the physician to identify. We all know that physicians are expert herpetologists. As a potential physician-herpetologist, you should be aware that dead snakes can still bite for at least 20 and perhaps as long as 60 minutes after their demise. There-

2

fore, the prudent physician will avoid coming in close proximity to the head of the dead snake.

Treatment

1. Incision and suction can remove substantial amounts of venom. Incise the skin longitudinally along the fang marks and use some sort of mechanical device for suction on the wound. Oral suction is certainly dramatic but carries a high risk of wound contamination and some risk of poisoning the rescuer.
2. Immobilize the bitten parts in a slightly dependent position and keep the patient quiet.
3. Apply a constricting band above the bitten area which is tight enough to occlude venous and lymphatic return but loose enough to preserve the distal arterial pulse. The band may need to be adjusted or moved proximally as the swelling progresses.
4. Do not apply ice to the wound. (There is disagreement on this.)
5. Treat any systemic effects with standard medical techniques.
6. Administer tetanus prophylaxis.
7. Perform surgical debridement of affected tissues.

Although most authorities on snake bite believe that antivenom is the mainstay of treatment, the decision to use antivenom in the a-symptomatic person who has been bitten by a snake may be difficult. Most available antivenoms are horse serum, which can cause anaphylaxis in some people and will cause serum sickness in 30 to 75 per cent of patients. Since poisonous snakes do not always inject venom when they bite, antivenom may not be necessary. Therefore, the clinician must weigh the likelihood of adverse effects from the antivenom against the possibility of the eventual development of adverse effects from the snake bite.

Further information on the location of antivenom for rare species of poisonous snakes and the names and phone numbers of experts on venomous bites can be obtained from the Oklahoma City Poison Control Center, telephone 405-271-5454.

Reference: Abramowicz, M., et al. (Eds.): The Medical Letter, *20*:101, 1978.

MUSHROOM POISONING (Mycetismus)

Identification of the type of mushroom eaten is essential in treating a patient suspected of suffering from mushroom poisoning. A mushroom similar to the type ingested should be brought in with the patient so proper identification can be made. A list of the important points to appreciate when evaluating a patient with mycetismus is provided.

TYPE OF MUSHROOM	SYNDROME PRODUCED	TOXIN	TREATMENT
Amanita phalloides	Mycetismus choleriformis 1. Cramps, diarrhea, vomiting 10–15 hours after ingestion 2. Liver, kidney damage	Phallotoxins Amatotoxins	Thioctic acid (experimental, but no other known antidote)
Gyromitra esculenta	Mycetismus sanguinarius 1. Central nervous system symptoms	Monomethylhydrazine formed from hydrolysis of gyromitrin	Thioctic acid Pyridoxine 25 mg/kg
Amanita muscaria *Amanita pantherina* *Clitocybe illuldens* *Clitocybe dealbata* *Inocybe species*	Mycetismus nervosus 1. Headache, nausea, vomiting 2. Symptoms of excess parasympathetic discharge — salivation, lacrimation, diffuse perspiration, miosis, visual disturbances, bronchoconstriction, bradycardia 3. Shock associated with vasodilation and bradycardia	Muscarine Muscimol Ibotenic acid	*Atropine* is the specific antidote for *Inocybe* and *Clitocybe* poisonings. It is contraindicated in *A. muscaria* and *A. pantherina* poisonings. There is no antidote for the latter two poisonings.
Many species	Mycetismus gastrointestinalis 1. Nausea, vomiting, diarrhea 2. Usually not fatal	Unknown	Supportive
Coprinus atramentarius	Disulfiram reactions 1. Symptoms of disulfiram toxicity occur if this mushroom is eaten and alcohol is also consumed	? Disulfiram (Antabuse)	Supportive

Reference: Gray, W. D.: Drug Therapy, September 1978, p. 103.

2

I SPOUT A VEIN

You are "on call" in the emergency room when John Doe is brought in comatose. You must latch onto whatever details are available: his age, nutritional state, hygiene, and dress; how and where he was discovered; clues in his wallet or pockets. A thorough physical exam, with a careful neurologic exam including calorics, is imperative. Some causes of rapid brain death are remediable, so therapy should precede diagnosis: check for a pulse, secure an airway, administer oxygen, and establish a large bore intravenous line, maintained with an infusion of 5 per cent dextrose in water. Immediately give three drugs by IV bolus: Naloxone, 0.4 mg; Thiamine, 100 mg; and 50 per cent dextrose, 25 to 50 grams.

The chart on pages 44 and 45 offers a mnemonic for recalling the essentials in differential diagnosis, the tests that must be done immediately, and the emergency therapy that must be given. After these initial things are done, more complex, time-consuming, or invasive tests can be performed.

EMERGENCY MANAGEMENT OF ACUTE PULMONARY EDEMA (M–O–S–T D–A–M–P–V^2)

Goals of Therapy

1. Reduction of pulmonary congestion.
2. Improvement of gas exchange.
3. Improvement of ventricular performance.
4. Recognition of underlying diseases.
5. Treatment of precipitating factors.

See table on pages 46 and 47.

A good heart and kidneys can surmount all but the most willfully incompetent fluid regimen.

	DISEASES	TEST	THERAPY
I	Insulin — Too much: Too little: Hypoglycemia Ketoacidosis Hyperglycemia	Blood sugar	25 ml–50 ml $D_{50}W$ Intravenous line
S	Shock Hypoperfusion Cardiac arrythmias Pulmonary embolus	EKG/monitor Arterial blood gases	Airway Insure circulation
P	Psychogenic Hysteria, malingering	Raise arm and release; if true coma, forearm will strike patient's face	
O	Opiates and other drugs Aspirin, Doriden, Quaalude, barbiturates, heroin, morphine, phenothiazines	Serum and urine toxic drug screen Urine ferric chloride	Naloxone: 0.4 mg IV; Physostigmine 1–4 mg IV (may repeat)
U	Uremia and other metabolic derangements Uremia, myxedema coma anoxia, CO_2 narcosis, hepatic insufficiency, Addison's disease, hyper-calcemia, hypothermia, hyperthermia, electrolyte imbalance, hypoglycemia	Blood urea nitrogen Electrolytes Arterial blood gases Calcium Temperature	Urinary catheter Oxygen Normalize body tempera-ture where appropriate

T	Trauma	Epidural hematoma, subdural hematoma, cerebral lacerations, cervical spine trauma	Skull x-rays Cervical spine x-rays	Stabilize neck
A	Alcohol	Acute intoxication, Wernicke's encephalopathy	Blood alcohol level	Thiamine 100 mg IV (to precede the glucose therapy)
V	Vascular	Cerebral-vascular accident hemorrhage, arteriovenous malformation, berry aneurysm, carotid occlusion, sub-arachnoid bleed, underperfusion		
E	Encephalopathy	Hypertensive, post-infectious, viral, post-ictal	Blood pressure	
I	Infection	Brain abscess, epidural abscess, meningitis, gram negative sepsis	Complete blood count Blood cultures Lumbar puncture	
N	Neoplasm	Primary or metastatic tumor, hypercalcemia, electrolyte imbalance		

M-O-S-T

Emergency Measures	Rationale
M	Morphine sulfate 5 to 10 mg IV slowly to avoid hypotension	Relieves hyperventilation and dyspnea by reducing respiratory reflexes and the work of breathing; sedative effect allays anxiety and tachycardia and reduces cardiac oxygen demand; decreases sympathetic tone; venous dilatation reduces venous return; relieves pain
O	Oxygen administration	Reduces dyspnea and hypoxemia
S	Sit the patient up	Relieves dyspnea by reducing venous return to the right heart, thereby diminishing pulmonary blood volume and congestion
T	Rotating tourniquets occlude the venous return but not the arterial pulse; apply to three limbs and rotate every 15 minutes	Reduction of venous return reduces pulmonary blood volume; beneficial in patients with normal or increased blood pressure; do not use in patients with hypotension or shock

D-A-M-P

D	Digitalis Give intravenously if patient has not been previously digitalized; Digoxin 0.5 to 0.75 mg or a rapidly acting digitalis glycoside	Improves myocardial contractility (positive inotropic effect); monitor digitalization with electrocardiography for signs of toxicity
A	Aminophylline 5.6 mg per kilogram IV in 30 to 50 ml of solution slowly (10 to 20 minutes); if necessary, follow up with a continuous infusion	Bronchodilating effect in cardiac asthma; inotropic effect improves myocardial contractility; mild diuretic effect

M Mercurials (diuretics in the old days) or furosemide, 1 to 2 mg per kilogram IV or sodium ethacrynate, 50 to 150 mg IV

Reduction of blood volume reduces venous return; furosemide increases peripheral venous capacitance; monitor potassium levels

P Phlebotomy

Consider 250 ml phlebotomy if there is no response to the above measures after 30 minutes; phlebotomy is contraindicated in the presence of hypotension or shock

Rapidly lowers pulmonary arterial and venous pressures and decreases left ventricular workload

$\underline{V^2}$

V Vasodilator therapy

Nitroglycerin

Isosorbide dinitrate

Predominantly dilates the venous capacitance vessels but also dilates the peripheral arterioles

Venous dilators reduce venous tone and venous return to the right heart, thereby reducing left ventricular filling and diastolic pressure (preload effect)

Nitroprusside

Phentolamine

Predominantly dilates the arteriolar bed

The arterial dilators reduce systemic vascular resistance and lower impedance to left ventricular ejection, thus facilitating ventricular emptying and increasing cardiac output (afterload effect)

V Ventilation (mechanical)

Facilitates removal of secretions; allows positive end expiratory pressure (PEEP); reduces preload

CARDIAC ASTHMA

When a patient over 40 develops wheezing, the "asthma" may be due to left-sided heart failure. In patients with pulmonary edema, the likelihood of developing bronchospasm varies. Frequently, patients with pre-existing chronic obstructive pulmonary disease, "real asthma," or a history of allergies will have an increased tendency to exhibit bronchospasm when they develop congestive heart failure.

It is of the utmost importance to discern the real cause for bronchospasm, since morphine is helpful in managing pulmonary edema (see preceding article) but is contraindicated in the true asthmatic.

Cardiac asthma usually occurs when the patient exerts himself, becomes excitable or anxious, or lies down to sleep. Once an attack begins, respirations become rapid, shallow, and laborious. The skin is cool and clammy, and the face ashen. There may be marked diaphoresis and neck vein distension. Blood pressure is usually elevated, and the pulse is rapid. Cyanosis becomes obvious as bronchospasm and fluid-filled alveoli impair oxygen exchange. Auscultation is difficult because wheezes and rhonchi mask cardiac sounds; however, an accentuated second heart sound and a gallop rhythm may be heard. Pulsus paradoxus may be found.

The clinical distinction between cardiac and pulmonary asthma is difficult unless the patient's history is known. In general, the paroxysmal and *recent* occurrence of these attacks, coupled with associated signs and symptoms of left heart failure (i.e., orthopnea, hemoptysis, paroxysmal nocturnal dyspnea, cardiomegaly, murmurs, pleural effusions, and interstitial edema), helps define cardiac asthma, whereas an extended history of respiratory difficulties, atopia, change in body habitus, and a chest x-ray showing the changes of a primary pulmonary problem define pulmonary asthma.

Occasionally, both cardiac *and* pulmonary asthma may be present, or the distinction may be impossible to make. In the latter cases, therapy for congestive heart failure is warranted to clarify the problem.

CARDIOPULMONARY RESUSCITATION

All physicians should be proficient in both basic and advanced cardiopulmonary resuscitation. Basic cardiac life support is a motor skill that can only be mastered by practice. The review of the essential steps in basic life support presented here (Fig. 2–4) will serve as a reminder of the appropriate sequence of action to follow in treating cardiac arrest. Proficient performance requires periodic "hands-on" practice with a mannequin.

Training programs in basic cardiac life support are given by the American Red Cross and the American Heart Association. The American Heart Association offers an excellent course in advanced cardiac life support that combines teaching of the background material with hands-on training. Your local chapter of the Red Cross or Heart Association will be able to provide you with details about the training programs.

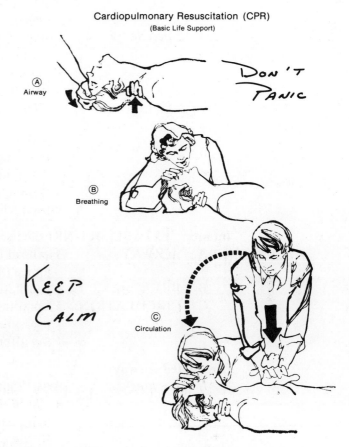

FIG. 2–4 The ABC's of CPR.

ESSENTIAL STEPS IN BASIC LIFE SUPPORT

Cardiac arrest is *apparent unexpected death* due to ventricular fibrillation, asystole, or electromechanical dissociation.

Adults: ESTABLISH UNRESPONSIVENESS (4 to 10 sec): c):
Shake shoulders, shout, "Are you OK?"
Call "help!" Turn victim prone if necessary.

A. AIRWAY:	Open airway; establish apnea.
B. BREATHE:	4 breaths of 1000 cc at 1/sec (if airway is obstructed, see below). Establish pulselessness (4 sec). Call for help again.
C. CIRCULATION:	Start closed cardiac compression: Firm surface, midline lower sternum, 1.5-inch chest movement.
1 person:	Compressions (80/min): "One and . . . two and," etc.

Rhythm: 15 compressions — 2 breaths. (Four cycles per minute.)

Recheck for pulse and respiration after four cycles.

2 people: Compressions (60/min): "One one-thousand ... Two one-thousand," etc.

Rhythm: 5 compressions — 1 breath. (On fifth upstroke, no pause.)

Change: Compressor says, "Change, on, *three,* next, time." Ventilator gives breath and moves hands to xiphisternum. After third compression, he moves hands and continues, "four one-thousand ... five one-thousand," etc.

Pulse rechecked by ventilator periodically.

Infants: ESTABLISH UNRESPONSIVENESS: Shake, shout.

    A. AIRWAY: Tip head back (no hyperextension); establish apnea (4 sec).

    B. BREATHE: 4 ventilations (puffs); establish pulselessness.

    C. CIRCULATION: 5 compressions — 1 breath; 80 to 100 compressions/min. Check for pulse and breathing after 30 seconds.

Obstructed Airway:

    If Conscious: Ask, "Can you *speak?"* If he cannot:

    4 sharp back blows (interscapular); other hand supports chest. Then 4 abdominal thrusts, or 4 chest thrusts (preferred in pregnant and obese patients). Repeat sequence until airway is cleared or patient becomes unconscious.

    Unconscious: ESTABLISH UNRESPONSIVENESS (see section on adults)

    A. AIRWAY: Open Airway; establish apnea

    B. BREATHE: Attempt ventilation; reposition head; try again.

    Then: To use back blows: Roll victim against your thigh for support. 4 back blows, then 4 abdominal thrusts or 4 chest thrusts. Fingerprobe mouth. If no response, repeat sequence until airway is cleared, or consider laryngoscopy, transtracheal catheter ventilation, or cricothyreotomy if equipment available.

    C. CONTINUE BASIC LIFE SUPPORT AS ABOVE.

Thanks to Dr. Alan Grogono for this concise summary of BLS.

ADVANCED LIFE SUPPORT IN A NUTSHELL

Advanced life support for a patient with cardiac arrest consists of the following elements:

1. Basic life support (A–Airway, B–Breathing, C–Circulation).
2. Use of adjunctive equipment for ventilation and circulation.
3. Cardiac monitoring for dysrhythmia recognition and control.
4. Defibrillation.
5. Establishing and maintaining an intravenous infusion lifeline.
6. Employing definitive therapy, including drug administration
   — to correct acidosis and hypoxemia.
   — to aid in establishing and maintaining effective cardiac rhythm and circulation.
7. Stabilization of the patient's condition.
8. Transportation with continuous monitoring.

Don't forget that it is crucial to maintain uninterrupted basic life support until spontaneous circulation is restored.

Advanced life support can be approached in the following sequence:

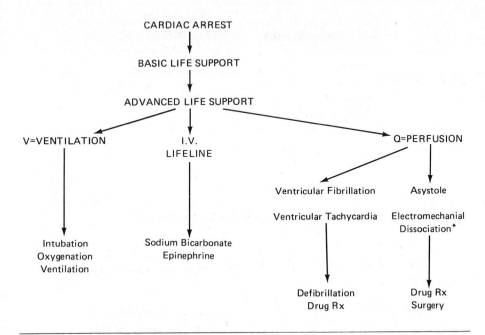

*See article on Electromechanical Dissociation, page 58.

After initiation of basic life support, ventilation (consisting of intubation, oxygenation, and ventilation) and an IV infusion lifeline are established, sodium bicarbonate and epinephrine are administered. Normal circulation is restored by means of countershock and/or drug therapy, depending on the rhythm disturbance seen with the "quick look" paddles. A blind defibrillation using the maximum output of the machine should be performed when a defibrillator becomes available before an EKG monitor.

Objectives of Drug Treatment

1. To correct hypoxia.
2. To correct metabolic acidosis.
3. To increase perfusion pressure during cardiac compression.
4. To stimulate spontaneous or more forceful myocardial contraction.
5. To accelerate cardiac rate.
6. To suppress ventricular ectopic activity.
7. To relieve pain and to treat pulmonary edema.

ESSENTIAL DRUGS	USEFUL DRUGS
Oxygen	Isoproterenol
Sodium bicarbonate	Propranolol
Epinephrine	Procainamide
Atropine	Dopamine
Lidocaine	
Morphine	
Calcium chloride	

Summary of Drug Therapy in Advanced Life Support

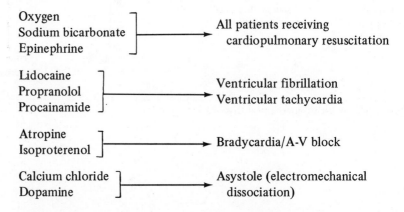

Oxygen
Sodium bicarbonate
Epinephrine
⟶ All patients receiving cardiopulmonary resuscitation

Lidocaine
Propranolol
Procainamide
⟶ Ventricular fibrillation
Ventricular tachycardia

Atropine
Isoproterenol
⟶ Bradycardia/A-V block

Calcium chloride
Dopamine
⟶ Asystole (electromechanical dissociation)

SELECTED ESSENTIAL DRUGS

Oxygen:
    Action   — Correction of hypoxia
    Dose   — 100% (never withhold O_2 in an arrest)

Sodium Bicarbonate:
    Action   — Reversal of metabolic acidosis
    Dose   — 1 mEq/kg IV at time 0
                 1 mEq/kg IV at 10 min
                 0.5 mEq/kg IV Q 10 min thereafter until circulation restored
    Remember — Must be combined with adequate ventilation to be effective

Epinephrine:
    Action   — Elevates perfusion pressure generated during CPR
                 Improves myocardial contractility
                 Stimulates spontaneous contractions
                 Converts fine to coarse fibrillation
    Dose   — 0.5 mg IV (5 ml of 1:10,000 solution) Q 5 min until circulation
                 restored (for effect on perfusion pressure)
    Remember — Epinephrine is not effective until acidosis is corrected
                 Can be administered via the tracheobronchial tree
                 Inactivated when administered simultaneously with alkaline
                 solutions

Atropine
    Action   — Acceleration of heart rate
    Dose   — 0.5 mg IV Q 5 min until desired heart rate is achieved or total
                 dose of 2 mg is given without effect

Lidocaine:
    Action   — Suppression of ventricular dysrhythmias
    Dose   — 1 mg/kg IV bolus, then 1 to 4 mg/min IV drip
    Remember — Need to repeat bolus when infusion rate increased (e.g., from
                 2 to 4 mg/min)
                 Can be given intramuscularly

Calcium Chloride:
    Action   — Increases force of myocardial contraction
                 Stimulates spontaneous contraction
    Dose   — 2.5 to 5.0 ml of 10% $CaCl_2$ IV (250 to 500 mg of $CaCl_2$; can
                 repeat Q 10 min)

SELECTED USEFUL DRUGS

Isoproterenol:
    Action   — Acceleration of heart rate ("chemical pacemaker")
    Dose   — 2 to 20 μg/min IV titrated according to heart rate and rhythm

Propranolol:
    Action   — Suppression of ventricular tachyarrhythmias
    Dose   — 1.0 mg IV slowly Q 5 min to total dose of 5 mg

TABLE CONTINUED ON THE FOLLOWING PAGE

SELECTED USEFUL DRUGS

Procainamide:

    Action   — Suppression of ventricular tachyarrhythmias

    Dose   — 100 mg IV slowly Q 5 min until:

            a. Arrhythmia resolved

            b. Total dose of 1 gram

            c. Toxicity occurs

                1. Hypotension

                2. Conduction disturbance (QRS prolongation)

Dopamine:

    Action   — Vasopressor

    Dose   — 2 to 20 μg/kg/min titrated according to clinical response

---

DEFIBRILLATION

A now defunct television program entitled "Marcus Welby, M.D.," used a defibrillation scene as its opening. An impeccably dressed Marcus Welby strolls into the room and is given the paddles by the nurse. The camera pans to the monitor, which shows sinus rhythm. The intrepid physician applies the paddles with the appropriate dramatic expression and shocks the patient. The patient makes an appropriately dramatic tonic contraction, and the camera then pans back to the monitor, which now shows ventricular fibrillation. In addition to knowing the difference between ventricular fibrillation and sinus rhythm, the physician needs to know a bit more about the fine points of electrical defibrillation.

Point 1. *Know your equipment.* There are a wide variety of defibrillators on the market, and although their basic controls (as outlined below) are similar, the location of the controls and the "frills" will vary from model to model. This get-acquainted session should be held some leisurely afternoon and not during the heat of a cardiac arrest.

    1. On/off switch.

    2. Charge device — activates storage of energy in the capacitor. On many units, one needs both to set a dial to the desired

energy and to press a switch or button to start the activation process.

3. Energy measurement — indicates either how much energy is stored in the capacitor or how much energy will be delivered. Delivered energy is always less than stored energy, and in some models, markedly less.

4. Firing mechanism — releases the energy stored in the capacitor through the defibrillator paddles.

5. Synchronizer. This can be a fooler. The synchronization mode is used during cardioversion of tachyarrhythmias. Synchronization insures that the electrical energy will be delivered during the QRS complex, and not during the vulnerable Q-T period when an electrical discharge is more likely to cause ventricular fibrillation. When the defibrillator is in the synchronization mode, it will not discharge until it senses an R wave. Thus, if one tries to treat ventricular fibrillation with the synchronization circuit on, the machine will not fire.

Point 2: *Know the procedure.*

1. Verify that there is cardiac arrest.

2. Turn the machine on.

3. Set the desired energy level. The current recommendations of the American Heart Association are:

   a. For patients weighing less than 50 kg, 3.5 to 6.0 watt seconds per kilogram.

   b. For patients heavier than 50 kg, the maximum output of the defibrillator.

   (There currently is a raging debate about the appropriate energy levels to use for defibrillation. Some experts advocate much higher energies and others advocate much lower energies. With higher energies, there is increased risk of myocardial damage. With lower energies, there is greater probability of unsuccessful defibrillation. At this time [1980] the controversy has not been resolved, and it is our practice to follow the recommendations of the American Heart Association.)

4. Reduce skin resistance. Saline-soaked gauze pads or electropaste may be used. Don't use alcohol unless you like your patient flambé.

5. Apply the paddles as shown in Figure 2–5. The paddles should not be over the sternum, as bone provides significant resistance to current flow.
6. Apply pressure.
7. Clear the area of personnel.
8. Fire. The patient's chest muscles should contract with the defibrillation. If they do not, no current has reached the patient, and you should check to assure that:
   a. The defibrillator is plugged in and turned on.
   b. The synchronizer circuit is turned off.
   c. The battery is charged (if the defibrillator is battery-powered).
   d. The operator knows what he is doing.
9. Check pulse and electrocardiogram. If there is no pulse, even with an EKG rhythm, immediately reinstitute basic life support

STANDARD PADDLE PLACEMENT

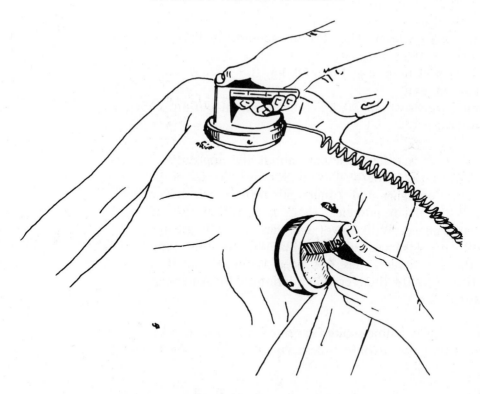

FIG. 2–5

Standard Paddle Placement for Cardiac Defibrillation.

and continue with the other aspects of advanced life support (see Advanced Life Support in a Nutshell).

Reference: Parker, M. R.: Defibrillation and synchronized cardioversion. In: Manual for Providers of Advanced Cardiac Life Support. Dallas, American Heart Association, 1977. Figure reproduced with permission of author and the American Heart Association, Inc.

Success covers a multitude of blunders.

AUTOMOTIVE RESUSCITATION

Battery failure almost always occurs at the worst time or place: on frigid mornings or late at night in the hospital parking lot. When the diagnosis is correct, a "jump start" from a normal battery is usually successful and by far the most convenient means of battery resuscitation. Carry your own set of booster cables. There are potential hazards in the method, and the proper technique insures the best results.

Caveats

1. Don't smoke, and beware of any sparks. Batteries generate hydrogen!
2. Check the dead battery to make sure it isn't frozen or dry. Don't try to start a frozen battery. A dry battery needs volume replacement with distilled water.
3. Make sure the booster and dead batteries are of the same voltage.
4. Make sure the cars aren't touching and the engines are off.
5. Remove the water filler clips (if any) from both batteries.

Procedure

1. Connect the cable clamp to the positive terminal of the dead battery first. Then clamp the other end to the positive terminal of the booster.
2. Connect the other cable to the negative terminal of the booster. Connect the other end of the cable to the engine block (not the negative terminal) on the side away from the dead battery. Make sure the cables clear any moving engine parts.
3. Start the engine of the car that has the good battery before attempting to start the disabled car.
4. After you get the disabled car going, remove the negative cable first, starting with the end connected to the engine block.
5. Remove the positive cable.
6. Replace the filler caps.

ELECTROMECHANICAL DISSOCIATION

Electromechanical dissociation (EMD) is a condition in which there is some semblance of normal cardiac electrical activity but no appreciable cardiac output. The various pathologic conditions that can result in electromechanical dissociation are listed below. With the exception of massive myocardial infarction, they all are potentially reversible if recognized and treated appropriately. Notice that the treatment is surgical in most instances. An asterisk denotes the conditions that may arise as a complication of cardiopulmonary resuscitation. A specific examination for these conditions should be conducted when a patient who has been electrically resuscitated following a cardiac arrest develops EMD.

1. Massive myocardial infarction
2. Exsanguination*
3. Pericardial tamponade*
4. Pulmonary embolism
5. Air embolism*
6. Tension pneumothorax*
7. Hypocalcemia

"Shock: a momentary pause in the act of death."

John Collius Warren

AIR EMBOLISM-VENOUS

The air embolism syndrome occurs when a breach in the vasculature allows air to enter the venous circuit and collect in the right ventricular outflow tract. This causes actual obstruction of blood flow out of the right ventricle. Although an uncommon occurrence, the condition must be recognized and treated immediately if a fatal outcome is to be avoided. The clinical settings in which one should suspect air embolism include:

1. CVP placement.
2. Chest trauma.
3. Neurosurgical operations (especially those performed in a sitting position).
4. Following cunnilingus (especially during pregnancy).

The development of shock in one of these settings should cause the physician to auscultate the heart to find out whether the characteristic mill wheel murmur of air embolism is present. The treatment consists of first placing the patient in the left lateral decubitus Trendelenberg position. This shifts the air away from the right ventricular outflow tract and toward the apex of the right ventricle. A central line may then be passed into the right ventricle, and the air removed by aspiration. In severe cases, it may be necessary to open the chest and aspirate the air from the right ventricle under direct vision.

> *Asphyxia* — From the Greek *a*, "without," and *sphyxis*, "pulse."

HYPERBARIC OXYGEN

Hyperbaric oxygen therapy is useful in the treatment of decompression sickness, arterial air embolism (especially cerebral air embolism), clostridial cellulitis with myonecrosis, carbon monoxide poisoning, and perhaps refractory decubitus ulcers and chronic osteomyelitis. The facilities for hyperbaric oxygen therapy are complex and not widely available. However, rapid treatment is essential, especially in cases of air embolism, decompression sickness, or carbon monoxide poisoning. When faced with one of these medical emergencies, further information on hyperbaric oxygen therapy and available facilities can be obtained by calling 512-536-3281 or 3278.

Reference: Medical Letter, *20*:11, 1978.

DRIPS

The table on the following pages should help you in preparing drug solutions for continuous intravenous infusion. These drugs should be administered with a metriset and a constant infusion pump to safeguard against inadvertent administration of a large bolus of the drug. In patients who will need fluid restriction, the final concentration of the drugs may be doubled by halving the amount of solution.

DRUG	RECIPE	CONCENTRATION	SUGGESTED STARTING DOSE	COMMENTS
Aminophylline	500 mg/500 ml D5W	1 mg/ml	Load with 5.6 mg/kg/½ hr Maintenance 0.9 mg/kg/hr	1. Reduce loading and maintenance dose to 60% if hepatic, renal, or cardiac dysfunction present 2. Therapeutic blood level 10 to 20 μg/ml
Dopamine	400 mg/500 ml D5W	800 μg/ml	2 to 5 μg/kg/min	1. Effects dose-related 2. Inactivated by $NaHCO_3$
Dobutamine	250 mg/500 ml D5W	500 μg/ml	2.5 μg/kg/min	1. Negligible vascular effects 2. Inactivated by $NaHCO_3$
Epinephrine	2 mg/250 ml D5W	8 μg/ml	1 to 2 μg/min	1. Occasional patient will respond to epinephrine but not dopamine 2. Inactivated by $NaHCO_3$
Glucagon	125 mg/250 ml NS	500 μg/ml	Load with 5 to 8 mg/15 min Maintenance 3 to 8 mg/hr	1. Inotropic effect augmented by aminophylline
Isoproterenol	1 mg/500 ml D5W	2 μg/ml	2 μg/min	1. Chemical pacemaker
Nitroglycerin	83 1/100 sublingual tabs/500 ml NS	100 μg/ml	0.33 to 0.5 μg/kg/min	1. Crush tabs, dissolve in saline, filter solution through 27 millipore filter 2. Primarily a venous dilator with weak arterial action

2

Drug	Preparation	Concentration	Dose	Comments
Nitroprusside	50 mg/250 ml D5W	200 μg/ml	0.5 μg/kg/min	1. Light sensitive — cover bottle and tape tubing. Change bottle every 4 hours; may get hypotension with new bottle at previous dose 2. More arterial than venous dilation 3. Metabolic acidosis sign of cyanide toxicity
Norepinephrine	4 mg/500 ml D5W	8 μg/ml	1 to 2 μg/min	1. Reduces renal blood flow
Pitressin (vasopressin)	200 units/500 ml D5W	0.4 units/ml	0.4 units/min	1. Peripheral IV route may be nearly as effective as direct intra-arterial route
Trimethaphan	500 mg/500 ml D5W	1 mg/ml	0.1 mg/min	1. Tachyphylaxis may develop

COMPATIBILITY OF IV SOLUTIONS AND BLOOD TRANSFUSIONS

Normal saline is the ideal solution to infuse with blood or to start a blood transfusion. Most solutions containing dextrose and water (5 per cent aqueous dextrose [D5W], 5 per cent dextrose in 0.9 per cent saline [D5/NS], 5 per cent dextrose in 0.225 per cent saline [D5/0.2S]) are *inappropriate*, since they induce erythrocyte aggregation and osmotic shock, which may lead to erythrocyte lysis *in vivo*. Lengthy retention of these solutions in intravenous tubing after transfusion has begun and blood-warming devices increase these erythrocyte alterations.

Lactated Ringer's solution is a physiologic isotonic solution. However, it contains a high concentration of calcium, which may neutralize the anticoagulant activity of the citrate anticoagulant that is used in the blood preservative solution. It may also lead to clot formation in the infusion lines. Clotting in intravenous tubing may be increased when infusion rates are slow and the ambient temperature is high. Hence, small fibrin clots may be produced in the intravenous tubing and be administered to the patients.

In summary, of the intravenous solutions commonly available, only physiologic saline (0.9 per cent) should be infused concomitantly with blood.

Reference: Reyden, S. E., and Oberman, H. A.: Transfusion, *15*:250, 1975.

HYDROCHLORIC ACID FOR THE TREATMENT OF METABOLIC ALKALOSIS

Metabolic alkalosis occurs commonly in the critically ill patient and may have serious adverse physiologic effects, including mental confusion, cardiac compromise, arrhythmias, gastrointestinal ileus, and hypoventilation. Etiologic factors include loss of gastric secretions through vomiting or nasogastric suctioning, potassium depletion, diuretic use, mineralocorticoid excess in response to hypovolemia, and bicarbonate excess produced by the large amounts of citrate in massive blood transfusions. Because of these adverse effects and a significant correlation between mortality rates and degree of alkalosis, it is important to treat metabolic alkalosis in the critically ill patient. In cases refractory to the usual forms of therapy, such as removal of etiologic factors and infusion of sodium and potassium chloride, the intravenous infusion of hydrochloric acid is an effective and safe method for correcting the problem rapidly. The dose of hydrochloric acid to be given can be

2

approximated by using the following equation to estimate the hydrogen ion deficit:

$$\text{mEq HCl} = \text{base excess} \times 0.4 \text{ (body weight in kg)}.$$

Fifty per cent of the calculated hydrogen ion deficit is then replaced over the first 12 hours. Plasma electrolyte levels and arterial blood gases should be monitored several times during this period of rapid infusion. Further doses of hydrochloric acid are then given as needed, depending on the response to the initial dose.

The hydrochloric acid solution is prepared by diluting concentrated hydrochloric acid to 0.2 N with distilled water. This solution is then filtered through a millipore filter and mixed with equal volumes of sterile 10 per cent dextrose in water to give a resultant solution of 0.1 N hydrochloric acid in 5 per cent dextrose. This solution has 100 mEq of HCl per liter. Solutions of 0.15 N or 0.2 N hydrochloric acid may be used when volume load may be a problem. The acid infusion should be given through a central venous catheter. The 0.1 N hydrochloric acid can also be added directly to the essential amino acid mixtures used in hyperalimentation, if desired.

Reference: Abouna, G. M., Veazey, P. R., and Terry, D. B.: Surgery, *75*:194, 1974; Harken, A. H., Gabel, R. A., Fencl, V., et al.: Arch. Surg., *110*:819, 1975.

DISSECTING AORTIC ANEURYSM: TEARING AROUND THE BEND

Acute aortic dissection is an emergency. Studies of its natural history show that approximately 25 per cent of the patients will die within the first day unless appropriate intervention is undertaken. The following outline will guide the clinician to early diagnosis and effective therapy.

I. Epidemiology
   A. *Occurence:* The fifth to seventh decade, predominantly in men.
   B. *Predisposing factors:* Atherosclerosis, hypertension, cystic medial necrosis, giant cell arteritis, Marfan's and Ehler's-Danlos syndromes, idiopathic kyphoscoliosis, coarctation of the aorta, Turner's syndrome, aortic hypoplasia, bicuspid aortic valves, pregnancy, and relapsing polychondritis.
II. Types of dissection — The DeBakey Classification (see Fig. 2–6)
   A. *Type I:* Dissection begins in ascending aorta and extends

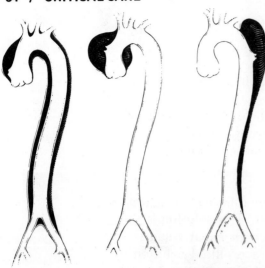

FIG. 2-6.

The DeBakey classification of acute aortic dissections. From left to right: Type I, Type II, Type III.

proximally and distally to involve the entire aorta. This is the most common type of dissection.

B. *Type II:* Dissection is limited to ascending aorta and the aortic arch. This type is most often associated with Marfan's syndrome.

C. *Type III:* Dissection begins distal to the left subclavian artery and extends more distally. Involvement of aortic branches is usually limited to innominate, iliac, and sub-clavian arteries.

III. Physiologic considerations

A. *Likelihood of propagation* of a dissection depends on shearing force, which in turn is a function of the blood pressure and the *rate of change* of blood pressure.

IV. Patient history

A. Abrupt onset of pain.

B. Pain limited to back is distinctive of Type III dissection.

C. The patient's general presentation is usually nonspecific. Aortic dissection should be considered in *every* acute thoracic or abdominal pain syndrome.

V. Physical exam — anatomic correlation

A. *Neurologic:* Syncope, coma, hemiplegia, and blindness are consequences of occlusion of carotid or vertebral branches or are secondary to hypotension associated with pericardial tamponade.

B. *Cardiovascular:*

1. There is a loss of peripheral pulses or blood pressure.

2. Differences in pressure or pulse between arms are secondary to peripheral artery occlusion.

3. Cardiac tamponade may be a result of dissection into the pericardial sac (hemopericardium).

4. Acute aortic regurgitation appears secondary to dissection into the valve ring.

5. Pulsation of sternoclavicular joint may be noted.

6. Acute myocardial infarction may result from exten-

sion of the dissection into the coronary arteries and subsequent occlusion.

C. *Pulmonary:* Hemothorax.

D. *Renal:* Oliguria, hypertension and hematuria secondary to dissection and occlusion of renal artery branches.

VI. Laboratory

A. *EKG:* The EKG is usually nonspecific; in 20 per cent of cases, evidence for myocardial injury is seen.

B. *Chest x-ray:* It may show widening of the mediastinum. That widening may be due to uncurling of the aorta. Hemothorax, pericardial effusion, or both may be seen.

C. *Aortogram:* The definitive test to diagnose dissection and to determine its extent. Prior to the aortogram, the patient should be stabilized, the hypertension controlled, and acute myocardial infarction excluded.

VII. Prognosis

A. *Factors predisposing to high mortality:* (1) extent of underlying medical disease; (2) severe neurologic involvement; (3) Type I and II dissections.

B. *Favorable prognosis:* (1) Type III dissection; (2) failure to opacify the false lumen at aortography.

VIII. Therapy

A. *General measures:*
   1. The patient requires an intensive care unit.
   2. An arterial line and Swan-Ganz catheter should be inserted for accurate and frequent monitoring.
   3. Treat left heart failure with appropriate agents.

B. *Acute medical therapy* to limit the dissection includes:
   1. Therapy aimed at reducing the shear force.
   2. Trimethaphan camsylate (Arfonad) or nitroprusside (Nipride) is used to lower blood pressure.
   3. Propranolol is used to reduce dp/dt of the left ventricle.

C. *Surgical therapy* is undertaken in the following circumstances:
   1. Delay surgery as long as possible to allow healing of the aortic wall, since there is a high operative mortality with immediate surgery.
   2. Indications for immediate surgery include:
      a. Leaking aneurysm (pericardial or pleural hemorrhage).
      b. Progression of the dissection.
      c. Vascular occlusion.
      d. Uncontrollable left heart failure from aortic valvular incompetence.
      e. Rarely uncontrollable hypertension or pain.
   3. Elective surgical repair is undertaken after three weeks in all Type I and II dissections.*

D. *Chronic therapy* entails maintaining patients on antihypertensives and propranolol to prevent further dissection.

---

*At present it is not clear whether patients with stable Type III dissections should undergo elective surgery at a later date.

References: Anagnostopoulos, C. E., Probhaka, M. J. S., and Kittle, C. F.: Am. J. Cardiol., *30*:263, 1972; Slater, E. E., and DeSanctis, R. W.: Am. J. Med., *60*:625, 1976; Wheat, M. W.: Prog. Cardiovasc. Dis., *16*:87, 1973; McFarland, J., et al.: N. Engl. J. Med., *286*:115, 1972; Parker, F. B., et al.: Ann. Thorac. Surg., *19*:436, 1975.

Figure reproduced with permission of author and publisher. From Anagnostopoulos, C. E.: Acute Aortic Dissections, University Park Press, 1975, p. 42.

NO MORE

This note was written by a 39-year-old woman with long-standing metastatic breast carcinoma. She had undergone radical mastectomy, left upper lobectomy, oophorectomy, radiotherapy, and multiple chemotherapeutic regimens. The note was written one day after she had been taken to the intensive care unit, intubated, and put on mechanical ventilation for pulmonary failure secondary to lung metastases, pneumonia, and sepsis. She was in severe pain from her bone metastases at the time but was fully alert and oriented.

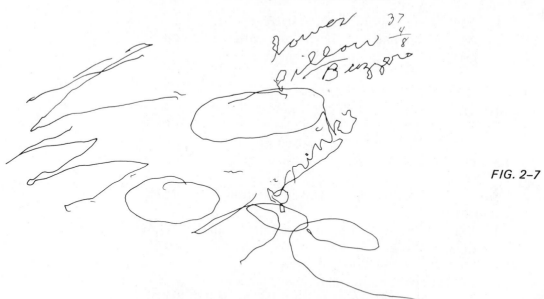

FIG. 2–7

The technology of critical care medicine, in some cases, serves only to prolong the suffering and dying process, rather than to preserve life. Critical care medicine is extensively oriented to machines and procedures and it is often easy to forget that there is a thinking, feeling, suffering patient involved. It is important to remember that in some instances intensive care is not justified — and perhaps even cruel.

Reference: Clouser, K. D.: Ann. Intern. Med., *89*:622, 1977.

3
DERMATOLOGY

SKIN: THE TOP TWENTY

The twenty most common skin conditions seen by the general physician are listed below. Organize a "mini-course" in dermatology for yourself, focusing on these common problems. Include a review of history, regional diagnosis, and current therapy.* You'll find it extremely easy to learn (or relearn) scraping, staining, and culture techniques. Inexpensive disposable biopsy punches are now available. Getting skin for the pathologist has become a benign and technically simple procedure. You should be able to diagnose each disease with ease.

The Twenty

Acne
Pigmented nevi
Warts
Actinic keratosis
Seborrheic keratosis
Seborrhea
Pityriasis rosea
Psoriasis
Drug eruptions
Tinea versicolor

Urticaria
Alopecia
Dyshydrosis
Contact dermatitis
Atopic dermatitis
Neurodermatitis
Xerosis
Basal cell carcinoma
Fungal infections
Bacterial infection

*A skin atlas is essential.

References: Sauer, G. C.: Manual of Skin Diseases, 3rd Edition. Philadelphia, J. B. Lippincott Company, 1972; Stewart, W. D., et al.: Synopsis of Dermatology, 2nd Edition. St. Louis, The C. V. Mosby Company, 1970.

HOMEMADE FUNGAL STAIN

You can examine skin scrapings for fungi by using your own homemade fungal stain:

1. Dissolve 6 grams of potassium hydroxide (KOH) pellets in 60 ml of Parker permanent blue-black ink. Do not substitute.
2. Centrifuge at 3000 rpm in an ordinary laboratory centrifuge to remove residual crystals.
3. Remove the blue supernatant fluid and store in a clean plastic bottle. It will keep indefinitely.

To use, add a drop or two of this stain to your sample under a cover slip. Heat gently. This preparation will dissolve most of the confusing debris and stain the fungal forms very clearly.

Reference: McMillan, J., Stockman, J., and Oski, F.: The Whole Pediatrician Catalog, Vol. 2: Philadelphia, W. B. Saunders Company, 1979, p. 178.

SYNDROMES ASSOCIATED WITH A GENERALIZED INCREASE IN PIGMENTATION

Generalized hyperpigmentation (melanin) may occur in a variety of clinical syndromes, including those listed below:

I. *Nutritional*
   Vitamin B_{12} deficiency
   Folic acid deficiency
   Chronic liver disease (cirrhosis, Wilson's disease, hemachromatosis)
   Nontropical sprue
   Whipple's disease
   Malnutrition
II. *Endocrine*
   Addison's disease (ACTH-, MSH-mediated)
   Nelson's syndrome (ACTH-, MSH-mediated)
   Endocrine and nonendocrine malignancies
   Myxedema
   Graves' disease
III. *Drugs*
   Busulfan
   Arsenicals
   Dibromomannitol
   Estrogen excess (including pregnancy)
IV. *Metabolic*
   Porphyria (cutanea tarda, erythropoietica, variegata)
V. *Collagen-vascular*
   Systemic scleroderma
   Felty's syndrome

Reference: Greipp, P. R.: Arch. Intern. Med., *138*:356, 1978.

A YELLOW BAGATELLE

The skin and sclera are yellowed in jaundice. The skin, but not the sclera, is stained when the pigmentation is due to carotonemia or quinacrine (Atabrine) ingestion.

ALOPECIA SECONDARY TO NONCUTANEOUS DISEASE

There are a host of conditions that may cause either diffuse or patchy hair loss. The most common form of baldness is physiologic or androgenic alopecia seen in aging men. It occurs on the vertex and frontal areas of the scalp, with recession of the anterior hair line. The following is a listing of the various conditions associated with alopecia.

Infectious

Secondary syphilis (patchy)
Leprosy

Metabolic

Iron deficiency
Homocystinuria
Orotic aciduria

Endocrine

Hypopituitarism
Hypothyroidism
Hyperthyroidism
Hypoparathyroidism
Pregnancy (usually postpartum)

Idiopathic

Alopecia areata (patchy)
Systemic lupus erythematosus
Scleroderma (may be patchy)
Sarcoidosis (patchy)
Myotonic dystrophy
Turner's syndrome

Drugs

Antineoplastic agents
Hypervitaminosis A
Colchicine
Heparin
Coumarins
Thallium reaction

Psychogenic

Trichotillomania

References: Thorn, W. G., Adams, R. D., and Braunwald, D. (Eds.): Harrison's Principles of Internal Medicine, 8th Edition. New York, McGraw-Hill Book Company, 1977, 287; Alopecia. In: Roche Handbook of Differential Diagnosis, Hoffman-LaRoche, Inc., 1978.

GREEN HAIR

Green hair is as amazing to the physician as it is to the patient. Green hair was noted as early as the 1800's, when there were scattered reports of it occurring in copper workers. In the early 1970's a small epidemic was reported at a state college in Framingham, Mass. The majority of patients were women with "blond" hair whose "condition" occurred after the town had fluoridated its water supply. The fluorine acidified the water, which subsequently leached copper from piping. The copper was then deposited onto the hair during routine showering. The condition may be produced by chlorinated pool water in which copper-based algicides are used or by water that has a pH level so low that it leaches appreciable amounts of copper from the piping. Brass and mercury have also been associated with green hair.

> *Jade* — The stone was brought to Spain from the New World by the early explorers. It was named *piedra de i jada,* or "stone of the side," because it was reputed to cure colic. In French the word became *l'ejade* and later *le jade.*

You can suggest assaying the hair and water for copper content. Normal hair copper values range between 4 to 128 mg/kg hair. However, there is a simpler and less expensive alternative: Tell your patient to stop swimming or showering in the offending water, and the green color will gradually fade from the hair with daily shampooing in copper-free water.

References: Lampe, R. M., Henderson, A. L., and Hansen, G. H.: J.A.M.A., *237*:2092, 1977; Parish, L. C.: New Engl. J. Med., *292*:483, 1975; Cooper, R., and Goodman, J.: New Engl. J. Med., *292*:483, 1975; Goldsmith, L. W., and Holmes, L. B.: New Engl. J. Med., *292*: 484, 1975.

EXCESSIVE SWEATING (HYPERHIDROSIS)

1. Emotional stress
2. Fever and post lysis of fever
3. Thyrotoxicosis
4. Pheochromocytoma

5. Menopause
6. Withdrawal of addictive drugs (opiates, alcohol, depressants)
7. Drugs (hypothalamic action of aspirin in fever; anticholinesterases)
8. Acromegaly
9. Central nervous system or spinal disorders
10. Chronic illness (e.g., lymphoma, Hodgkin's disease, tuberculosis, brucellosis), often at night
11. Dumping syndrome
12. Hypoglycemia
13. Dyskeratosis congenita (Probably a recessive trait associated with hyperhidrosis of palms and soles, atrophy, hyperkeratosis and hyperpigmentation, loss of fingernails, keratosis of mucus membranes, ectropion of eyelids, splenomegaly, mental retardation, and aminoaciduria. Onset in childhood or during puberty. Often fatal).
14. Pachydermoperiostosis (An autosomal dominant trait characterized by periosteal new bone formation, particularly at distal ends of long bones, resulting in enlargement and clubbing of fingers and toes. Onset in early adult life).
15. Familial dysautonomia (Riley-Day syndrome. Onset in infancy).
16. Autonomic dysfunction of the Guillain-Barre syndrome.

Reference: Hyperhidrosis. In: Roche Handbook of Differential Diagnosis, Hoffman-LaRoche, Inc., 1978.

PUZZLING PRURITUS: THE INVISIBLE ITCH

Evaluation of the patient complaining of severe pruritus yet having no skin rash is difficult at best. The clinician should be aware of the medical conditions associated with itching before dismissing the complaint as psychogenic.

Psychogenic pruritus usually occurs during periods of stress and frequently affects the skin of the scalp. Other sensory complaints, such as burning of the tongue, may be present. There is usually no loss of sleep from psychogenic pruritus. The following tables will assist you in completing an evaluation of pruritus without a rash.

Medical Conditions Associated with Pruritus

CONDITION	COMMENT
1. Dry skin	— Blacks more frequently than whites — Most common cause of pruritus — Increasing frequency with advancing age — Aggravated in winter, especially if dry air heating used — Also called senile pruritus, pruritus hiemalis, asteatosis
2. Obstructive biliary disease — intra- or extrahepatic	— From any cause including stones, stricture, carcinoma of ducts, primary biliary cirrhosis, viral hepatitis, drug-induced cholestasis
3. Uremia	— More common with chronic, rather than acute, nephropathy — Usually relieved with dialysis
4. Hyperthyroidism	— Disappears with effective anti-thyroid therapy
5. Hypothyroidism	— May be related to dry skin occurring with this endocrinopathy
6. Hyperparathyroidism	— Relief of itching with return of calcium and phosphorus to normal levels
7. Diabetes mellitus	— Rare cause — May be related to cutaneous yeast or bacterial infection to which diabetics are more susceptible

Medical Conditions Associated with Pruritus

CONDITION	COMMENT
8. Malignancy	— Hodgkin's disease most common of the malignancies to cause itching — Pruritus responds to disease control — Return of pruritus may be earliest sign of relapse — In mycosis fungoides, itching may precede skin lesions — May occur with non-Hodgkin's lymphoma — Rare with carcinoma
9. Intestinal parasitosis	— Hookworm (*Ancylostoma duodenale* or *Necator americanus*) during constitutional phase of disease — Pinworm (*Enterobius vermicularis*) is common cause of pruritus ani
10. Subclinical drug reactions	— Most common with histamine-liberating drugs, including opium derivatives (opium, heroin, morphine), codeine, aspirin, polymyxin B
11. Pregnancy	— Approximately 65 per cent of all pregnant women have modest bilirubin elevations (0.75–3.0 mg/100 ml) during last trimester — Intensity of pruritus generally parallels serum bilirubin level — Should abate in immediate postpartum period; if not, suspect underlying liver disease
12. Polycythemia vera	— Induced or aggravated after a hot bath — Responds to disease control (i.e., phlebotomy) — Reappears with elevation of red cell mass

> *Idiosyncratic* — A private mixture. From the Greek *idio* "private," *syn* "together and *krasis*, "mixture.

Laboratory Evaluation of Pruritus of Undetermined Etiology

1. Complete blood count with eosinophil count
2. Liver function tests — bilirubin, alkaline phosphatase, SGOT, SGPT
3. Fasting blood sugar and two-hour-postprandial glucose
4. Thyroid function tests
5. Serum calcium and phosphorus
6. BUN
7. Pregnancy test

This list is not sufficiently exhaustive to cover all the diagnostic possibilities, and it should not be considered a routine evaluation for all cases of pruritus. Naturally, good clinical judgment will dictate the extent of the evaluation. However, if the cause of the pruritus remains undiagnosed even after basic procedures, more extensive examinations, such as stool tests for ova and parasites, a search for malignancy, and formal psychiatric evaluation, may be required.

There is no satisfactory therapy for generalized pruritus. A topical preparation of 0.5 per cent menthol and 1 per cent phenol in Nivea oil may give relief temporarily. Avoid topical anesthetics containing benzocaine, because of the risk of allergic sensitization. Antihistamines are useful only in cases of pruritus secondary to urticaria. Cimetidine has recently been reported to be helpful in the pruritus of polycythemia vera. In both polycythemia vera and Hodgkin's disease, the pruritus responds to therapy controlling the disease. Reappearance of this symptom may be the first sign of relapse.

References: Friedman, H. H., and Papper, S. (Eds.): Problem-Oriented Medical Diagnosis. Boston, Little, Brown and Company, 1975, pp. 21–25; Wintrobe, M. M., et al. (Eds.): Harrison's Principles of Internal Medicine, 8th Edition. New York, McGraw-Hill Book Company, 1977, pp. 272–273.

THE HELLISH HIVE, OR UNEASY WITH URTICARIA

The erythematous pruritic wheal that characterizes urticaria results from mast cell degranulation in response to various stimuli. This is followed by the release of substances that mediate vascular permeability and eosinophil chemotaxis, among other effects. Usually the patient with hives does not seek medical attention unless the urticaria is severe or persistent.

Acute urticaria is defined as recurrent episodes of less than six weeks' duration. Management is directed at determining the offending agents by a thorough investigation of the patient's history and appropriate elimination of these agents from the environment. Treatment consists of epinephrine, antihistamines, or both, depending on the severity of the attack.

Chronic urticaria (longer than six weeks duration) is a challenge to the clinician because this diagnosis often requires a systematic search for the causal agent. Although the etiology is established in only 20 per cent of cases of chronic urticaria, a consideration of known causative factors will help direct the investigation.

The causes of urticaria may be classified under the following major categories:

I. *Immunologic causes* — distinguishable antigen and reaginic antibody (usually of the IgE class) may act directly or by way of a complement-dependent antigen-antibody reaction and mediate mast cell degranulation.

II. *"Paraimmunologic" causes* — same as I, but the relationship between antigen and antibody is less obvious.

III. *Nonimmunologic causes* — these include physical or emotional stimuli that may result in urticaria.

Immunologic Causes

ETIOLOGY	COMMENT
1. Yeast hypersensitivity (*Candida albicans*)	— Cross-reaction occurs with certain foods and inhaled yeast — Diagnosis suspected if beer exacerbates urticaria
2. Foods	— Fresh fruit, strawberries, nuts, tomatoes, chocolate, shellfish, cottonseed, soybean, egg, wheat, milk, corn are most common
3. Insect bites	— Bees usually, but may also occur with mosquitoes, bed bugs, lice, scabies
4. Drugs	— Penicillin is most common — In yeast-sensitive individual, antibiotics derived from yeasts may incite lesions
5. Serum sickness	— From any cause

"Paraimmunologic" Causes

ETIOLOGY	COMMENT
1. Infection	— Virus, bacteria, and fungi implicated — Occurs during prodrome of HAA positive hepatitis or infectious mononucleosis
2. Infestation	— Most common with the nematodes (trichinosis, ascarisis, oxyuriasis, hookworm disease)
3. Endocrinopathy	— Hypothyroidism, hyperthyroidism, diabetes mellitus — Mechanism unknown
4. Malignancy	— Hodgkin's and non-Hodgkin's lymphoma more common than carcinoma
5. Collagen-vascular disease	— Occurs more commonly in systemic lupus erythematosus, juvenile rheumatoid arthritis, and dermatomyositis
6. Chemicals	— Beware of food additives (especially sodium benzoate and its congeners) — Synthetic food dyes

3

Nonimmunologic Causes

ETIOLOGY	COMMENT
1. Cold	— May be familial — Ice cube application may be diagnostic — Occurs only on parts exposed to cold — May be associated with cryoglobulins
2. Heat	— Immersing hand in 100.5°F water with subsequent wheal formation is diagnostic
3. Sunlight	— Usually only specific spectra are inciting — Effectively treated with sunscreens
4. Trauma	— Dermographism is accentuation of normal triple response — May respond to hydroxyzine — Rarely caused by systemic mast cell disease (urticaria pigmentosa)
5. Cholinergic urticaria	— Typical lesion is a 1–2 mm wheal surrounded by large red flare — Heat, exercise, emotional stress trigger urticarial reaction — Other parasympathomimetic manifestations (abdominal cramps, salivation, sweating) may occur — Methacholine skin test is diagnostic
6. Drugs	— Most commonly morphine, quinine, polymyxin B, curare, hydralazine, meperidine, heroin — Aspirin (in individuals with aspirin-induced asthma)
7. Emotion	

References: Beeson, P. B., and McDermott, W. (Eds.): Textbook of Medicine, 14th Edition. Philadelphia, W. B. Saunders Company, 1975, pp. 117–119; Friedman, H. H., and Popper, S. (Eds.): Problem-Oriented Medical Diagnosis. Boston, Little, Brown and Company, 1975, pp. 27–31.

CUTANEOUS REACTIONS TO DRUGS

The Boston Collaborative Surveillance Program estimated the rates of allergic skin reactions to commonly employed drugs in 22,227 patients admitted consecutively to participating hospitals. Reactions to penicillin or blood products affected 38 per cent of the patients and accounted for 70 per cent of the skin reactions observed.

Once these patients were subtracted from the data base, the detection of individual drugs that produced skin reactions was based on two criteria: The frequency of reactions in the patients receiving the drug in question had to be at least twice as high as the frequency of reactions in the remaining patients at large, and a characteristic cluster of rashes had to appear in the days after the first exposure to the drug.

Clearly the data are firmer for the drugs received by at least 1000 patients. The list is also a good indication of drug utilization in a hospitalized population.

Reference: Arndt, K. A., and Jick, H.: J.A.M.A., *235*:918, 1976.

DRUG	NO. OF REACTIONS	NO. OF RECIPIENTS	REACTION RATE PER 1000 PATIENTS
Trimethoprim-sulfamethoxazole	10	169	59
Ampicillin	156	2988	52
Semisynthetic penicillin	27	760	36
Whole blood	32	908	35
Corticotropin	3	106	28
Platelets	4	145	28
Erythromycin	11	481	28
Sulfisoxazole	8	462	17
Penicillin G	51	3286	16
Practolol	2	128	16
Gentamicin sulfate	10	607	16
Cephalosporins	17	1308	13
Plasma protein fraction	3	245	12
Quinidine	8	652	12
Dipyrone	10	876	11
Mercurial diuretics	6	630	9.5
Nitrofurantoin	2	219	9.1
Packed red blood cells	11	1366	8.1
Chloramphenicol	2	292	6.8
Trimethobenzamide hydrochloride	5	752	6.6
Phenazopyridine hydrochloride	1	153	6.5
Methenamine	1	157	6.4
Nitrazepam	7	1118	6.3
Cyanocobalamin	3	486	6.2
Barbiturates	22	4658	4.7
Glutethimide	1	221	4.5
Indomethacin	1	229	4.4
Chlordiazepoxide	9	2161	4.2
Metoclopramide hydrochloride	1	247	4.0
Diazepam	18	4692	3.8
Propoxyphene	10	2976	3.4
Isoniazid	2	675	3.0
Guaifenesin and aminophylline	7	2440	2.9
Nystatin	1	342	2.9
Chlorthiazide	2	707	2.8
Furosemide	9	3497	2.6
Isophane insulin	1	777	1.3
Phenytoin	1	905	1.1
Phytonadione	1	1111	0.9
Flurazepam hydrochloride	1	1862	0.5
Chloral hydrate	1	4809	0.2

AMPICILLIN RASH

Ampicillin is one of the most common causes of drug-induced skin rash (see preceding article). Deciding what should be done may be difficult, particularly when ampicillin is the drug of choice for the infection being treated. The pediatricians have looked at the problem rather closely and offer some help in decision-making.

1. Seven to 10 per cent of children who receive ampicillin develop a rash. Children who have infectious mononucleosis and are treated with ampicillin will develop a rash 70 to 95 per cent of the time. There is also an increased incidence of rash in patients who have cytomegalovirus infection or acute lymphocytic leukemia and receive ampicillin.

2. The rash is likely to be maculopapular, mildly pruritic, and unaccompanied by systemic symptoms. In this case it is safe to continue with therapy. If the rash is of the florid or urticarial type, discontinue therapy immediately. This type of rash may also be accompanied by fever, periarticular swelling, and/or lymphadenopathy.

3. Truncal involvement almost always occurs first in the ampicillin rash. The face and extremities are involved more than one half the time. There is usually sparing of palms, soles, and mucosal surfaces.

4. The onset of the rash may occur any time from 24 hours to 16 days after beginning treatment with ampicillin.

5. The patient with a personal history of atopic manifestations is *not* more likely to develop a rash when given ampicillin.

6. Lack of response to penicillin skin testing is no assurance that the patient will not develop an ampicillin rash. The mild maculopapular rash described above is not thought to be related to penicillin allergy; however, the patient who develops an urticarial reaction to ampicillin may have a true penicillin sensitivity.

Reference: Kerns, D. L., Shira, J. E., Go, S., et al.: Am. J. Dis. Child., *125*:187, 1973.

COUMARIN NECROSIS

A rare, and therefore often unappreciated, adverse reaction to coumarin derivatives is the syndrome of coumarin necrosis. The syndrome characteristically occurs in middle-aged obese females receiving oral coumarin compounds. The lesion begins as a *painful* erythematous patch, which rapidly progresses to produce an indurated red-blue-black discoloration. The lesion may become necrotic, can involve the entire

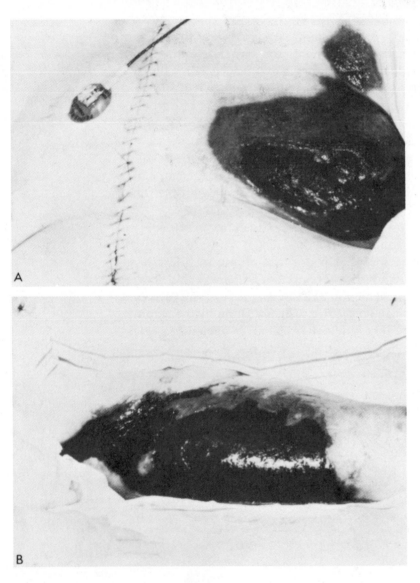

FIG. 3-1

Extensive necrosis of the chest wall secondary to coumarin.

skin, and may extend deeply into the subcutaneous tissue. The lesion usually occurs in areas with abundant subcutaneous fat, such as the breasts, thighs, buttocks, and abdomen (Fig. 3–1). Multiple areas of involvement are uncommon.

Coumarin necrosis appears between days 3 and 10 of therapy. More than 90 per cent of cases begin on days 3 to 5. It occurs in 0.01 per cent to 1 per cent of patients receiving oral coumarin derivatives. Surprisingly, continuing the drug does not seem to influence the course and healing of the lesion nor cause new lesions to appear. The cause of this adverse reaction is unknown.

References: Koch-Weser, J.: Ann. Intern. Med., *68*:1366, 1968; Lacy, J. P., and Goodin, R. R.: Ann. Intern. Med., *82*:381, 1975. Figure reproduced from DiCato et al.: Ann. Intern. Med., *83*:234, 1975 with permission of publisher.

RASH ON THE PALMS AND SOLES

You are at a loss! The lab just called to inform you that the serology you ordered on the patient with a rash on his palms and soles is negative. If it isn't syphilis, what is it?

Acute

Hand, Foot, and Mouth disease (Coxsackie A-16 and others): Fever, conjunctivitis, linear or oval vesicles on hands and/or feet, erosions on soft palate and tonsillar pillars.

Mononucleosis: Nonspecific macular erythema and urticaria associated with upper eyelid edema, palatal petechiae, and pharyngeal inflammation.

Rocky Mountain fever: First, pink and macular, blanches on pressure; then, maculopapular, red, finally, petechiae that do not fade with pressure.

Erythema multiforme: Distinctive circular erythematous and edematous lesions with a depressed center ("target" or iris lesions). May become bullous. Begins distally, spreads proximally. Mucosal lesions may be present (Stevens-Johnson syndrome).

Secondary syphilis: Nonpruritic erythematous macules or papules on palms and soles. (But the serology should have been positive at this stage).

Gonococcemia: Purpuric, tender pustules occasionally found on palms and soles.

Drug reaction: May look like anything.

Chronic

Reiter's syndrome: Pinpoint vesicular lesions leading to erythematous pustular eruptions on palms and soles. Associated with urethritis, arthritis, conjunctivitis, balanitis, and buccal mucosal lesions. The fancy name for the rash is keratodermia blenorrhagica.

Pustular psoriasis (of Barber): Discrete erythematous plaques studded with uniform 1 to 3 mm pustules and older, pruritic, exfoliative brown crusted lesions.

Dyshidrotic eczematous dermatitis: Discrete skin-colored vesicles, which may have an erythematous halo. Markedly pruritic. Often follows an inflammatory dermatitis.

Pustular bacterid: Vesicles that rapidly become purulent, associated with severe pain and pruritus. May be an "id reaction" to localized infection elsewhere.

Darier-White disease: Hyperkeratotic, minute papules on palms and soles. A genetic disease transmitted as an autosomal dominant.

Hyperlipoproteinemia (type III, and florid obstructive liver disease): Yellow, orange, or brownish-yellow "palmar striae."

Fungal infection: Asymptomatic erythema and hyperkeratosis with accentuation and fissuring of the palmar creases.

Arsenic poisoning: Warty, keratotic lesions and ulcers in palmar creases. Malaise, anorexia, diarrhea, and peripheral neuritis.

Mercury poisoning: Acrodynia (painful, pink hands and feet). May look like erythema multiforme or fixed drug reaction.

Halogen poisoning: Unusual, but may cause acneiform and tumor-like lesions on palms and soles.

Stigma — In Greek it meant a brand made by a pointed instrument. Seventeenth century England actually stigmatized criminals with a hot iron.

ERYTHEMA NODOSUM

Although erythema nodosum is a benign dermatologic entity that heals without ulceration or scarring in the majority of cases, its recognition should lead to a search for the underlying cause. It may be confused with nodular liquefying panniculitis, Weber-Christian panniculitis, and various types of vasculitis, all of which may present as tender subcutaneous nodules. Therefore, biopsy may be required in those instances in which the clinical presentation alone does not lead to a specific diagnosis.

Erythema nodosum occurs most frequently in young adults. The incidence is three times greater in females. Erythema nodosum is thought to be a pattern of allergic skin reaction to various blood-borne antigens. The following list enumerates the sources of the antigen and the various inciting disease entities.

Infectious Etiologies

Beta-hemolytic streptococcal infection
Tuberculosis
Histoplasmosis
Blastomycosis
Coccidioidomycosis
Leprosy (lepromatous form)
Lymphogranuloma venereum

3

Drugs

Penicillin
Sulfonamides
Bromides
Iodides
Sulfonylureas
Oral contraceptives (those containing ethinyl estradiol or norethynodrel)

Miscellaneous

Behçet's disease
Systemic lupus erythematosus
Sarcoidosis
Inflammatory bowel disease (ulcerative colitis, Crohn's disease)

References: Wintrobe, M. M., et al. (Eds.): Harrison's Principles of Internal Medicine, 8th Edition. New York, McGraw-Hill Book Company, 1977, p. 269; Erythema nodosum. In: Roche Handbook of Differential Diagnosis. Hoffman-LaRoche, Inc., 1975.

CUTANEOUS MANIFESTATIONS OF MALIGNANCY

The skin can sometimes be a mirror, reflecting the presence of an internal malignancy. Some cutaneous markers are highly specific, such as the association of Gardner's syndrome with malignant small and large bowel polyps. Other skin conditions may be less specific, with a differential diagnosis that includes numerous malignancies as well as normal variants (i.e., acanthosis nigricans). Recognition of the cutaneous manifestations of malignancy will allow for early diagnosis and treatment. The associations noted in most cases are neither specific nor invariable, so avoid the overly expensive and unduly extended search.

Cutaneous Manifestations of Internal Malignancy

MANIFESTATION		ASSOCIATED CANCER
Vascular erythema	Localized	
	Pinch purpura	Multiple myeloma, dysproteinemia, amyloid
	Purpura (petechiae, ecchymoses)	Polycythemia vera, thrombocytopenia secondary to malignancy, leukemia
	Thrombophlebitis (unusual variants)	Pancreas, lung, stomach, gallbladder, colon, uterus, ovary
	Ischemic leg ulcers	Polycythemia vera, dysproteinemia (hyperviscosity syndrome), cryoglobulinemia
	Caput medusa	Gastric carcinoma
	Superior vena caval syndrome	Cancerous invasion of mediastinum
	Diffuse and variable erythemas	
	Erythroderma (exfoliative dermatitis)	Hodgkin's disease, lymphoma, leukemia, adenocarcinoma of stomach, liver, prostate gland, tongue, and lung
	Telangiectasia	Lymphoma (ataxia-telangiectasia)
	Bloom's syndrome	Leukemia, squamous cell carcinoma of skin
	Vasculitis	Leukemia, lymphoma, multiple myeloma, lymphosarcoma
	Erythema perstans*	Breast, lung, cervix, metastatic carcinoma
	Flush (carcinoid)	Gastrointestinal tract — appendix; liver; bronchial; rarely, endocrine organs
Urticaria and bullous states	Urticaria	Choriocarcinoma
	Erythema multiforme	Leukemia, lymphoma, carcinomas
	Pemphigoid	Gastric, pancreatic, and pulmonary (bronchial) carcinoma, melanoma
Hyperpigmentation	Acanthosis nigricans	Adenocarcinoma of gastrointestinal tract, liver, uterus, ovaries, pancreas, prostate gland, and kidney; pituitary tumors; pinealoma; lymphoma; choriocarcinoma; squamous cell carcinoma
	Addisonian states	Adrenal gland invasion, usually lymphoma or carcinoma (esp. bronchogenic)

MANIFESTATION		ASSOCIATED CANCER
	Peutz-Jeghers syndrome	Rare malignant degeneration of polyp of small intestine, stomach, and colon (disputed)
	Chronic arsenicalism	Squamous cell carcinoma, mainly in the mouth, gastrointestinal and urinary systems, respiratory tract, liver, reticuloendothelial system, endocrine system, breast, and eye
	Diffuse generalized	Rarely, an expression of cutaneous melanin deposition in malignant melanoma; hepatoma in hemochromatosis
Endocrine and metabolic	Hirsutism Hypertrichosis lanuginosa Hypertrichosis	Bladder or bronchial carcinoma Arrhenoblastoma, hilus cell, and adrenal rest tumors of ovary, virilizing adrenal tumor
	Cushing's syndrome	Lung (oat cell), pancreatic islet cell, thyroid gland, parotid glands, testes, ovary, colon, gallbladder, breast parathyroid gland, brain tumor (pituitary), thymoma-like and mediastinal tumors, neuroblastoma, pheochromocytoma, malignant bronchial carcinoids
	Hepatic estrogenic effect	Metastatic disease to liver causing hepatic dysfunction
	Painful gynecomastia	Endocrine tumors, pulmonary carcinoma
	Metastatic calcification of dermis	Paget's disease, multiple myeloma, leukemia, metastatic carcinoma (destructive bone disease with excessive osteoclastic activity)
	Nonendocrine neoplasms with cutaneous markers	Secreting gonadotropin-like peptides from trophoblastic elements in tumors, choriocarcinoma, teratoma, embryonal cell carcinoma, rare nonendocrine tumor secreting antidiuretic hormone, thyroid-stimulating hormone, parathormone
	Nodular fat necrosis	Pancreatic carcinoma (lipase)
Miscellaneous	Pruritus — unexplained by other cutaneous lesions	Polycythemia vera, Hodgkin's disease, pancreas, stomach, lymphoma (esp. m. fungoides), leukemia, brain tumors

3

Cutaneous Manifestations of Internal Malignancy

MANIFESTATION		ASSOCIATED CANCER
	Herpes zoster; unusual, recurrent, or chronic herpes simplex; candidiasis	Hodgkin's disease, lymphoma, chronic granulocytopenia, thymoma
	Cryoglobulinemia	Carcinoma of breast or colon, leukemia, lymphoma, multiple myeloma
	Acquired ichthyosis	Lymphoma (Hodgkin's), multiple myeloma, lung (oat cell), breast
	Herpes-like syndrome	Lymphoreticular (Wiskott-Aldrich syndrome)
	Hypertrophic osteoarthropathy (clubbing and pachydermoperiostosis)	Intrathoracic tumor, bronchogenic carcinoma, mesothelioma and metastatic cancer); see Clubbing (Chapter 1)
	Paget's disease and extra mammary Paget's disease	Adenocarcinoma of breast, rectum, urethra, exocrine and apocrine glands
	Diffuse xanthomatosis	Multiple myeloma, leukemia
	Dermatomyositis	Lung, gastrointestinal tract carcinoma, carcinoma of the breast, lymphoma, sarcoma, melanoma, rarely in any other organ
	Bizarre (psoriasis and eczema-like)	Gastrointestinal tumors or metastasis with malabsorption, squamous carcinoma, mycosis fungoides
	Subcutaneous or dermal metastatic nodules	Breast, lung, ovary, uterus, gastrointestinal tract
	Adenoma sebaceum	Rhabdomyosarcoma (esp. cardiac in tuberous sclerosis)
Benign cutaneous	Tylosis-keratoderma (palms and soles)	
	Acquired	Questionable relationship to esophageal carcinoma
	Hereditary	Esophageal carcinoma
	Multiple mucosal neuromas	Medullary thyroid cancer, pheochromocytoma (multiple endocrine adenomatosis, type II)
	Gardner's syndrome[†]	Malignant degeneration of polyps of small and large bowel

Reference: Table modified from Kierland, R. R.: South. Med. J., *65*:563, 1972 with permission of The Southern Medical Journal (*65*:563, 1972).

4
NEUROLOGY

SENSATION!

It's important to have when you need it...

Dermatome Areas

Dermatome Areas

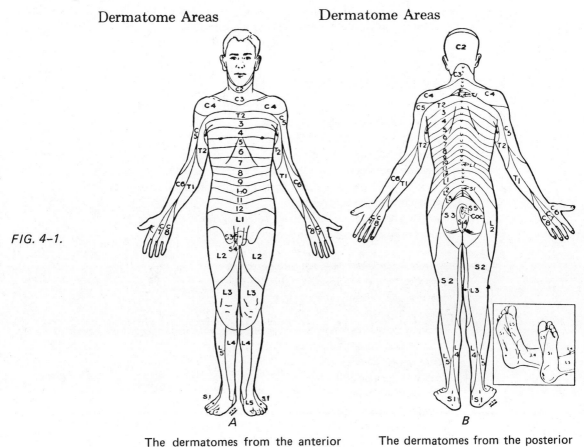

FIG. 4–1.

A

The dermatomes from the anterior view.

B

The dermatomes from the posterior view.

Reference: McMillan, J. A., Niebury, P. I., and Oski, F. A.: The Whole Pediatrician Catalog. Philadelphia, W. B. Saunders Co., 1977, p. 363.

DEMENTIA

Dementia is a deterioration of intellectual and cognitive function without a disturbance of perception. Repeated poor performance on the mini mental status exam (see following article) should lead to the consideration of a diagnosis of dementia. Don't forget that many patients may have transiently poor performance on the mental status exam because of their illness and/or the drugs we give them. A useful classification of dementia is listed in the following table. Your patients will be grateful if you eliminate the possibility of any correctable etiology (e.g., hypothyroidism, chronic subdural hematoma) before you consign them to a nursing home.

Communicating hydrocephalus is an important reversible cause of dementia and one that must be considered because of the marked improvement possible with surgical shunting of the cerebrospinal fluid. The diagnosis of communicating hydrocephalus is confirmed by dynamic radionuclide scanning of spinal fluid distribution and absorption. The following table summarizes the important differences between this syndrome, Alzheimer's disease, and vascular dementia, the latter two being the commonest causes of dementia.

Classification of Dementia

Dementia Associated with Clinical and
Laboratory Signs of Medical Disease
  Hypothyroidism
  Cushing's syndrome
  Nutritional deficiency (Wernicke-Korsakoff, pellagra, vitamin B_{12})
  Chronic meningoencephalitis
  Familial and acquired hepatolenticular degeneration
  Bromism and chronic barbiturism

Dementia Associated with Neurologic Signs
  Thrombotic and embolic vascular disease
  Primary and metastatic neoplasm
  Abscess (brain)
  Trauma, including cerebral contusions and chronic subdural hematoma
  Communicating or obstructive hydrocephalus
  Huntington's chorea
  Lipid storage disease
  Myoclonic epilepsy
  Creutzfeldt-Jakob disease
  Spastic paraplegia

Dementia As the Only Evidence of Neurologic Disease
  Alzheimer's disease
  Pick's disease

4

Differential Findings in Dementia

	ALZHEIMER'S DISEASE	VASCULAR DEMENTIA	COMMUNICATING HYDROCEPHALUS
Onset/course	Slow and progressive; may take years to develop	Stepwise and episodic	Rapidly progressive; may take days to weeks
Background	Occasionally positive family history	History of vascular disease, hypertension, and diabetes	Recent trauma, meningitis, or subarachnoid hemorrhage; occasionally no antecedent history
Common signs	Memory loss, agitation, disorientation, language disturbance	Mental symptoms with associated hemiparesis, pathologic reflexes, pseudobulbar palsy, cerebellar signs	Rapidly progressive signs and symptoms of dementia with mutism, apraxia, ataxia, urinary incontinence
CAT scan findings	Ventricular enlargement and diffuse cerebral atrophy	Distinct areas of infarction; occasionally, ventricular enlargement and cortical atrophy	Enlargement of all ventricles *without* cerebral atrophy; brain surface smoother than normal
Dynamic radionuclide scan	Normal	Normal	Abnormal, shows failure of absorption and ventricular accumulation of radioactive material

Reference: Dreyfus, P. M.: Consultant, January 1979, p. 31. (Table reproduced with permission.)

THE MINI MENTAL STATUS EXAM

The examination presented below is a quick, reliable, quantitative, and reproducible test of the patient's mental status. A score of 20 or less is indicative of dementia, delerium, schizophrenia, or an affective disorder.

> *Delirium* — From the Latin, *de,* "off," and *lira,* "track" or "furrow."

Mini Mental Status Exam

Maximum Score	Score	
		ORIENTATION
5	( )	What is the (year) (season) (date) (day) (month)?
5	( )	Where are we: (state) (county) (town) (hospital) (floor).
		REGISTRATION
3	( )	Name 3 objects: 1 second to say each. Then ask the patient all 3 after you have said them. Give 1 point for each correct answer. Then repeat them until he learns all 3. Count trials and record.

Trials _____

ATTENTION AND CALCULATION

5	( )	Serial 7's. 1 point for each correct. Stop after 5 answers. Alternatively spell "world" backwards.

RECALL

3	( )	Ask for the 3 objects repeated above. Give 1 point for each correct.

LANGUAGE

9	( )	Identify a pencil and watch. (2 points) Repeat the following, "No *ifs, ands,* or *buts.*" (1 point) Follow a 3-stage command: "Take a paper in your right hand, fold it in half, and put it on the floor." (3 points) Read and obey the following: Close your eyes. (1 point)

Write a sentence. (1 point)
Copy a design. (1 point)

_____ **Total score**

Assess level of consciousness along a continuum

_____

Alert   Drowsy   Stupor   Coma

Instructions for Administration of Mini-Mental Status Examination

ORIENTATION

1. Ask for the date. Then ask specifically for parts omitted, e.g., "Can you also tell me what season it is?" One point for each correct.

2. Ask in turn "Can you tell me the name of this hospital?" (town, county, etc.). One point for each correct.

REGISTRATION

Ask the patient if you may test his memory. Then say the names of three unrelated objects, clearly and slowly, about one second for each. After you have said all three, ask him to repeat them. This first repetition determines his score (0–3), but keep saying them until he can repeat all three, up to six trials. If he does not eventually learn all three, recall cannot be meaningfully tested.

ATTENTION AND CALCULATION

Ask the patient to begin with 100 and count backwards by 7. Stop after 5 subtractions (93, 86, 79, 72, 65). Score the total number of correct answers.

If the patient cannot or will not perform this task, ask him to spell the word "world" backwards. The score is the number of letters in correct order (e.g., dlrow = 5, dlorw = 3).

RECALL

Ask the patient if he can recall the three objects you previously asked him to remember. Score 0–3.

LANGUAGE

Naming: Show the patient a wrist watch and ask him what it is. Repeat for pencil. Score 0–2.

Repetition: Ask the patient to repeat the sentence after you. Allow only one trial. Score 0 or 1.

Three-Stage command: Give the patient a piece of plain blank paper and repeat the command above. Score 1 point for each part correctly executed.

Reading: On a blank piece of paper print the sentence "Close your eyes" in letters large enough for the patient to see clearly. Ask him to read it and to do what it says. Score 1 point only if he actually closes his eyes.

Writing: Give the patient a blank piece of paper and ask him to write a sentence for you. Do not dictate a sentence; it is to be written spontaneously. It must contain a subject and verb and be sensible. Correct grammar and punctuation are not necessary.

Copying: On a clean piece of paper, draw intersecting pentagons, each side about 1 inch, and ask him to copy it exactly as it is. All 10 angles must be present and two must intersect to score 1 point. Tremor and rotation are ignored.

Estimate the patient's level of sensorium along a continuum, from alert, on the left, to coma, on the right.

Reference: Folstein, M. F., Folstein, S. E., and McHugh, P. R.: J. Psychiatr. Res. *12*: 196–198, 1975. Reprinted with permission of author and publisher. Copyright 1975, Pergamon Press, Ltd.

VASCULAR HEADACHES

The migraine headache (common and classic), cluster headache, and the headache of temporal arteritis are classified as vascular headaches. The evaluation of vascular headaches includes a careful review of the patient's history and a physical exam, coupled with a thorough clinical investigation to exclude organic neurologic disease. The historic highlights of the four major categories of vascular headaches are presented below.

The pain of the **common migraine** headache is located behind the eyes and/or over the forehead. This headache is associated with photophobia and a tender scalp. Recurrent headaches, dizziness, and blackouts (blindness or syncope) are usually present. There is often a family history (usually the mother) of a similar type of headache pattern. Characteristically, the patient has also suffered at least one classic migraine. A good response to anti-migraine therapy is usually seen.

The **classic migraine** appears to be related to serum serotonin levels, which drop 12 hours prior to the headache. The headache is preceded by an aura (i.e., scintillating scotoma) and is accompanied by nausea, vomiting, photophobia, a tender scalp, diuresis, and some loss of the visual field on the side opposite the headache. There may be aphasia or contralateral neurologic deficits (hemiplegia, hemiparesis). Although this headache is classically unilateral, it may switch sides. The patient is headache-free except for occasional major headaches. Therapy is discussed below. Medicine can be taken either daily as a prophylactic measure or during the aura as a suppressive measure.

The **cluster headache** has no aura. It starts abruptly and intensely, lasts 20 to 40 minutes, and leaves gradually. It is located over one eye and is accompanied by hyperemia of the conjunctiva and the periorbital skin, unilateral tearing, and miosis of the pupil. It may have a trigger, such as chocolate, ice cream, smoking, or intense concentration. The headache may occur day or night, usually on a definite schedule (i.e., at 4 a.m. every day for four weeks). Between clusters the patient is headache-free. Most therapy is dismally unsuccessful. An ergot preparation may be tried either an hour before the headache is expected or daily in morning and evening doses. Patients have been known to pound their head against the wall, maim themselves, or even commit suicide because of cluster headaches!

Temporal arteritis affects the elderly. The pain is located over the temporal area. There is often a burning sensation which may be accompanied by claudication of the jaw. Examination may reveal a low-grade fever and palpable tender, beaded, or fusiform swellings of the temporal artery. Skip areas are common. The Westergren sedimentation rate is characteristically greater than 100. The diagnosis is confirmed by a temporal artery biopsy.

The main complication of untreated temporal arteritis is occlusion of the ophthalmic artery which leads to irreversible blindness. The main risk of treatment is the side effects of continuous high-dose corticosteroids. Thus, temporal arteritis is clearly a disease that must be diagnosed accurately. Temporal arteritis frequently accompanies, or is accompanied by, polymyalgia rheumatica (fever, malaise, arthralgias, and proximal muscle weakness and discomfort).

Current therapy for temporal arteritis is 100 to 140 mg of prednisone daily (not every other day!). The Westergren sedimentation rate is closely monitored as the steroid dose is reduced to maintenance levels.

DOC, THESE HEADACHE PILLS DON'T WORK!

You have arrived at a diagnosis of **migraine headache** by history, physical exam, and careful laboratory investigation. Your satisfaction at having established a diagnosis is short-lived, however, since there are very few therapeutic problems as frustrating as the treatment of migraine headaches. To maintain the trust and cooperation of the patient, you must inform him or her that proper therapy is arrived at by trial and error.

Chocolate, alcohol, ice cream, exhaustion, smoking, and emotional upset are a few of the well-known migraine headache "triggers." You should help your patient identify and avoid these personal triggers. Trials of numerous drugs in different doses may be required before the headaches are suppressed with minimal drug side effects. Prescriptions should be written initially for small amounts of medication (enough for three or four headaches), since the therapy will probably be changed often. Medication should be readily accessible so the patient can begin therapy at the first sign of the aura or headache.

Drugs to Try

DRUG	DOSE	COMMENT
Bellergal (ergotamine phenobarbital, belladonna)	3 to 4 tablets/day	Good for patients with dizziness accompanying headache
Periactin (cyproheptadine)	4 mg tablets 2 to 8 tablets/day	Gradually increase dose. Works on dizziness, too. Can make patient drowsy. Atropine-like side effects.
Propranolol	80 to 120 mg/stat 80 to 240 mg/day	For the rare headache For four or more per month
Dilantin (diphenylhydantoin)	300 to 400 mg/day	Chronically, for patients with frequent migraines
Cafergot (ergotamine, caffeine)	2 to 4 tablets at onset. Repeat one every half-hour if needed. Maximum dose: 6/day, 15/week	Ergot alkaloids are vaso-constrictive. They may be contraindicated in peripheral vascular disease, coronary artery disease, and hyper-tension. They may induce labor in pregnancy.
Ergomar (ergotamine)	2 mg sublingual	Expensive
Ergotamine	2 to 4 whiffs at onset; one whiff every half-hour	60 whiffs in a container, expensive but quick and convenient
Antidepressants		Use if depression is the trigger factor. "Tricyclic" antidepressants before bed-time may be helpful.
Sansert (methysergide)	2 mg tablets 4 to 8 mg/day	Gradually increase dosage. It works, but it has many significant side effects: thrombophlebitis, adductor cramps, edema, paresthesias, retroperitoneal fibrosis, and pleuropulmonary and cardiac valvular fibrosis

If a patient has an ongoing, established migraine, the therapy above rarely works. *One* of the following treatments is suggested:

Ergotamine (Gynergen)	0.5 mg subcutaneously (vomiting 20 minutes after the shot)	
or		
Ephedrine	50 mg intravenously	
or		
Demerol	100 to 125 mg intramuscularly.	

Arrange an appointment to initiate prophylactic therapy when the patient has recovered.

"DIZZY"

Vertigo is an hallucination of motion. "Subjective vertigo" is when the patient feels that he is spinning. "Objective vertigo" is the sensation that the surroundings are spinning. There is no clinical difference between subjective and objective vertigo. Vertigo must be differentiated from light-headedness, weakness, and dizziness.

About 80 per cent of the causes of vertigo are peripheral in origin, yet central lesions can be life-threatening and must be considered. One establishes a diagnosis of vertigo by reviewing the patient's history and verifying the presence of nystagmus. The following are three tables that list the different kinds of central and peripheral lesions, the tests necessary to differentiate central from peripheral lesions, and the specific diseases associated with vertigo.

Reference: Marlowe, F. I. and Wolfson, R. J.: Vertigo. In Schwartz et al.: Principles and Practice of Emergency Medicine. Vol. I. Philadelphia, W. B. Saunders Co., 1978, p. 581. Tables reproduced with permission of author and publisher.

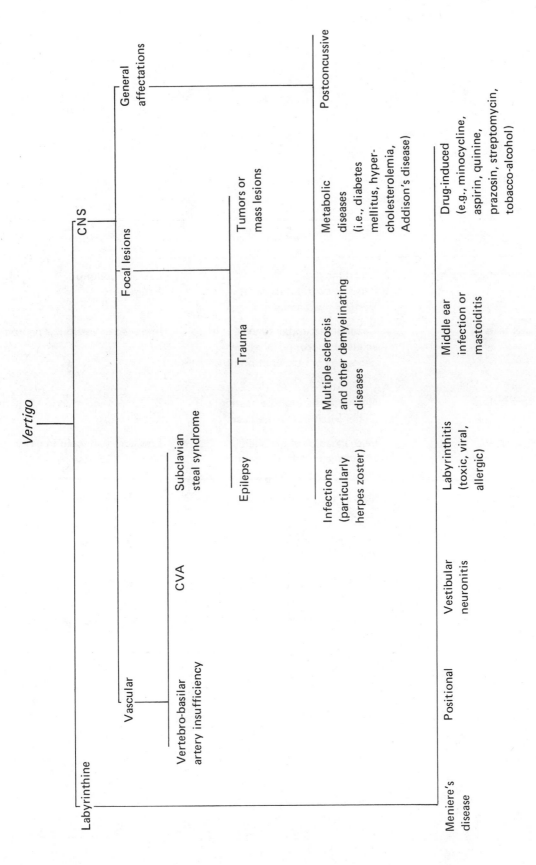

4

ORIGIN

Test	Central	Peripheral
Electronystagmography	No latency Persistence (nonfatigable) Vertical nystagmus	Latency common Fatigability
Caloric tests	Generally unimpaired except in acoustic neuroma, in which depressed or nonfunctioning on affected side	Impaired in vestibular neuronitis
Tuning fork	No diplacusis (double hearing higher pitch in involved ear)	Diplacusis common in Meniere's disease
Audiometry	Unchanged or diminished High tone loss more common in early acoustic neuroma	Low tones affected in early Meniere's disease
Visual fields	May be altered from central lesion	Usually normal
Angiography	May show mass lesion or vascular lesion	Usually normal
EEG	May show diffuse or focal abnormality	Usually normal
Lumbar puncture	Protein generally mildly elevated in neuroma	Normal findings expected

4

DISEASE OR CONDITIONS	VERTIGO	NYSTAGMUS	CALORIC RESPONSE	COCHLEAR SYMPTOMS AND SIGNS	ASSOCIATED SYMPTOMS AND SIGNS	COMMENTS
1. Endolymphatic hydrops (Meniere's disease)	Severe attacks with nausea and vomiting, which last hours (not days or weeks)	Spontaneous during critical stage; postural in 25% of patients during first few weeks after an attack	Usually depressed in involved ear(s); progressive with recurrent episodes	Tinnitus (louder during attacks) Sensori-neural hearing loss Recruitment and diplacusis usually present	Fullness in the ear during an attack; may also be noted before attack begins (as an aura)	Unilateral in 90% of patients Recurring attacks typical Interval is variable (days to years)
2. Benign positional vertigo	Always positional — provoked by certain head positions	Always positional, with latency, brief duration, and fatigability	Normal	Absent	None	
3. Viral labyrinthitis or vestibular neuronitis	Severe 3 to 5 days, with nausea and vomiting; regresses over 3 to 6 weeks, usually	Spontaneous during severe stage; may be postural during recovery phase	Depressed in the involved ear, usually	Absent	Antecedent or concomitant acute febrile disease	Does not recur
4. Acoustic neuroma	Usually late; more often a progressive feeling of imbalance May be provoked by sudden head movements	Spontaneous type frequently present	Depressed or nonfunctioning labyrinth	Usually appear first Unilateral high-tone sensori-neural hearing loss and tinnitus Very poor discrimination; rapid tone decay; recruitment usually absent	Decreased corneal sensitivity (ipsilateral) Facial weakness Diplopia Headache Positive x-ray findings Elevated CSF protein	Early diagnosis essential while lesion is small and may be removed with minimal sequelae
5. Vertebro-basilar insufficiency	Usually positional — provoked by certain head positions	Usually accompanies the vertigo	Normal	Absent	Arteriosclerosis	Usually seen in older age group with other symptoms of brain-stem ischemia. Visual symptoms common.

A GUIDE TO THE USE OF ANTIEPILEPTIC DRUGS

The table on the opposite page lists the class, indications and the generic and trade names for the commonly employed antiepileptic drugs.

Drugs should be employed in such a manner that steady-state concentrations are effective and no more than minimally toxic. Generally, these agents should be administered at periods shorter than their half-lives to avoid a fall in drug concentration to ineffective levels. Steady-state concentrations are closely approached after 5 to 7 half-lives on a fixed dosage schedule. Serum levels can be obtained and should be employed as a:

1. Baseline in the seizure-free patient.

2. Means of determining toxic levels and their distinction from episodes of CNS dysfunction.

3. Guide to dose adjustment in the patient having continued seizure activity.

4. Guide to dose adjustment when multiple drugs are being employed.

4

CLASS	INDICATIONS	GENERIC NAME	TRADE NAME	COMPANY
Hydantoins	Generalized convulsive seizures; all forms of partial seizures	Phenytoin Mephenytoin Ethotoin	Dilantin Mesantoin Peganone	Parke-Davis Sandoz Abbott
Barbiturates Desoxybarbiturates	Generalized convulsive seizures; all forms of partial seizures	Phenobarbital Mephobarbital Metharbital Primidone	Luminal Mebaral Gemonil Mysoline	Winthrop Winthrop Abbott Ayerst
Oxazolidinediones	Generalized nonconvulsive seizures (absences)	Trimethadione Paramethadione	Tridione Paradione	Abbott Abbott
Succinimides	Generalized nonconvulsive seizures (absences)	Phensuximide Methsuximide Ethosuximide	Milontin Celontin Zarontin	Parke-Davis Parke-Davis Parke-Davis
Acetylurea	Partial seizures with complex symptoms	Phenacemide	Phenurone	Abbott
Dibenzazepine	Partial seizures with complex symptoms; generalized convulsive seizures	Carbamazepine	Tegretol	Geigy
Benzodiazepine	Generalized nonconvulsive seizures (absences)	Clonazepam	Clonopin	Roche
Branched-chain carboxylic acid	Clonic seizures; absences; generalized tonic-clonic seizures; all forms of partial seizures	Valproic acid	Depakene	Abbott

DRUG	DOSAGE	EXPECTED BLOOD LEVEL		TIME TO REACH STEADY-STATE BLOOD LEVELS	SERUM HALF-LIFE	EFFECTIVE BLOOD LEVEL	TOXIC BLOOD LEVEL	PROTEIN BOUND
		Average	Range					
	mg/day	µg/ml	µg/ml	days	h	µg/ml	µg/ml	%
Phenytoin	300	10	5–20	5–10	24 ± 12	>10	>20	90
Phenobarbital	120	20	10–30	14–21	96 ± 12	>15	>40	40–50
Primidone	750	8	5–15	4–7	12 ± 6	>5	>12	0–50
phenobarbital	Derived	24	5–32	14–21	. . .	. . .	. . .	. . .
Carbamazepine	1200	6	3–12	2–4	12 ± 3	>4	>8	70
Valproic acid	1500	50	40–70	2–4	12 ± 6	>50	>100	90
Ethosuximide	1000	60	40–100	5–8	30 ± 6	>40	>100	0

Reference: Penry, J. K., and Newmark, M. E.: Ann. Intern. Med., *90:207*, 1979. Tables reproduced with permission of author and publisher.

The table on the opposite page provides a guide to the pharmacologic properties of the most common antiepileptic drugs. Note that the recommendations for optimal blood levels are slightly different in the following article and may vary from lab to lab.

INSTRUCTIONS TO SEIZURE PATIENTS

Compliance is a difficult problem for people on long-term drug therapy for chronic diseases. (The author was recently on a 10-day course of antibiotics. After two days, he was missing approximately 50 per cent of the prescribed doses, even though he is an otherwise reliable, well-informed physician.) Patients who understand their diseases and their medications are more likely to follow a drug program than are patients who are given a bottle of pills without adequate explanation or instructions on the drug's actions and side effects. The "Instructions to Seizure Patients" that follows is a simple, easy-to-understand aid for the patient who requires anticonvulsant medication. Dr. John Wolf has been kind enough to allow us to provide this adaptation.

4

> *Faint* — Both the French words *faint* and *feint* meant "pretended" or "feigned" and derive from *feindri,* which means to "be cowardly," "pretend," or "avoid one's responsibility."

Seizure control is related directly to the concentration of anticonvulsant medications in the blood. The most common cause of failure of seizure control is either that the person is missing his pills or that his doctor has not prescribed enough medication. These sheets will provide information for you so you can understand the process of seizure control better. You must know something about how your medications work. You may want to use some of the tricks that other people use to maintain their proper dose. You may be concerned about some of the common problems with anticonvulsant medications. If there are other areas that need to be covered, please tell us.

Anticonvulsant Pharmacology.

You must understand two important facts: The first is that excellence of seizure control depends on the amount of anticonvulsants in your blood. The second is that anticonvulsants are "slow" medications.

Because most anticonvulsants are absorbed and handled slowly in your body, they are not fully effective for several weeks after you begin taking them. This also means that if you forget any particular dose, you do not completely lose all the anticonvulsant activity in your body. Rather, the blood concentration drops slightly and then must build itself up over the next few days to the previous level. This also means that we will not change your dose of anticonvulsant more frequently than about every two weeks. If you continue to have seizures after two weeks on a given dose, you should be calling us so that we can change the dose and get seizure control as rapidly as possible.

As blood concentrations are rising during the first few weeks of treatment with phenobarbital, Mebaral, or Mysoline, you may find that you have some sleepiness. Be persistant and take your medications *regularly*. If you are on a correct dose, this sleepiness will disappear, and you can have seizure control with the fewest number of side effects. People who take anticonvulsants irregularly frequently complain that they are always sleepy when they take their medication. This is because they have rapidly rising and falling blood levels and are never stabilized. If you are on a correctly prescribed dose and if you take your medication every single day, you should not have continuing sedation unless yours is a particularly difficult seizure problem.

There is now a laboratory examination that determines how much anticonvulsant you have in your blood. This test has revolutionized the process of seizure control because the concentration of anticonvulsant in the blood is directly related to seizure control. This means if your "blood level" is too low, you will be having seizures. If it is too high, you may be toxic, and we can discover this. If it is just right, you should have a minimum of side effects and no seizures.

The following medications should be maintained at approximately the blood levels listed below:

Dilantin:	2.0–3.0 mg/100 ml	(20–30 μg/ml)
phenobarbital:	2.0–3.0 mg/100 ml	(20–30 μg/ml)
	(Many people can have much higher pheno-barbital levels without signs of toxicity.)	
Zarontin:	4.0- 10.0 mg/100 ml	(40–100 μg/ml)
Tridione (measured as DMO):	over 10.0 mg/100 ml	(over 100 μg/ml)
Mysoline:	0.4–1.2 mg/100 ml	(4–12 μg/ml)
Mesantoin:	15–25 μg/ml	

Tegretol: This medication has only recently been released for use in seizure disorders. At present, we have no great experience with it. It is recommended only for aid in controlling severe seizure disorders that are not controllable with the routine medications. Published dosage schedules vary from 200 mg per day to 1200 mg per day. Tegretol has side effects that involve the bone marrow. We are more wary of it than we are of Dilantin and phenobarbital. Published therapeutic blood levels are in the range of 0.2 to 0.8 mg per hundred ml (2 to 8 μg/ml).

Tricks to be Sure You Always Get the Proper Dose

1. *Missed Doses*

   Because anticonvulsants are "slow" the total week's dose is as important as any particular day's dose. This means that you must make up missed doses, but do *not* miss any doses intentionally!

2. *Single Dose Per Day*

   Adults may take Dilantin, phenobarbital, Zarontin, Tridione, and Mesantoin on a once-a-day dosage schedule because of the "slow" nature of these medications. You need not split your daily dose into three or even into two separate portions. An easy schedule would be to take all medications just before retiring at night or just on arising in the morning. Children under 10 may need to take these medications more frequently. You should discuss this question as your child grows. Mysoline is "faster." Because of this, Mysoline itself disappears very rapidly from the blood, even though it becomes phenobarbital. Mysoline should be taken on a three-dose-per-day schedule.

3. *The One-Week Bottle Trick*

   People are sometimes unaware that they are missing doses of their medications. It is easy to keep yourself informed if you simply put a full week's supply of each medication into a small bottle every Sunday. By the next Sunday the entire week's dose will be *gone.* If you have any stray tablets left over at the end, take those on Sunday. If you are not sure in the middle of the week, you can easily count out and discover whether you are on schedule. Some people put the entire week's dose in individual sections of an egg carton. This is more clumsy, but it is more certain.

   Whatever technique you use, be *certain* that you get the entire week's dose each week spaced as regularly as possible so your blood levels will be stable.

Problems

1. *Toxicity*

   "Toxicity" usually means symptoms caused by too much medication. If you become toxic on phenobarbital, Mysoline, or Mebaral, you are likely to become sleepy or irritable. You may have a difficult time waking up in the morning. Children sometimes become hyperactive. Toxicity to Dilantin is more likely to cause blurred vision, double vision, and then staggering. If you develop symptoms that you think are related to toxicity, you should call us and probably plan to have a blood level drawn to determine which medication is causing your particular toxic symptoms.

2. *Pregnancy*

   Recent reports have suggested that women taking anticonvulsants are more likely to have babies with various kinds of malformations. Because of this, it is difficult to advise a general policy. It seems, however, that the consequences of having seizures are so devastating that the best advice would be for pregnant women to be on the smallest dose of medication that will control their seizures. This is especially true during the first three or four months of pregnancy. Secondly, babies that are born to women on Dilantin and phenobarbital occasionally have trouble with bleeding immediately after birth. If you go into labor and are taking either of these medications, you should ask your obstetrician for an injection of Vitamin K during labor. This should prevent that problem.

3. *Children*

Very small infants should have anticonvulsants given in divided doses at least three to four times a day. Children between the ages of 2 and 5 should probably have at least three doses a day. Between the ages of 5 and 10, depending upon the size of the child, phenobarbital could be decreased to one or two doses a day. After the age of 10 or 12, most children may take their anticonvulsants on a once-a-day schedule.

4. *Special Problems With Dilantin*

The body handles Dilantin in a more irregular manner than it does the other medications. Many medications interfere with the body chemistry of Dilantin. If you are taking Dilantin, you would be best advised to stay away from all other medications as much as possible — even aspirin! Such things as tranquilizers, antituberculous drugs, aspirin, and many other medications can change your blood level of Dilantin and may cause you either to have a seizure or to become toxic. If you absolutely *must* take other medications, then you should establish the correct dose of Dilantin in your particular case while you are taking that particular medication.

Questions

1. *Alcohol*

   In general, a seizure patient who is under control should lead a normal life at all times except that he takes his medications once a day. Alcoho*lism* causes seizures, but usually the modest use of alcohol does not affect a seizure disorder.

2. *Addiction*

   You need not worry about becoming addicted to anticonvulsants. Naturally, if you stop your anticonvulsants, you will have seizures. However, true addiction in the usual sense of the word does not occur with the anticonvulsants.

3. *If You Have A Seizure*

   If you have a seizure, you will need to know why it occurred. You should come into the laboratory with a copy of these *Instructions* and ask for blood to be drawn for accurate blood level determination. You must do this within 24 hours of the seizure so the blood levels will be the same as they were when you had your seizure. Do not take extra medication before the blood level is drawn. This is vitally important, because from the result of the blood level, you and we can determine whether the cause of the seizure was inadequate prescription or inadequate taking of the prescribed medication. Some people have seizures that are simply not controllable. Blood levels can help establish this diagnosis as well.

   You should have the results of your blood level within a week. If you do not get the results, call us, or write to us, because you need to be informed as much as we do.

   Finally, wear a "medical alert" bracelet, indicating that you have a seizure disorder. One can be obtained by writing Medical Alert; Turlock, California 95380.

TREMORS

Classification of Abnormal Tremors According to their Relationship to Rest and Voluntary Movement

TYPE OF TREMOR	PRESENT	TEST
Static tremor Parkinsonism	At rest	Inspection
Postural tremor	In sustained posture	Arms outstretched or over head

1. Accentuated physiologic tremor
  Action tremor of parkinsonism
  Epinephrine-induced tremor
  Thyrotoxic tremor
  Anxiety tremor
  Tremor of fatigue
  Essential tremor
  Alcoholic tremor
2. Cerebellar tremor
3. Asterixis
		Hands extended at the wrist
		
		Standing

Intention tremor Brachium conjunctivum lesions (cerebellar)	During coordinated movement	Finger to nose Heel to shin
Miscellaneous tremors 1. Tremors of Wilson's disease	During coordinated movement, at rest, and in sustained posture	
2. Tremors due to poisonings	In sustained posture and at rest	
3. Tremors in acute infectious states	In sustained posture	
4. Spasmus nutans	In sustained upright posture (infants, ages 6–18 mos.)	

Tremors Commonly Encountered in Various Disease States

DISEASE STATE	TYPE OF TREMOR			
	Tremor at Rest (Static Tremor)	*Tremor During Sustained Posture (Postural Tremor)*	*Tremor During Coordinated Movement (Intention Tremor)*	*Other Types of Tremors*
Parkinsonism	++++	++	0	0
Essential Tremor	+	++++	++	0
Cerebellar Disease Hemisphere	0	++++	0	0
Brachium conjunctivum	0	0	++++	0
Wilson's disease	+	++++	+++	Wing-beating
Multiple sclerosis	0	+++	++++	0
Metabolic diseases	0	++++ (Asterixis)	0	0
Alcoholism	0	++++	0	0
Thyrotoxicosis	0	++++	0	0
Anxiety	0	++++	0	0
Fatigue	0	++++	0	0

0   Not present
+   Rarely present
++   Occasionally present
+++ Frequently present
++++ Characteristically present

Reference: Fahn, S.: Differential diagnosis of tremors. Med. Clin. of North Am., *56*:1363, 1972. Tables reproduced with permission of author and publisher.

CEREBRAL EDEMA

Understanding the three types of cerebral edema can lead to correct therapy. An increase in the blood volume of the brain is called brain engorgement. Brain engorgement is caused by obstruction of the cerebral veins and venus sinuses or arterial vasodilatation, as in hypercapnea. If unrelieved, brain engorgement may be associated with vasogenic cerebral edema.

Vasogenic edema is characterized by increased permeability of brain capillary endothelial cells. It is associated with brain engorgement, brain tumor, brain abscess, hemorrhage, infarction, and contusion — conditions usually associated with a positive brain scan. In addition, it is associated with lead encephalopathy and purulent meningitis. The characteristic increase in permeability of brain capillary endothelial cells allows the collection of extracellular edema fluid containing plasma proteins. Vasogenic edema is responsible for most cerebral herniations.

Swelling of the glial, neuronal, and endothelial cells of the brain is called **cytotoxic edema**. Cytotoxic edema can be caused by purulent meningitis in which the lysosomal elements of intracerebral leukocytes are released, causing cellular swelling. Cytotoxic edema may also be caused by water intoxication, hypo-osmolality, and hypoxia. The cellular swelling may compress the cerebral vascular supply, causing ischemia. In general, people with cytotoxic edema have a normal brain scan and normal cerebral spinal fluid protein.

Interstitial edema is caused by communicating or noncommunicating obstructive hydrocephalus, pseudotumor cerebri, and purulent meningitis. The continued production of cerebral spinal fluid worsens this condition.

The table shown on the opposite page characterizes the features of cerebral edema. Acetazolamide may be useful in interstitial edema, as it decreases the production of cerebral spinal fluid.

Features of the Three Types of Brain Edema

FEATURES	VASOGENIC	CYTOTOXIC	INTERSTITIAL
Characteristics:			
Pathogenesis	Increased capillary permeability	Cellular swelling — glial, neuronal and endothelial	Increased brain fluid because of block of cerebrospinal-fluid absorption
Location of edema	Chiefly white matter	Gray and white matter	Chiefly periventricular white matter in hydrocephalus
Edema-fluid composition	Plasma filtrate, including plasma proteins	Increased intracellular water and sodium	Cerebrospinal fluid
Extracellular-fluid volume	Increased	Decreased	Increased
Capillary permeability to large molecules	Increased	Normal	Normal
Clinical Disorders:			
Syndromes	Brain tumor, abscess, infarction trauma, hemorrage, lead encephalopathy	Hypoxia or hypo-osmolality (water intoxication, etc.)	Obstructive hydrocephalus, pseudotumor cerebri (?)
	Purulent meningitis	Purulent meningitis	Purulent meningitis
Electroencephalographic changes	Focal slowing common	Generalized slowing	Tracing often normal
Therapeutic Effects:			
Steroids	Beneficial in brain tumor and abscess	Controversial May be useful in hypoxia	Uncertain effectiveness
Osmotherapy (e.g., mannitol)	Reduces volume of normal brain tissue only (acutely)	Reduces brain volume acutely in hypo-osmolality	Rarely useful
Acetazolamide	No effect	No effect	Minor usefulness
Surgery	Beneficial	Not indicated	Beneficial

Reference: Adapted from Fishman, R. A.: New Engl. J. Med., *293*:706, 1975 with permission of author and publisher.

"Our knowledge of the mysterious complexities of clinical medicine grows with the experience we digest, the understanding we master and disciplined inquiry we make. We find what is there only if we sacrifice that part of ourselves which is expended with complete attention and concentration. We see and hear what is before us only if we look, listen, and focus. Often we find what we think of, sometimes what we search for, but rarely what we look at."

William Bean

WHAT THE MIND DOES NOT KNOW THE EYE WILL NOT SEE

The intern is very excited — his new patient appears to have papilledema! But the medical student has many questions: How does one recognize papilledema? What else could this be? If it is papilledema, what caused it? They turn to you for wisdom.

Criteria for the Diagnosis of Papilledema

1. Elevation of the optic disc (record the elevation in number of diopters).
2. Enlargement, dilatation, and tortuosity of venules.
3. Absence of venular pulsations.
4. Deflection of vessels over the edge of the elevated optic disc.
5. Blurred disc margins (many healthy patients have blurred nasal margins).
6. Reddish discoloration of optic disc.
7. Flame-shaped hemorrhages on or near the optic disc.
8. Few exudates.
9. Folds in the retina (corrugated retina); edema of the retina.
10. Usually bilateral.
11. In advanced cases, transitory obscuration of vision and constriction of visual fields.

The patient may have optic neuritis — called papillitis — if the disc is involved but the retina is spared, or neuroretinitis if both are involved. The following checklist will sort things out:

	PAPILLEDEMA	OPTIC NEURITIS
Location	Usually bilateral*	Unilateral†
Visual acuity	Normal	Decreased
Visual fields	Increased blind spot	Central scotoma
Pain on motion	Absent	Present
Disc elevation	May be 2 diopters	2 diopters or less
Venous pulsations	Absent	Present

*May be unilateral in some situations.
†May be bilateral.

4

CAUSES OF PAPILLEDEMA

Cranial	Increased intracranial pressure: — space-occupying lesions: edema, tumor, brain abscess, hemorrhagic infarct, etc. — meningitis — pseudotumor cerebri — leukemia or lymphoma with CNS involvement
Orbital and ocular (may be unilateral)	Tumors Graves' disease Glaucoma Uveitis Injuries
Toxic	Methanol Lead poisoning CO poisoning
Systemic	Hypertension Anemia, acute blood loss CO_2 retention (e.g., polio, chronic bronchitis, Guillain-Barre syndrome, cystic fibrosis) Uremia Hypercalcemia Hypoparathyroidism (in juveniles)

GAZE ABNORMALITIES

The following chart shows gaze abnormalities in isolated cranial nerve lesions.

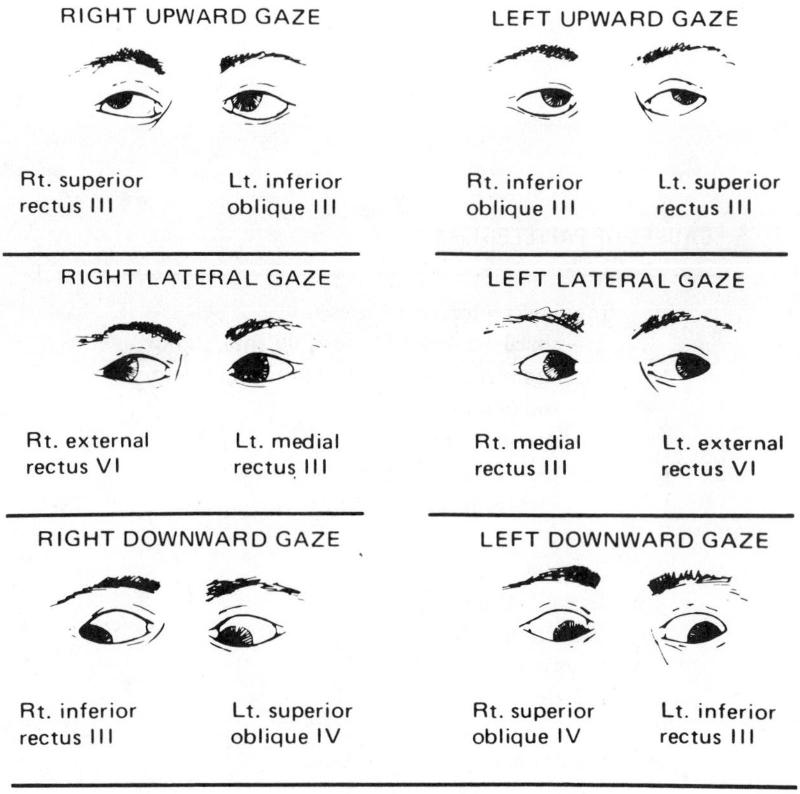

RIGHT UPWARD GAZE

Rt. superior   Lt. inferior
rectus III   oblique III

LEFT UPWARD GAZE

Rt. inferior   Lt. superior
oblique III   rectus III

RIGHT LATERAL GAZE

Rt. external   Lt. medial
rectus VI   rectus III

LEFT LATERAL GAZE

Rt. medial   Lt. external
rectus III   rectus VI

RIGHT DOWNWARD GAZE

Rt. inferior   Lt. superior
rectus III   oblique IV

LEFT DOWNWARD GAZE

Rt. superior   Lt. inferior
oblique IV   rectus III

FIG. 4–2

Belladonna — From the Renaissance ladies of Italy who found that a drop of extract of the deadly nightshade plant placed in the eye produced mydriasis and a "beautiful lady."

4

Reference: Dodge, P. R.: Neurologic history and examination. In Farmer, T. W. (Ed.): Pediatric Neurology. New York, Harper & Row, Publishers, Inc., 1975, p. 18.

PUPILS FOR THE PUPIL

Abnormal Pupils

DESCRIPTION	NAME	DIFFERENTIAL DIAGNOSIS
Shape:		
Absent iris	Aniridia	Wilms' tumor
Scalloped or asymmetrical retraction	Irregular iris	Adhesions, old iritis, persistent pupillary membrane, trauma
Tearing the root of the iris from ciliary attachment	Iridodialysis	Trauma
Loss of circular shape	Coloboma	Congenital or operative
Movement and Size:		
Loss of light reflex, preservation of accommodation, miosis	Argyll Robertson pupil	Syphilis, also seen occasionally in encephalitis, multiple sclerosis, CNS tumor
Very slow light reflex, preservation of accommodation, mydriasis	Adie's pupil	Benign
Preservation of light reflex, loss of accommodation	Reverse Argyll Robertson pupil	Bilateral: Diabetes mellitus, syphilis, basilar meningitis, tumor of the corpora quadrigemina Unilateral: Diphtheria, intoxication (alcohol), syphilis
Loss of all reflex movements of the pupil	Ophthalmoplegia interna	Third nerve nucleus damage, diabetes mellitus, syphilis, diphtheria, tumor, trauma
Loss of ipsilateral light reflex, loss of contralateral consensual reflex	Optic nerve lesion	Lesion between chiasma and globe
Loss of psychic or sensory mydriasis (may be associated with Horner's syndrome)	Sympathetic pupil	Syringomyelia, paralysis of cervical sympathetic

Abnormal Pupils

DESCRIPTION	NAME	DIFFERENTIAL DIAGNOSIS
Miosis, preservation of light and accommodation reflexes	Miotic, reactive pupil	Neonates, the elderly, stimulation of pupillary sphincter, paralysis of dilater pupillae (encephalitis, syringomyelia, CNS abscess) tumor or hemorrhage irritating the center for constriction. Opiates, organic phosphates, pilocarpine.
Mydriasis*, preservation of light and accommodation reflexes	Mydriatic, reactive pupil	Mania, schizophrenia, irritation without destruction of cervical sympathetics (i.e., aneurysm, tumor, blood infection), LSD
Pupil alternately dilate and contract rapidly ("tremor of the iris")	Hippus	Multiple sclerosis, drug/alcohol overdose, homocystinuria, central scotoma with macular damage or disease or injury to axial fibers of optic nerve
More than one pupil in an eye	Polycoria	Congenital, traumatic, surgical
Inequality of size of pupils	Anisocoria	Variation of normal, iritis, diabetes mellitus, cervical sympathetic lesion, eye drops, glaucoma, unilateral damage to third nerve fibers, syphilis, trigeminal neuralgia, carotid or aortic aneurysm, cranial lesion, cerebral herniation, artificial eye
Pupils dilate under light stimulus	Paradoxical pupil (rare)	Syphilis
With strong deviation of the eyes, the pupil of the abducted eye is larger than that of the adducted eye	Tournay's sign	Normal

*The atropines cause cycloplegia; dilatation and *paralysis* of the iris.

AUTONOMIC NEUROPATHY OF THE GUILLAIN-BARRE SYNDROME

The neuromuscular aspects of the Guillain-Barre syndrome are well known. Until recently respiratory muscle paralysis had been the main cause of death from this syndrome. As improved respiratory care has prolonged survival in the most severe cases, it has become apparent that autonomic dysfunction occurs frequently and is often a factor in deaths. The degree of autonomic dysfunction does not necessarily correlate with the degree of paralysis. The types of autonomic dysfunction that may occur include:

Sympathetic Hyperactivity

1. Hypertension — transient, but may be severe*
2. Wide fluctuations in blood pressure*
3. Agitated irrational behavior
4. Profuse diaphoresis
5. Peripheral vasoconstriction
6. Sinus tachycardia*

Sympathetic Hypoactivity

1. Postural hypotension*
2. Absent "fright reaction"

Parasympathetic Hyperactivity

1. Facial flushing*
2. Bradycardia*

Parasympathetic Hypoactivity

1. Adynamic ileus
2. Bladder dysfunction*

---

*Indicates common occurrences.

Many patients will have several kinds of autonomic dysfunction during their illness. Sudden death may occur and is associated with severe hypertension or wide swings in blood pressure. Appropriate drug therapy to correct life-threatening abnormalities — such as atropine for bradycardia — should be employed. Short-acting preparations of drugs are to be preferred due to the unpredictable and paroxysmal nature of the autonomic dysfunction. Patients with severe bradycardia should have a prophylactic transvenous pacemaker.

Reference: Lictenfeld, P.: Am. J. Med., *50*:772, 1971.

AN APPROACH TO MUSCLE WEAKNESS

4

LOCATION OF PRIMARY LESION	ATROPHY	TENDON REFLEXES	SENSORY INVOLVEMENT	PAIN	MUSCLE TENDERNESS	ELECTROMYOGRAM	COMMENTS
I. Central nervous system							
A. Cerebral cortex and projections	–	Hyperactive	–	–	–	–	Some atrophy if sensory cortex also involved
B. Spinal cord—anterior horn cell							
Poliomyelitis	+	Absent	–	–	–	Positive sharp waves, Fibrillation	
Amyotrophic lateral sclerosis							
Spinal	+	Absent	–	–	–	Fasciculations	Fasciculations are prominent
Bulbar	+	Absent	–	–	–		
Combined	+	Absent (arms)	–	–	–		
II. Peripheral nerve (e.g., Guillain-Barre syndrome)	+	Absent	Usual	Sometimes	Sometimes	Fibrillation, Positive sharp waves	
III. Muscle							
A. Progressive muscular dystrophy	+	Disappear with progression	–	–	–	Myopathic pattern, brief low-voltage action potentials	May have pseudohypertrophy early in Duchenne type. Various modes of inheritance
B. Myotonia	+ (Especially facial, temporalis and sternocleidomastoid)	Characteristic delayed relaxation	–	–	–	Normal pattern, but failure to relax	Autosomal dominant; diabetes mellitus, frontal baldness, cataracts, and genital atrophy associated findings
C. Dermatomyositis/polymyositis	+ (Less than with denervation)	Decreased	–	In 15%	+	Myopathic pattern	Systemic signs and symptoms common, especially rash. May be associated visceral malignancy (esp. > 40 years of age)
D. Myasthenia gravis	–	Present	–	–	–	Decrease in amplitude with repetitive stimuli	Diagnosis with Tensilon test
IV. Metabolic disturbances							
A. Periodic paralysis	–	Absent with attack	–	–	–	Refractory to stimulation	Hypo- and normokalemic forms
B. Hypothyroidism	Volume increased	Delayed relaxation	–	–	–	Pseudomyotonia	Respiratory muscles spared
C. Hyperthyroidism	+	Normal to hyperactive	–	–	–	Normal	Check for exogenous iodine in medications
D. Hyperadrenalism/high-dose corticosteroid therapy	–	Usually normal	–	–	–	Myopathic pattern	Recovery with discontinuation of corticosteriods

+ = Present   – = Absent

CRAMPS

A cramp is a spasmatic (painful), involuntary contraction of a muscle sustained for more than a few seconds. The vast majority of cramps are not caused by metabolic muscle disease. Most muscle cramps are caused by overexertion, repetitive motion, electrolyte imbalance, vascular insufficiency and/or the combination of caffeine, nicotine, and exhaustion.

Important clues to etiology are available from the patient's history and laboratory tests, as indicated in the following table. At times, the diagnosis is obvious. The physical and neurologic exam should include examination for Chvostek's and Trousseau's signs and myopercussion. In more complex cases, attention should be paid to calcium, magnesium, phosphorus, and electrolyte data, as well as renal and thyroid function.

Reference: Layzer, R. B., and Rowland, L. P.: New Engl. J. Med., *285*:31, 1971. Table reproduced by permission of author and publisher.

4

KIND OF CRAMP	MUSCLE		NERVE			CENTRAL	
	Contracture	*Myotonia*	*Neuromyotonia*	*Tetany*	*Ordinary Muscle Cramps*	*Tetanus*	*Stiff-man Syndrome*
Differential diagnosis or examples of disease	Deficiency of muscle phosphorylase or phosphofructokinase	Myotonia congenita, myotonic dystrophy, paramyotonia, hyperkalemic periodic paralysis and chondrodystrophic myotonia	Pseudomyotonia, myokymia with delayed muscular relaxation, quantal squander, and armadillo syndrome	Hypocalcemia, hypomagnesemia, (relative or absolute), alkalosis	After hard exercise, pregnancy, dehydration, salt depletion, hypothyroidism, thyrotoxic myopathy, uremia, hypomagnesemia, clofibrate therapy, partially denervated muscle, or vascular insufficiency		
Provoking factors	Exertional only	Delayed relaxation of voluntary contraction; percussion or electrical stimulation of muscle	Delayed relaxation of voluntary contraction	Spontaneous; provoked by hyperventilation; nerve compression	Exertional; with minor movement; in sleep	Movement and emotional or sensory stimuli	Movement and emotional or sensory stimuli
Painful cramps	Yes	No	No	Variable	Yes	Yes	Yes
Continuous stiffness at rest	No	No	Yes	No	No	Yes	Yes
Electromyogram	Little or no electrical activity in muscle affected by contraction	Myotonic bursts after contraction, percussion, or needle movement	Continuous electrical activity at rest; after discharge, contraction; potentials range from single muscle fibers to motor units	Regularly repetitive motor-unit discharge in doublets or triplets at 10/sec	Irregular, high-frequency, high voltage, profuse bursts of motor-unit potentials	Persistent normal motor-unit discharges at rest; heightened during spasm	Persistent normal motor-unit discharges at rest; heightened during spasm
Effect of curare	None	Myotonia persists, evoked by direct stimulation of muscle	Blocked	Blocked	Not known	Blocked	Blocked
Effect of nerve block	None		Activity reduced, not abolished	Activity persists	Evoked by stimulation distal to block	Not known	Activity blocked
Effect of sleep or narcosis	Not known	Persists	Persists	May persist	May begin during sleep, but awakens subject	Abolished	Abolished or reduced
Probable site of disturbed physiology	Sarcoplasmic reticulum	Muscle membrane	Distal motor nerve	Motor-nerve fibers with lowered threshold	? Motor nerve fibers; ? hyperexcitable motorneurons in spinal cord	Loss of inhibitory postsynaptic potentials in spinal cord	Unknown; may be similar to tetanus or hyperactivity of fusimotor system
Treatment	? Carbohydrate in phosphorylase deficiency; ? isoproterenol in phosphofructokinase and phosphorylase deficiency	Quinine, procainamide, cortisone, diphenylhydantoin	Diphenylhydantoin, carbamazepine	Calcium or correction of alkalosis; diphenylhydantoin, phenobarbital	Passive stretch of muscle; correction of metabolic disturbance; quinine, diphenylhydantoin	Tetanus antitoxin; chlorpromazine; phenobarbital, diazepam, and curare, with assisted respiration	Diazepam

CARPAL TUNNEL SYNDROME

The patient's complaint is nocturnal hand paresthesias or pain. The diagnosis may be carpal tunnel syndrome, which may be a clue to the presence of systemic disease. Typically, numbness, tingling, or pain in the first three digits of the hand occurs first at night, then during the day. A sensory deficit may follow, and eventually weakness of the adductors of the thumb and atrophy of the thenar eminence may occur. Pain may be felt up the arm. The syndrome, which may be unilateral or bilateral, is caused by pressure on the median nerve as it passes through the carpal tunnel between the bones of the wrist and the transverse carpal ligament.

Physical examination may reveal pain or tingling elicited by (1) tapping the median nerve at the carpal tunnel (Tinel's sign) or (2) sustained flexion of the wrist. A sensory deficit or diminished motor strength may be found. The diagnosis can be confirmed with nerve conduction studies.

Treatment depends on the etiology of the syndrome. When occurring in pregnancy, the syndrome usually disappears following delivery. It may occur in subsequent pregnancies. Casting the wrists in a neutral position provides symptomatic relief. The acute onset of carpal tunnel syndrome may indicate arterial thrombosis. Symptoms occurring during exercise may be related to muscular hypertrophy. If symptoms are persistent or neurologic findings show sensory deficit or weakness, surgery may be indicated; surgery is usually curative. The causes of the carpal tunnel syndrome are listed below.

Factors that Increase the Volume in the Carpal Tunnel

Synovitis* — trauma,* including excessive use
Rheumatoid arthritis*
Edema — pregnancy*
Amyloidosis
Hypothyroidism*
Acromegaly
Tumors
Muscular hypertrophy
Gout, pseudogout
Hyperparathyroidism
Multiple myeloma (amyloid)

Conditions that Alter the Contour of the Carpal Tunnel

Arthritis
Dislocation
Fracture
Cysts (ganglion)

Neuropathies

Diabetes mellitus or other peripheral neuropathy
Collagen-vascular diseases
Arterial thrombosis
Vasospasm

---

*Indicates most common causes.

4

CORRECTING THE BLOODY SPINAL TAP

All too often when the cerebrospinal fluid (CSF) white cell count and protein concentration are needed to help establish a diagnosis, the spinal tap seems traumatic. Is it traumatic? Can you salvage some information from it?

Actual hemorrhage into the subarachnoid space will cause the number of red cells present in the first and last samples of cerebrospinal fluid to be similar. In addition, the cerebrospinal fluid will appear xanthochromic after centrifugation, if blood has been present in the subarachnoid space for any period of time. If there has been a traumatic tap, the supernatant will be clear.

To estimate the number of white cells in the spinal fluid after a traumatic tap, the following corrections can be applied:

1. As a rule of thumb, 1000 RBCs/mm^3 will contribute 1 WBC/mm^3.

2. $\dfrac{\text{Patient's peripheral white blood cell count/mm}^3}{\text{Patient's peripheral red blood cell count/mm}^3} = \dfrac{\text{number of WBCs introduced}}{\text{number of RBCs in CSF}}$

   number of WBCs introduced $= \dfrac{(\text{Patient's peripheral WBC}) \times (\text{RBCs in CSF})}{\text{Patient's peripheral RBC count}}$

For example:

Patient's peripheral WBC = 15,000/mm^3 μl

Patient's peripheral RBC = 5,000,000/mm^3

Patient's spinal fluid WBC count = 350/mm^3

Patient's spinal fluid RBC count = 30,000/mm^3

Number of WBCs introduced $= \dfrac{(15,000) \times (30,000)}{5,000,000}$

$= \dfrac{(15) \times (30)}{5}$

$= \dfrac{450}{5}$

Number of WBCs introduced = 90 WBCs/mm^3

Therefore, the patient has 350-90, or 260 cells/mm³ in the spinal fluid. To estimate the spinal fluid protein concentration, similar corrections can be made:

1. As a rule of thumb, *1000 RBCs/mm³* in the spinal fluid will *raise* the spinal fluid *protein 1.5 mg/dl.*

2. Protein introduced $= \dfrac{\text{serum protein (mg/dl)} \times \text{RBCs in CSF}}{\text{patient's peripheral RBC count}}$

For example:

Patient's serum protein is 8.0 grams/dl (8000 mg/dl)

Patient's peripheral RBC count = 5,000,000/mm³

Patient's spinal fluid protein = 110 mg/dl

Patients spinal fluid RBC count = 30,000/mm³

Protein introduced $= \dfrac{8{,}000 \times 30{,}000}{5{,}000{,}000}$

$= \dfrac{8 \times 30}{5}$

Protein introduced $= \dfrac{240}{5} = 48$ mg/dl

Patient's actual spinal fluid protein is 110-48, or about 62 mg/dl.

Reference: Adapted from McMillan, J., Stockman, J., and Oski, F.: The Whole Pediatrician Catalog, Vol. 2. Philadelphia, W. B. Saunders Company, 1979, p. 402.

WHEN TO ORDER SKULL X-RAYS

A skull x-ray series is expensive and time-consuming. Fear of litigation, inexperience, or demands by consulting services (often before they arrive on the scene) make the skull series the most over ordered test in the emergency room. Bell and Loop classified 1500 patients into high-yield groups and low-yield groups based on the number of fractures discovered. In the high-yield group, 92 of 1065 patients were found to have skull fractures, as compared to one fracture detected in 435 patients in the low-yield group. The tables on the opposite page summarize their data.

Findings Not Significantly Associated With Skull Fractures

SOURCE	FINDING
History	Hospitalized or outpatient
	Sex
	Age
	Confusion or drowsiness
	Headache
	Visual disturbance
	Seizure
	Time since injury
Physical examination	Hematoma
	Laceration
	Swelling
	Intoxication

High-Yield Findings

SOURCE	YIELD	
	Fracture per Number of Examinations	*Per Cent of Fractures Associated with Findings*
History:		
>5 min of unconsciousness	1/8	41
>5 min of retrograde amnesia	1/7	44
Vomiting	1/8	20
Nonvisual focal symptoms	1/9	16
Accident at work or gunshot wound	1/5	15
Physical examination:		
Palpable bony malalignment	1/6	15
Discharge from ear	1/3	30
Discharge from nose	1/9	14
Ear-drum discoloration	1/4	23
Bilateral black eyes	1/7	8
Neurologic examination:		
Stupor, semiconsciousness or coma	1/6	43
Breathing irregular or apneic	1/4	16
Babinski reflex present	1/5	24
Other reflex abnormality	1/7	18
Focal weakness	1/9	15
Sensory abnormality	1/9	10
Anisocoria	1/7	19
Other cranial-nerve abnormality	1/5	21

Reference: Bell, R. S. and Loop, J. W.: New Engl. J. Med., *284*:236, 1971.

5
CARDIOLOGY

A BASIC APPROACH TO THE HYPERTENSIVE PATIENT

Hypertension is one of the most common clinical problems the clinician faces. Assessment of the hypertensive patient includes *determining the severity of hypertension,* the *extent of complications* and the *diagnosis of curable causes.* The scope of the initial laboratory investigation is still the subject of much debate in the literature. However, it is generally agreed that a thorough search for remediable causes is warranted in hypertension *refractory* to appropriate therapeutic trials.

The lists below enumerate the surgically correctable causes of hypertension, suggest appropriate initial laboratory studies, and outline a graded approach to therapy. It should be understood that the choice of therapy ultimately depends upon the severity of the disease, the susceptibility of the patient to side effects of particular drugs, and the presence of cardiac or other complications.

Remediable Causes of Hypertension

Pheochromocytoma
Coarctation of the aorta
Cushing's syndrome
Primary hyperaldosteronism
Renal artery stenosis
Unilateral renal parenchymal disease

Laboratory Evaluation

EKG
Chest x-ray
Urinalysis
Serum electrolytes
Serum creatinine
Intravenous pyelography*
Renal scan*

Graded Approach to Therapy†

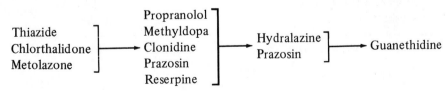

---

*Optional; indicated in young hypertensives, in patients with flank or abdominal bruits, and in the sudden onset or sudden exacerbation of hypertension particularly following trauma.
†See following article for commercial names and dose of agents.

References: Vidt, D.: Drug Therapy, August 1978, p. 33; Ayer, C. R., Slaughter, A. R., and Smallwood, H. D.: Am. J. Cardiol., *32*:533, 1973; American College of Physicians: Medical Knowledge Self-Assessment Program IV, 1977, pp. 45–50.

COMMONLY USED ANTIHYPERTENSIVES

Antihypertensives can be categorized according to their mechanism of action: diuretics, adrenergic blocking agents, and direct vasodilators. The following lists include agents frequently used in practice and their suggested dosages.

ANTIHYPERTENSIVE	DAILY DOSE (mg) (Approximate Range)
Thiazide Diuretics	
Bendroflumethiazide (Naturetin)	10–15 QD
Benzthiazide (Exna, Hydrex)	50–75 BID
Chlorothiazide (Diuril)	500–750 BID
Hydrochlorothiazide (Esidrix, Hydrodiuril)	50–75 BID
Hydroflumethiazide (Saluron)	50–75 BID
Methyclothiazide (Enduron)	10–15 QD
Polythiazide (Renese)	2–4 QD
Loop Diuretics	
Furosemide (Lasix)	20–100 BID
Ethacrynic acid (Edecrin)	50–75 BID
Potassium-sparing Diuretics	
Spironolactone (Aldactone)	50–100 TID or QID
Triamterene (Dyrenium)	100–150 BID
Miscellaneous Diuretics	
Chlorthalidone (Hygroton)	50–100 QD
Quinethazone (Hydromox)	50–75 BID
Metolazone (Zaroxolyn)	2.5–5.0 QD
Adrenergic Blocking Agents	
Reserpine (Serpasil)	0.1–0.5 QD
Alseroxylon (Rantenoin)	2–4 QD
Guanethidine (Ismelin)	10–100 QD
Methyldopa (Aldomet)	250–500 TID or QID
Clonidine (Catapres)	0.1–0.2 BID
Propranolol (Inderal)	10–100 QID
Peripheral Vasodilators	
Hydralazine (Apresoline)	10–40 QID
Prazosin (Minipress)	1.5–10 BID

Reference: Vidt, D. G.: Drug Therapy. August 1978, p. 34.

ADVERSE EFFECTS AND INTERACTIONS OF ANTIHYPERTENSIVE AGENTS

The chemotherapy for hypertension is usually extremely effective in lowering blood pressure. Nonetheless, antihypertensive agents have a substantial number of adverse effects and carry with them the potential for further adverse drug interactions. These side effects are of such consequence that the risk/benefit rates must be considered in each case and are of particular import when a decision must be made about the treatment of a "mild" hypertensive patient (i.e., one with diastolic pressures of 90 to 104 mmHg).

Thiazides

Adverse Effects

General

Hypokalemia
  Weakness
  Muscle cramps
  Night cramps
  Digitalis potentiation (toxicity)
Hyperglycemia

Hyperuricemia
Hypercalcemia
Confusion
Orthostatic hypotension
Renal insufficiency

Gastrointestinal

Anorexia
Gastric irritation
Vomiting
Cramping
Diarrhea

Constipation
Cholestatic jaundice
Pancreatitis
Sialadenitis

Central Nervous System

Dizziness
Vertigo
Paresthesias
Xanthopsia

Hematologic

Leukopenia
Agranulocytosis
Thrombocytopenia
Aplastic anemia

Hypersensitivity

Purpura
Photosensitivity
Rash
Urticaria
Vasculitis
Fever
Respiratory distress
Anaphylactoid reaction

Notes

1. Additive to other antihypertensives.
2. Potentiates digitalis effects (hypokalemia).
3. Increases aminoglycoside ototoxicity.
4. Potentiates tubocurarines.
5. Inhibits uricosuric and hypoglycemic agents.
6. With steroids, enhances potassium loss.
7. Cholestyramine binds thiazides.
8. Retards methenamine conversion to formaldehyde.
9. Quinidine absorption increased.

Spironolactone

Adverse Effects

Hyperkalemia
Gynecomastia
Postmenopausal bleeding
Inability to achieve or maintain
  erection (impotence)
(Cancer of breast reported; cause-effect
  relationship not established)

Cramping, diarrhea	Headache
Lethargy, confusion	Urticaria
Skin eruptions	Drug fever
Hirsutism	Ataxia
Deepening voice	

Notes

1. Enhances hypotensive effect of thiazides.
2. When used with ganglionic blockers, reduce ganglionic blocker dose by 50 per cent.
3. Do not use with potassium salts or other potassium-sparing diuretics.

Triamterene

Adverse Effects

Hyperkalemia	Dry mouth
GI disturbances	Anaphylaxis
Weakness	Photosensitivity
Headache	Cytopenias

Notes

1. Use potassium supplements or salt substitutes cautiously, if at all.
2. May elevate uric acid in patients predisposed to gouty arthritis.

Reserpine

Adverse Effects

Depression
Increased gastric acidity
Impotence
Nightmares
GI symptoms
Edema (weight gain)

Nasal congestion
Flushing
Bradycardia
Gynecomastia (pseudolactation,
  mammary tumors)

Deafness
Glaucoma, uveitis, optic
  atrophy
Rash, pruritus
Dry mouth

5

Notes

1. When administered with tricyclic antidepressants, may produce reserpine reversal; mania may occur.
2. Decreases cardiovascular effects of ephedrine.
3. May increase arrhythmias with cardiac glycosides or quinidine.
4. Lowers seizure threshold.
5. Orthostatic hypotension and bradycardia with guanethidine.
6. Potentiates norepinephrine.
7. Potentiates hypotensive effects of MAO inhibitors.
8. May aggravate "sick sinus" syndrome due to bradycardia.

Methyldopa

Adverse Effects

Sedation, depression
Edema, weight gain
Vertigo
Nightmares
Impotence
Dry mouth
Nasal stuffiness
GI symptoms

Hypotension (postural, exercise)
Prolactin release
Extrapyramidal signs
Paradoxical hypertension
Positive Coombs' test

Hepatitis
Hemolytic anemia?
Drug fever
Granulocytopenia
Thrombocytopenia

Notes

1. Hypotensive effect with phenothiazines.
2. Enhances pressor effect of amphetamines and norepinephrine.

3. Additive effect with propranolol, methotrimeprazine, procainamide, quinidine, procarbazine, and thioxanthines.

4. May aggravate "sick sinus" syndrome due to bradycardia.

Propranolol

Adverse Effects

Congestive heart failure
Bradycardia
Intensification of AV block
Raynaud's phenomenon
Bronchospasm in asthmatics
GI disturbances
Masks hypoglycemic symptoms
Sleep disturbances

Lightheadedness	Aching
Depression	Hallucinations
Lassitude	Visual disturbances
Weakness	Catatonia
Fatigue	Acute, reversible disorientation
Pharyngitis	Agranulocytosis
Erythematous rash	Thrombocytopenia
Fever	Reversible alopecia

Notes

1. Additive effect with long-acting nitrates for angina.

2. Enhances antihypertensive action of methyldopa, guanethidine, and hydralazine.

3. Exaggerates digitalis bradycardia.

4. Concurrent use with alpha-adrenergic blockers (phenoxybenzamine or phentolamines) prevents serious blood pressure rise in pheochromocytoma.

5. Potentiated by diphenylhydantoin.

6. Desipramine's anticholinergic action may block myocardial effects of propranolol.

7. Synergistic with quinidine in arrhythmias.

8. Blocks isoproterenol action in asthma.

9. Use cautiously with catechol-depleting drugs (reserpine).

10. Do not use with drugs that depress myocardium (ether, chloroform), epinephrine, and adrenergic-augmenting psychotropics, including MAO inhibitors.

11. Enhances tubocurarine neuromuscular blockade.

12. Synergistic hypotensive with phenothiazines.

13. May aggravate "sick sinus" syndrome secondary to bradycardia.

14. May produce hypoglycemia.

Hydralazine

Adverse Effects

Common

Headache
Palpitation
Angina
Tachycardia
Dizziness

Anorexia
Nausea
Sweating
Diarrhea

Less Common

Depression
Disorientation
Anxiety
Psychotic reaction
Paresthesias
Peripheral neuritis
Muscle cramps

Nasal congestion
Flushing
Lacrimation
Conjunctivitis
Postural hypotension
Tremors
Edema

Rare

Drug fever
Urticaria
Skin rash
Polyneuritis
GI hemorrhage

Anemia
Lymphadenopathy
Pancytopenia
Agranulocytosis
Paralytic ileus

Note

1. High doses of this drug may induce an acute rheumatoid state, disseminated lupus with positive LE cells, or a paradoxical pressor response.

Guanethidine

Adverse Effects

Orthostatic hypotension
Edema/congestive failure
Bradycardia
Retrograde ejaculation (impotence?)
Diarrhea
Weakness, fatigue
Dyspnea, asthma
Nausea, vomiting
Nocturia
Incontinence
Dermatitis
Scalp hair loss
Dry mouth

Ptosis
Blurred vision
Parotid tenderness
Myalgia
Depression
Nasal congestion
Mild hypoglycemia

Notes

1. Postural hypotension, bradycardia, and depression are exaggerated by rauwolfia (reserpine).
2. Thiazides enhance hypotensive effect.
3. Norepinephrine response may be enhanced.
4. Antagonized by amphetamines, ephedrine, and tricyclic antidepressants.
5. Contraindicated with MAO inhibitors and methylphenidate.
6. Phenothiazines in large doses may block action.
7. Methotrimeprazine exaggerates orthostatic hypotension.
8. Epinephrine hypersensitivity.
9. When tricyclics are withdrawn in patients receiving guanethidine, a profound hypertensive episode may occur.
10. Amphetamines stimulate release of guanethidine from adrenergic neurones, rapidly reversing adrenergic blockade.
11. Hypotensive effect delayed 2 to 3 days and persists 7 to 10 days after withdrawal.

Clonidine

Adverse Effects

Sedation	Pruritus
Impotence	Dizziness
Postural hypotension	Headache
Dry mouth	Fatigue
Constipation	Angioneurotic edema
Allergic rash	

Notes

1. Tricyclic antidepressants counteract its hypotensive action.
2. Alcohol and sedatives increase the central nervous system depression.
3. Hyperirritability and rebound hypertension are common when the drug is discontinued.

Prazosin

Adverse Effects

Syncope (first dose effect)
Tachycardia (first dose effect)
Dizziness
Headache
Drowsiness
Lack of energy

GI upset	Urinary frequency
Edema	Blurred vision
Diaphoresis	Red sclera
Depression	Epistaxis
Nervousness	Tinnitus
Paresthesias	Nasal congestion
Pruritus, rash	Dry mouth
Impotence	

Note

1. The dose must be reduced when it is used in combination with other hypotensive drugs.

Reference: Moses, C.: Ann. N.Y. Acad. Sci., *304*:84, 1978.

DON'T MAKE THE CURE WORSE THAN THE DISEASE

Originally entitled "Trials and tribulations of a symptom-free hypertensive physician receiving the best of care," the following is reprinted with permission of the author and publisher from Lancet, August 6, 1977. The author now states that "BP has remained 120/80 with weight stationary and diuretics being used only sparingly after salt-intake excess, such as Chinese dinner":

The wisdom of treating people over 60 with asymptomatic hypertension is being questioned. The arguments in favor of such treatment seem to prevail, and in ever greater numbers patients with mild to moderate hypertension receive a variety of drugs and go on their way with instructions to return for checkups in a few weeks or months, or at even longer intervals. Drugs may be prescribed in combinations, although little is known of drug interactions — for example, between methyldopa (Aldomet), propranolol hydrochloride (Inderal), and/or triamterene-plus-hydrochlorothiazide (Dyazide).

Having been the recipient of such therapeutic regimens for a number of years with variable results and side effects, this physician concludes that an account of his own experience could benefit his colleagues and their patients. Lest his motives be misinterpreted, let it be clear that he has the highest regard for all the physicians who have seen him, all of whom are excellent doctors, associated with teaching institutions of high repute.

The patient is a white male aged 61 years, and during the span of this story he weighed from 226 to 250 lb., which he carried on a massive frame of 6 ft, 2 in. He is married, has neither children nor major illnesses in his history, and he is leading an active, even hectic, life as a researcher and medical administrator. His family history includes gout in his mother's father and diabetes in his father's mother. Since 1944 he has been aware that his blood pressure was occasionally raised (140–150/90–100 mmHg), especially when he was examined in unusual circumstances, such as for a blood donation, army physical examination, or examination for life insurance, or before appointment to a job. On the other hand, at most of his routine annual physical examinations done regularly since 1944, the blood pressure was normal.

This changed in 1970, when a urologist, during an annual physical examination, obtained blood pressure readings of 160/95. The patient had also had for a few months recurrent episodes of cardiac arrhythmia, and he decided to consult a cardiologist. The raised blood pressure was confirmed, and phenobarbitone was prescribed for one week; at the end of a week the pressure would be rechecked, and if it remained high, admission to hospital would be arranged for complete investigation. The patient faithfully took the drug and had daily pressure readings at home, where they never exceeded 120/80. He decided that the combination of the cardiologist's personality and the possibility of admission to hospital was detrimental to his blood pressure, inducing temporary hypertension, and he changed physicians.

The next consultant, an expert on hypertension, found a pressure of 150/90 on repeated visits, even though readings taken at the same time at the patient's place of work and at home never exceeded 125/85. Aldosterone and renin studies, as well as urine analysis and hematological and biochemical investigations, were done. All were normal (except for a blood cholesterol of 350 mg/dl). The patient refused a proposed intravenous pyelogram (recalling two necropsies he did in the early 1940s on victims of catastrophes caused by that procedure), and he walked out of a scheduled kidney scan when he overheard technicians calculating the tracer dose and making decimal mistakes.

On clinical grounds, it was decided that the patient had essential hypertension in a labile phase and ought to be treated. First, he was given sodium chlorothiazide (Diuril), which led rather quickly to leg cramps and hypokalemia. The physician saw the patient every other week and carefully adjusted therapy. An evil-tasting potassium supplement was taken, and shortly arrhythmias, which had been absent for several months, reappeared. Joint pains made themselves felt and the serum uric acid rose to around 10 mg/dl. The diuretic was discontinued and a trial was begun with methyldopa. The pressure fell, but so did the patient's interest in sex and in the world around him. He became impotent but did not care. As a researcher, he concluded that methyldopa might well be an ideal drug for sex offenders.

He was not asked about his sex life by his physician and did not volunteer to talk about it until after a few months it came up casually during consultation. The drug was immediately discontinued, and reserpine (Serpasil) was given instead. The blood pressure remained normal, but after a few weeks severe depression set in. The patient now was not merely sexually neutered, but suicidal. Fortunately the physician spotted this and suggested that·reserpine be replaced by propranolol (Inderal). A small dose, 10 mg three times a day, proved ineffective, because readings of 140/95–100 recurred in the physician's office, even though at work and at home readings remained normal. Now a combination of triamterene and hydrochlorothiazide was added to propranolol. Blood pressure readings, even in the physician's office, became normal, no serum chemistry anomalies were noted (except the persistently raised cholesterol), and arrhythmias and gouty symptoms disappeared. The regimen was maintained, with periodic reviews, for more than three years.

Then the patient noted that gradually he became apathetic and indifferent to anything that went on in the world. He once again became disinterested in sex, for which he had re-established a normal urge, and he lived contentedly a placid and flaccid life. Then he noted that it became impossible to control the end phase of the urinary stream and that he invariably wet his pants during urination. When he asked the urologist about this at the annual prostate palpation session, he was told that weakening of certain urethral muscles was a normal phenomenon of aging and had to be accepted by many old men. Still later he noted that on the rare occasions when he ejaculated, the process was strangely slow and ended in an empty, disappointing feeling rather than in the usual climactic sensation. On several occasions a strange curtain-like opacity obliterated his field of vision. The disturbing symptom made him seek the advice of an ophthalmologist, who found no physical explanation. The old professor explained that at worst it might be temporary hypotension and advised the patient not to worry about it.

The patient was curious about the cumulation of these usual and annoying symptoms and he read the descriptive literature on the drugs he was taking. Propranolol occasionally may produce hypotension... lightheadedness, mental depression, lassitude, visual disturbances, clouded sensorium ...

The patient discussed this and his misgivings about his sympathetic nervous system with his doctor, and they decided to omit propranolol and to reduce the dose of the triamterene-hydrochlorothiazide combination to one capsule a day. This regimen has now continued for well over a year. The blood pressure has remained normal. An occasional rise of blood pressure in the physician's office is now disregarded. In all the years since 1944, although this phenomenon has been known, no changes have been seen in the patient's retinal vessels and no electro-cardiogram anomalies have been recorded, in spite of a history of occasional arrhythmias.

Within days of stopping propranolol the patient perked up and became once more his old self, with normal genitourinary functions. Shortly after the end of antihypertensive therapy (except for a small dose of diuretic) the patient went on six weeks' vacation and on his own initiative embarked upon a program of strenuous hiking and diet control. He lost 10 per cent of his body-weight and became quite fit. He continues to walk at least 7 miles each weekend throughout the year and deliberately parks his car away from his destination to enjoy brisk walks whenever possible. Thus weight, blood pressure, and serum cholesterol are now being maintained close to where they ought to be. The patient now wonders whether he could do without the diuretic and whether his regimen of diet control and exercise might not have spared him the drug-induced miseries he endured.

The story (which the patient has seen repeated in some of his own friends) is not an argument against treating the symptom-free hypertensive. On the contrary, it might encourage physicians to follow up more closely all hypertensive patients under treatment and to make every effort to reduce the level of medication to the smallest effective dose — not forgetting, of course, the patient as a whole and how he can benefit from simple measures such as diet control, exercise, and (sometimes) psychotherapy. Specific questions must be asked in order to discover early any side effects, without, however, suggesting each side effect to apprehensive patients. Above all, his experience has instilled in him a greater respect for the power of drugs.

PLEASE FEEL THE BEATING HEART

The characteristic of the cardiac apex impulse is an integral part of the bedside cardiovascular exam. The apex impulse should be evaluated with the patient in the supine position. The absolute displacement of the impulse is assessed most accurately by palpating with the fingertips rather than with the entire hand or palm. The size of the apex impulse is evaluated by determining the number of interspaces in which the impulse is palpated. The duration of the impulse during systole is measured by simultaneous auscultation and palpation or by observing stethoscope motion while auscultating over the apex.

A holosystolic impulse correlates with increased left ventricular mass, as does an impulse occupying two or more interspaces. A normal left ventricular chamber volume and mass can be predicted if the apex displacement occupies only one interspace and is less than one half of systole.

With cardiac angiography serving as the ultimate judge, the accuracy of predicting left ventricular hypertrophy is greater by palpation (88 per cent) than by the chest x-ray (81 per cent) or the electrocardiogram (60 per cent).

Reference: Conn, R. D., and Cole, J. S.: Ann. Intern. Med., *75*:185, 1971.

"HANDY" HEART SOUND SIMULATOR

The following is a simple but elegant technique for teaching cardiac auscultation, and one that does not require complicated electronic equipment or a bevy of patients. The basic technique involves grasping a stethoscope chest piece so that the diaphragm is against the palm. "Heart sounds" are then produced by using the index or middle finger of the free hand to tap the back of the forearm of the hand holding the stethoscope diaphragm. The frequency and intensity of the sound are dependent on the vigor of the tap and the distance of the tap from the diaphragm. Murmurs are produced by rubbing the back of the hand in various ways. For example, a cardiac cycle containing the murmur of mitral regurgitation can be simulated by tapping the back of the hand with the middle finger, lightly dragging the finger across the back of the hand (the murmur), and then terminating with a tap by the index finger.

Reference: Sanderson, J. N.: Am. J. Card., *36*:925, 1975.

THE SECOND HEART SOUND

The second heart sound is formed from the vibrations produced by closure of the aortic and pulmonic valves. Normally the aortic valve closes slightly before the pulmonic (physiologic splitting). Factors that favor ventricular filling and/or prolong ventricular ejection time or that delay ventricular activation or depolarization will delay closure of the corresponding heart valve. Conversely, rapid activation or ejection will result in "early" closure of the heart valve. As a consequence, the normal physiologic splitting of the second heart sound varies in a variety of situations.

I. **Intensity**
    A. *Increased:* Systemic or pulmonary hypertension
                      Thin chest wall
                      Dilatation of the pulmonary artery
                      Pulmonary regurgitation (with pulmonary hypertension)
    B. *Decreased:* Semilunar valvular stenosis or regurgitation

II. **Splitting**
    A. *Physiologic* (about 0.4 second): Slight asynchrony in ventricular contraction with respiration (wider in inspiration)

                      Posture: In normal children and young adults, expiratory splitting may sometimes be heard in recumbency but almost always disappears on sitting or standing

---

Sounds near S_2 that may confuse the listener

Opening snap (.06 to .10 second after S_2)
S_3 (.12 to .16 second after S_2, low pitch, dull character)
Pericardial knock (.06 to .10 second after S_2, sharp)
Late systolic click
Pulmonary hypertension

B. *Pathologic:*   Delay in closure of the pulmonary valve (wide splitting):
   Right bundle branch block (width of splitting increases slightly on inspiration)
   Obstruction to right ventricular outflow
Early atrioventricular closure:
Decreased left ventricle outflow due to mitral regurgitation or ventricular septal defect

C. *Parodoxical:* Obstruction to left ventricle outflow at valvu-
(wider in   lar or subvalvular level
expiration)

                Left ventricular failure
                Severe aortic regurgitation
                Left bundle branch block

D. *Fixed:*   Atrial septal defect
                Severe right ventricle failure, cardiomyopathy
                Massive pulmonary embolism

E. *Single:*   Old age (splitting less than 0.3 second)
                Aortic stenosis
                Pulmonic stenosis
                Common truncus arteriosus

DIFFERENTIAL DIAGNOSIS OF CARDIAC MURMURS

The interpretation of cardiac murmurs may be a vexing task (assuming one has heard the murmur in the first place; if one hasn't heard the murmur, then ignorance is bliss). The following chart summarizes several bedside diagnostic maneuvers and their characteristic cardiac effects. These manipulations often prove extremely useful in determining the nature of the murmur. Find the pathologic condition that you suspect. Under each condition, arrows will indicate the change in the murmur that is produced by the suggested maneuver. The "classic" changes are indicated. In practice the findings are somewhat more variable than in text.

MANEUVER	INNOCENT SYSTOLIC MURMURS	ATRIAL SEPTAL DEFECT	TRICUSPID STENOSIS	TRICUSPID INSUFFICIENCY	PULMONARY STENOSIS	PULMONARY INSUFFICIENCY	VENTRICULAR SEPTAL DEFECT	MITRAL STENOSIS	MITRAL INSUFFICIENCY	MITRAL PROLAPSE	AORTIC STENOSIS	IHSS*	AORTIC INSUFFICIENCY
Inspiration (Müller's maneuver)	↓	↑	↑	↑	↑	—	—	—	—		—	—	—
Valsalva's maneuver			↑ (with release)						↓	↑	↓	↑	—
Post PVC (or long R-R in A-Fib)	↑				↑				—↓		↑	↑	
Standing	↓	↓	↓	↓	↓	—			—	↑		↑	
Squatting	↑	↑	↑	↑	↑		↑	↑	↑	↑	↑	↓	↑
Amyl nitrate	↑	↑	↑	↑	↑	↑	Variable	↑	↓	Variable	↑	↑	↓
Hand-grip	—↓				—		↑	↑	↑	Variable	—↓	↓	↑

↑ = Increase
↓ = Decrease
— = No change
*Idiopathic hypertrophic subaortic stenosis

THE "INNOCENT" HEART MURMUR

A physical finding that frequently leads to anxiety in the patient and unwarranted investigation by the physician is a functional or innocent murmur. They are found in approximately 30 to 40 per cent of normal children at school age and may persist through adolescence and into early adulthood. Two of the innocent murmurs of childhood are *mid-systolic* and originate in the *right side* of the heart.

The innocent vibratory murmur of Still is a short, buzzing, medium-frequency murmur that probably originates from vibrations of the pulmonary valve. It is best heard at thoracic sites overlying the body of the right ventricle. This murmur is usually confined to the first third or half of systole and has a low frequency of vibration, in the range of 80 to 120 cycles per second. The wave form is similar to a musical tone.

The other right-sided functional murmur is thought to be an exaggeration of normal ejection vibrations within the pulmonary trunk. This murmur is less uniform in composition, is usually higher pitched, and tends to have a blowing, rather than a musical, quality, as compared to Still's murmur. Both murmurs are usually grade I or II in intensity and can be accentuated by elevation of the legs.

Mid-systolic murmurs may also occur during rapid ejection of blood into a normal aorta or pulmonary artery in conditions such as anemia, pregnancy, fever, or thyrotoxicosis. These murmurs are usually grade II or less in intensity, are heard at the base of the heart, are heard when the heart rate is fast, and vary greatly with position or respiration. There is an exaggerated splitting of the first heart sound. There may also be a third heart sound.

Pectus excavatum, the straight-back syndrome, and kyphoscoliosis can cause early and mid-systolic murmurs, best heard at the left sternal border and over bony prominences. These murmurs are relatively pure in tone and seldom louder than grade II. At times a rare diastolic murmur can also be detected.

5

EASY ECHOES

Echocardiography is a noninvasive diagnostic procedure that employs ultrasound to create images of the heart. At present, the information that may be obtained is definitive for some diseases and supports the diagnosis of others. Diseases for which echocardiography has a highly reliable diagnostic role in the present state of the art are included in the following table.

DIAGNOSES	CHARACTERISTICS OF THE ECHOCARDIOGRAM
Mitral stenosis	Delayed (slow) closure with decreased (E-F) slope Anterior motion of the posterior leaflet in diastole Heavy echoes of the mitral leaflets
Mitral valve prolapse	Posterior displacement of posterior or both leaflets in systole "Hammock" form
Idiopathic hypertrophic subaortic stenosis	Thick ventricular septum (the ventricular septum/LV wall ratio is 1.4 or more) There is systolic anterior motion of the mitral valve and mid-systolic closure of the aortic valve
Aortic stenosis	Dense echoes of the valve leaflets, diminished valve opening
Ruptured chordae	Instability of the mitral valve leaflets
Aortic insufficiency	Chronic—Fine flutter of anterior mitral leaflet in diastole Acute—Preclosure of mitral valve
Left atrial myxoma	Dense echoes are found behind the anterior mitral leaflet in diastole (they may be seen best in left atrial systole) There is a poor closing slope of the anterior mitral leaflet; the posterior leaflet moves correctly
Atrial septal defect	$\dfrac{\text{Left atrial size}}{\text{Aortic root size}} > 1.2$ or left atrial size > 4.5 cm
Pericardial effusion	An echo-free space anterior and posterior to the heart

Thanks to Dr. Willard Cohen for help with organization.

MITRAL VALVE PROLAPSE

Incidence Occurs predominantly in females in the younger population. Recent survey indicates an incidence of mitral valve prolapse of 6.3 per cent in 1169 healthy young women. An association with stroke has recently been made.

Pathophysiology Posterior protrusion of valve leaflets beyond the mitral ring during ventricular systole; often associated with mitral insufficiency. Redundancy of the posterior or both valve leaflets is associated with dilatation of the annulus and lengthening of the chordae.

Etiology The various hypotheses include:
1. Myxomatous degeneration of the valve.
2. Segmental cardiomyopathy of the left ventricle with secondary valvular changes.

Association
1. Congenital heart disease (especially secundum atrial defect).
2. Marfan's syndrome.
3. Collagen-vascular disorders.
4. Familial occurrence.
5. Thoracic deformities (pectus excavatum, straight-back syndrome, scoliosis).
6. Wolff-Parkinson-White syndrome.

Presentation
1. Majority asymptomatic (see incidence).
2. Palpitations; fatiguability; shortness of breath; atypical chest pain.
3. Symptoms seen in tall, slender females and in patients with developmental thoracic deformities.

Physical Exam Highly variable, even in the same patient. Apical midsystolic click followed by a late systolic murmur. Maneuvers that decrease left ventricular chamber size and consequently increase mitral leaflet malposition increase the intensity of the murmur (and vice versa).

When patient is sitting or standing, murmur is prolonged and click moves closer to S_1.

When patient is squatting, murmur becomes shorter, and click moves closer to S_2.

Holosystolic murmur of mitral insufficiency:

"Honk" or "whoop" may be heard because of resonation of leaflets and chordae.

X-ray Cardiac fluoroscopy normal except in the presence of mitral insufficiency, congenital heart disease, or thoracic abnormalities.

EKG Abnormalities in about a third of patients unless overt mitral insufficiency is present:
1. T wave inversion in II, III, AVF.
2. Supraventricular tachycardia.
3. Ventricular premature beats.

Abnormalities may be manifest only on exercise testing.

Echo/Phono Best test for documentation (see Easy Echoes, p. 150). A negative echostudy does *not* rule out mitral valve prolapse. Echocardiographic findings include:
1. Late systolic dip of the posterior or both valve leaflets occurring with the click.
2. Gradual "hammocking" of the mitral leaflets through systole.

Natural History Probably benign in the majority of asymptomatic patients. There is little evidence as yet to suggest the progressive development of mitral insufficiency. Sudden death may occur, presumably secondary to ventricular arrhythmias. Bacterial endocarditis may occur. A typical chest pain that is non ischemic in origin and refractory to therapy may be troublesome.

Management Reassurance for the asymptomatic patient without EKG abnormalities on rest and exercise. Prophylactic treatment of arrhythmias. Try propranolol for chest pain. Specific therapy of mitral insufficiency when present. Use of prophylactic antibiotics against the development of bacterial endocarditis is still uncertain.

References: Procacci, P. M., Savran, S. V., Schreiter, S. L., and Bryson, A. L.: N. Engl. J. Med., *249*:1086, 1976; Devereux, R. B., Perloff, J. K., Reichek, N., and Josephson, M. D.: Circulation, *54*:3, 1976.

PULSUS PARADOXUS

The presence of a paradoxical pulse (an exaggerated fall in blood pressure on inspiration during quiet breathing) is a valuable clue to serious cardiopulmonary disease. A specific examination for the condition should be conducted when *cardiac tamponade* is suspected. It is found in 50 per cent of patients with *constrictive pericarditis*. Patients with *severe airway obstruction*, as occurs in acute exacerbations of chronic obstructive pulmonary disease, or with acute asthma attacks may also demonstrate a pulsus paradoxus. Occasionally, a patient with primary disease of the myocardium will likewise exhibit pulsus paradoxus.

During an examination for a paradoxical pulse, the patient should be breathing as normally as possible and should *not* be made to inspire deeply. A blood pressure cuff is placed on the arm in a way that allows both the pressure gauge and the patient to be observed simultaneously. The cuff is *inflated* until *no* sounds are heard with the stethoscope bell over the brachial artery (i.e., it is inflated above systolic pressure), and then it is *slowly deflated* until sounds are heard in *expiration only*. The cuff pressure is then further lowered until sounds are heard *during both expiration* and *inspiration*. The *difference* between the two pressure levels represents the pulsus paradoxus. A difference of greater than 8 to 10 mm Hg represents a significant pulsus paradoxus.

References: Fowler, N. O.: Examination of the Heart — Part Two. American Heart Association, 1967, p. 28; McGregor, M., N. Engl. J. Med., *301*:480, 1979.

REVERSED PULSUS PARADOXUS

The term "reversed pulsus paradoxus" may be used to describe an *inspiratory rise* in the arterial systolic and diastolic pressures, presumably related to an inspiratory increase in left ventricular stroke output. Reversed pulsus paradoxus has been observed in three unrelated clinical circumstances: idiopathic hypertrophic subaortic stenosis, isorhythmic ventricular rhythms, and intermittent positive pressure breathing in the presence of left ventricular failure. These unusual respiration-related fluctuations of blood pressure must be differentiated from the "usual" pulsus paradoxus of cardiac tamponade.

Reference: Massumi, R. A., et al.: New Engl. J. Med., *289*:1272, 1973.

PERICARDITIS

The distinction between pericarditis associated with the early phase of myocardial infarction and pericarditis of other etiologies is a difficult but important one. A careful review of the patient's history and a physical exam are crucial. Laboratory investigation includes an electrocardiogram, an echocardiogram, roentgen studies, and monitoring of cardiac enzymes (see first table on the following page). Once a myocardial infarction with pericarditis has been eliminated from the differential diagnosis, the other causes of pericarditis can be explored (see second table on page 156).

Myocardial Infarction and Pericarditis

	PERICARDITIS	MYOCARDIAL INFARCTION
Age at onset	15 to 35	"Coronary age"
Preceding upper respiratory infection	Common	Infrequent
Pain syndrome onset	Sudden	Sudden
Quality	Sharp, stabbing, knife-like, infrequently squeezing	Predominantly pressure, squeezing, "vise-like"
Severity	Moderate to severe, rarely described as agonizing, fear of death infrequent	Severe, frequently described as agonizing, fear of death typical
Site	Wide area over base and precordium	Predominantly retrosternal
Radiation	Infrequent down right arm or to teeth or jaw	Frequent down both arms, goes to jaw
Movement	Aggravates pain	No effect
Pleuritic pain	Common	Rare in uncomplicated cases
Fever	Appears first day, erratic course, low grade	Rare in first 24 hours, gradually lyses, low grade
Pericardial rub	Appears first day with fever, wide distribution over chest, may persist 7 to 10 days	Appears after 24 to 36 hours, narrow area, frequently at apex, frequently transient, lasting 2 to 6 days
Heart sounds	Normal, except with effusion	Gallop (S_4)
Serum enzymes	LDH normal, SGOT rarely elevated	LDH and SGOT abnormal
Roentgen studies	May have dilated heart, pericardial effusion frequently present	May have dilated heart, effusion rare, abnormal left ventricular pulsation
Echocardiogram	Excellent noninvasive technique to show even small effusions; ejection fraction usually normal	Rare effusion, low ejection fraction, akinetic or dyskinetic areas of ventricular wall

5°

Classification of Pericarditis

CLINICAL CLASSIFICATION

    I. Acute pericarditis (6 weeks)
        A. Fibrinous
        B. Effusive (or bloody)

   II. Subacute pericarditis (6 weeks to 6 months)
        A. Constrictive
        B. Effusive-constrictive

  III. Chronic pericarditis (6 months)
        A. Constrictive
        B. Effusive
        C. Adhesive (nonconstrictive)

ETIOLOGIC CLASSIFICATION

    I. Infectious pericarditis
        A. Viral
        B. Pyogenic
        C. Tuberculous
        D. Mycotic
        E. Other infections (syphilitic, parasitic)

   II. Noninfectious pericarditis
        A. Uremia
        B. Neoplasia
            i. Primary tumors (benign or malignant)
           ii. Tumors metastatic to pericardium or heart
        C. Myxedema

    D. Cholesterol
    E. Chylopericardium
    F. Trauma
       i. Penetrating chest wall
       ii. Nonpenetrating
    G. Aortic aneurysm (with leakage into pericardial sac)
    H. Postradiation
    I. Associated with atrial septal defect
    J. Associated with severe chronic anemia
    K. Infectious mononucleosis
    L. Familial pericarditis (Mulibrey nanism*)
    M. Acute idiopathic

III. Pericarditis related to hypersensitivity or autoimmunity
    A. Rheumatic fever
    B. Collagen vascular disease
       i. Systemic lupus erythematosus
       ii. Rheumatoid arthritis
       iii. Scleroderma
    C. Drug-induced
       i. Procainamide
       ii. Hydralazine
       iii. Other
    D. Postcardiac injury
       i. Postmyocardial infarction
       ii. Postpericardiotomy
       iii. Dressler's syndrome

5

---

*An autosomal recessive syndrome characterized by growth failure, muscle hypotonia, hepatomegaly, ocular changes, enlarged cerebral ventricles, mental retardation, and chronic constrictive pericarditis.

MURRAY'S* APPROACH TO THE EKG DIAGNOSIS OF TACHYARRHYTHMIAS

The internist is often faced with the problem of diagnosing a tachyarrhythmia. A careful clinical examination, coupled with the following six-question examination of the electrocardiogram, should enable you to diagnose almost all tachyarrhythmias. To use this approach, you should begin with a 12 lead EKG and a generous length of the lead 2 or V_1 rhythm strip, a pair of calipers, a comfortable chair, and a good light. Then ask the following six questions:

1. What is the ventricular rate?
2. Is the rhythm regular or irregular?
3. Is the QRS configuration normal or abnormal?
4. Is there any atrial activity? You should search diligently for small, almost inapparent blips hidden in the QRS or T waves when looking for P waves in a tachyarrhythmia.
5. If there are P waves, are they related to the QRS complexes?
6. What response is there to carotid sinus massage?

Typical findings for five common tachyarrhythmias are provided in the accompanying table.

QUESTION	SINUS TACHYCARDIA	PAROXYSMAL ATRIAL TACHYCARDIA	ATRIAL FIBRILLATION	ATRIAL FLUTTER	VENTRICULAR TACHYCARDIA
Rate	100–200	160–190	160–190	140–160	100–230
Rhythm	Regular	Regular	Irregular	Regular	Slightly irregular
QRS shape	Normal[1]	Normal[1]	Normal[1]	Normal[1]	Abnormal
Atrial activity	Sinus P wave[2]	Absent or nonsinus P wave[2]	Absent	Flutter waves	Sinus P waves[2]
P-QRS relation	Yes	May be masked by rapid ventricular rate	No	May be masked by rapid ventricular rate	No
Carotid massage	Slows	No response, or converts to sinus rhythm	No response	Increased block	No response

[1]Unless intraventricular conduction disturbance.
[2]Sinus P waves are upright in lead II and occur at least 0.12 seconds before the QRS complex begins.

*Named for "Murray the G," who likes to dispense with work as quickly as possible.

POTASSIUM AND THE ELECTROCARDIOGRAM

The changes produced in the electrocardiogram by extremes of serum potassium concentration can be correlated with the degree of hypo- or hyperkalemia.

The progressive changes in the electrocardiogram seen with hypo- or hyperkalemia are shown in Fig. 5-1 and are enumerated below.

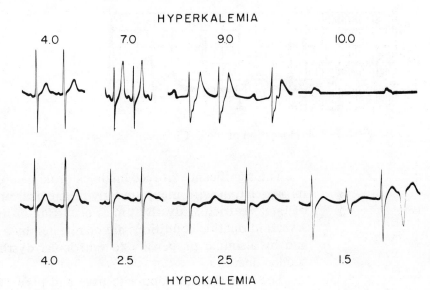

FIG. 5-1

Hypokalemia

Diminished amplitude of the T wave
Appearance of U waves
Depressed S-T segment
Arrhythmias — Atrial or ventricular ectopic beats
         — Atrial or ventricular tachycardia
         — Ventricular fibrillation

Hyperkalemia

Tall, peaked *symmetrical* T waves
Prolonged P-R interval
Widening of the QRS complex
Disappearance of the P wave — bradycardia
Arrhythmias — Sinus bradycardia
         — Sinus arrest
         — Nodal rhythm
         — Idioventricular rhythm
         — Ventricular tachycardia
         — Ventricular fibrillation
         — Complete asystole

Reference: Walker, W. G.: Disorders of potassium metabolism. In Harvey, A. M., Johns, R. J., Owens, A. H., and Ross, R. S. (Eds.): The Principles and Practice of Medicine. New York. Appleton-Century-Crofts, 1976, p. 102. Figure reproduced with permission of author and publisher.

PROLONGED Q-T INTERAL

The Q-T interval, which extends from the beginning of the QRS complex to the end of the T wave (Fig. 5-2), is a measure of ventricular repolarization time. Its length normally varies with the heart rate.

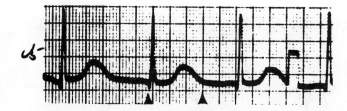

FIG. 5–2 Prolongation of the Q-T interval.

The significance of recognizing a prolonged Q-T interval lies both in its association with many underlying medical problems and in the risk of fatal ventricular dysrhythmias occurring in its presence. In addition, several idiopathic conditions are manifested by a prolonged Q-T interval and by a similar propensity to ventricular dysrhythmias, syncope, and sudden death.

The tables on the opposite page and page 162 provide a list of the conditions associated with a prolonged Q-T interval and normal variations of the Q-T interval.

Associated Conditions

ACQUIRED Q-T INTERVAL PROLONGATION

5

I. *Drugs*
   Quinidine
   Disopyramide
   Procainamide
   Phenothiazines
   Tricyclic antidepressants

II. *Electrolyte imbalance*
   Hypokalemia
   Hypomagnesemia
   Hypocalcemia

III. *Hypothermia*

IV. *Cerebral vascular disease*

V. *Neck surgery*

IDIOPATHIC Q-T INTERVAL PROLONGATION

I. *Jervell and Lange-Nielsen syndrome*
   Prolonged Q-T interval
   Syncope—sudden death
   Congenital deafness
   Autosomal recessive

II. *Romano-Ward syndrome*
   Prolonged Q-T interval
   Syncope—sudden death
   No deafness
   Autosomal dominant

III. *Sporadic prolonged Q-T interval*
   Prolonged Q-T interval
   Syncope—sudden death
   No congenital anomalies
   No heritable pattern

Normal Variations of the Q-T Interval

HEART RATE/MIN	R-R INTERVAL *(sec)*	LOWER LIMIT *(sec)*	UPPER LIMIT *(sec)* Men	UPPER LIMIT *(sec)* Women
40	1.50	0.44	0.51	0.52
43	1.40	0.41	0.50	0.51
46	1.30	0.40	0.49	0.50
48	1.25	0.39	0.48	0.49
50	1.20	0.38	0.47	0.48
52	1.15	0.37	0.47	0.48
55	1.10	0.36	0.46	0.47
57	1.05	0.36	0.45	0.46
60	1.00	0.33	0.44	0.45
63	0.95	0.34	0.43	0.44
67	0.90	0.33	0.42	0.43
71	0.87	0.33	0.40	0.43
75	0.80	0.32	0.40	0.41
80	0.75	0.31	0.39	0.40
86	0.70	0.30	0.38	0.37
93	0.65	0.40	0.37	0.38
100	0.65	0.29	0.36	0.37
109	0.55	0.26	0.35	0.35
120	0.50	0.27	0.33	0.34
133	0.45	0.26	0.30	0.32
150	0.40	0.25	0.30	0.30
172	0.35	0.24	0.28	0.28

References: Thanks to Thomas Fruehan, M.D., for furnishing the electrocardiogram and the table of normal variations of the Q-T interval. Moss, A. J., and Schwartz, P. J.: Am. J. Med., 66:6. 1977.

MULTIFOCAL ATRIAL TACHYCARDIA

Multifocal atrial tachycardia (MAT) is an irregular disturbance of heart rhythm defined by the following:

1. Recognizable P waves of varying morphology originating from three different foci.

2. Absence of a single dominant pacemaker site.

3. Irregular variation in P-P intervals and variable P-R and R-R intervals.

Usually the overall ventricular rate is rapid, but in one series 11 of 31 patients had ventricular rates between 56 and 100 beats per minute; thus chaotic atrial mechanism has been suggested as a more accurate name for this disorder. EKG departments may see 20 to 40 tracings per year (approximately one per 1000 tracings) with this arrhythmia. Because of the irregular rate, this rhythm is sometimes confused with atrial fibrillation. The distinction between the two is very important.

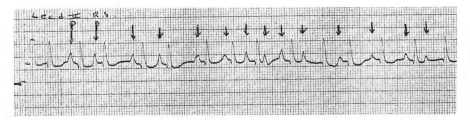

FIG. 5-3

Multifocal atrial tachycardia — Standard lead II. Atrial activity is indicated by arrows. Note the three different P wave forms and the variable P–P and P–R intervals. An occasional P wave is not conducted. Ventricular rate 110–120/min.

MAT affects the older population; the average age of patients is 72. The arrhythmia is associated with advanced heart disease, which is common in all series, and chronic obstructive pulmonary disease (COPD) or acute pulmonary disease, which is reported in 35 to 84 per cent of cases. When the arrhythmia is seen with COPD, cor pulmonale is often present. One series reported a high incidence of diabetes mellitus. The hospital mortality rates reported for patients with this arrhythmia has been between 37 and 58 per cent. Almost all patients have premature atrial contractions on the EKG when MAT is not present, and many have atrial fibrillation prior to or after the episode of MAT. Episodes of MAT have lasted from a few days to more than a year in a few cases.

The relationship of MAT to digitalis therapy is important. Many patients have not been on digitalis when the arrhythmia occurred. In reported cases, those on digitalis did not improve when the drug was withheld. When digitalis was increased to try to control the heart rate, digitalis toxicity frequently occurred with a high mortality rate. In some cases, the MAT seemed to be related to aminophylline or sympathomimetic drugs (e.g., isoproterenol), which were given for obstructive pulmonary disease. In some cases, stopping those drugs resulted in cessation of the MAT.

Treatment is difficult. Digitalis should be used only if heart failure is present. The dose of digitalis should not be increased to control the heart rate. Procainamide, diphenylhydantoin, quinidine, and lidocaine have failed to terminate the arrhythmia and control the heart rate. Cardioversion has been unsuccessful in all cases. Propranolol, in small doses (5 to 10 mg every 4 to 6 hours orally), has been useful in some cases when used alone or combined with quinidine. Propranolol either slowed the atrial rate or produced AV block, with a controlled ventricular response. In these low doses, it did not seem to aggravate the underlying pulmonary disease. Other therapeutic measures to correct the underlying diseases (e.g., acute or chronic respiratory problems or heart failure) seem to be helpful.

References: Wang, K., Goldfarb, B. L., Gobel, F. L., Richman, H. C.: Arch. Intern. Med., *137*:161, 1977; Kones, R. J., Phillips, J. H., and Hersh, J.: Cardiology, *59*:92, 1974.

"BE STILL MY FLUTTERING HEART"

Delirium tremens (DTs) reflects a total body derangement. It's not surprising, then, to see DTs of the heart, "delirium corus," as one manifestation. On an electrocardiogram, one may see paroxysmal atrial fibrillation, paroxysmal atrial tachycardia, atrial flutter, and premature atrial contractions with aberrant conduction. If ascites is present, you may find an S_1-Q_3-T_3 pattern similar to that seen with pulmonary embolus. Usually no specific cardiac therapy is necessary; in fact, antiarrhythmic drugs usually are unsuccessful. Pay particular attention to the therapy of associated metabolic derangements that might be present (e.g., hypokalemia, alkalosis).

QUICK GUIDE TO THE THERAPY OF CARDIAC ARRHYTHMIAS

The table on the following page is intended to provide general guidelines for the treatment of some common cardiac arrhythmias. The list is not exhaustive and the guidelines will not apply to every case, but the list will provide a good basis for therapy in the most frequently encountered arrhythmias. (See the chart on antiarrhythmic agents [p. 169] for a guide to dosages.)

5

ARRHYTHMIA	THERAPY	COMMENT
Atrial fibrillation	Cardioversion	—Start low (10 to 25 joules)
		—Useful if hemodynamic compromise is present
		—Useful in setting of acute infarct with rapid ventricular response precipitating chest pain
		—If atrial size is less than 4.5 cm by echo, there is a high probability the patient will remain in sinus rhythm
		—Anticoagulate patient with heparin prior to cardioversion if the fibrillation has persisted more than several days
	Digitalis	—Will control ventricular response
		—Propranolol is a useful adjunct in further slowing ventricular response, especially in mitral stenosis
		—Type I antiarrhythmics may be used to *maintain* sinus rhythm
		—May have adverse effect in patients with Wolff-Parkinson-White syndrome
Atrial flutter	Cardioversion	—Same as atrial fibrillation
	Digitalis	—Same as atrial fibrillation
Supraventricular tachycardia	Cardioversion	—If hemodynamic compromise is present
	Vagotonic maneuvers	—Includes carotid sinus massage, Valsalva, gagging, and the diver's reflex
	Edrophonium (Tensilon)	—May be diagnostic according to response of arrhythmia
		—May convert paroxysmal atrial tachycardia (PAT) to sinus rhythm
	Digitalis, Propranolol	—Both will slow ventricular rate or restore sinus rhythm
Premature ventricular contractions (PVCs)	Lidocaine	—Drug of choice in setting of acute infarction
		—Reduce dosage in liver disease and heart failure

ARRHYTHMIA	THERAPY	COMMENT
	Type I antiarrhythmics	—Procainamide can be given IV in setting of acute MI if lidocaine fails —All can be used orally for chronic suppression
	Propranolol	—Small IV doses excellent for acute suppression when other drugs fail —Can be used orally on chronic basis
Ventricular tachycardia	Cardioversion	—Initial agent if hemodynamic compromise present —Can try precordial thump in monitored arrest
	Lidocaine	—If cerebral perfusion is present, may use as initial agent
	Type I antiarrhythmics Propranolol Bretylium	—Same as PVC —Same as PVC —Try when all else fails —Don't forget CPR if needed!
Ventricular fibrillation	Defibrillation	—Lidocaine and procainamide may enhance effectiveness of defibrillation
	Bretylium	—If defibrillation, lidocaine, propranolol, and procainamide fail
Digitalis-induced tachyarrhythmias	Lidocaine	—Avoid cardioversion and bretylium
	Phenytoin	—Exacerbated by hypokalemia, hypomagnesemia, and hypercalcemia —Propranolol, procainamide, and hyperkalemia may exacerbate A-V block —Usually have a finite duration —If D/C countershock necessary, start with 5 joules and administer lidocaine or phenytoin beforehand

Reference: Abramowicz, M., et al. (Eds.): The Medical Letter, *20*:113, 1978.

ANTIARRHYTHMIC DRUGS

Arrhythmias arise from disorders of both automaticity (myocardial irritability) and conduction (re-entrant arrhythmias). All antiarrhythmic drugs available correct problems of automaticity by suppressing impulse generation. Arrhythmias caused by conduction disturbances are corrected by type I drugs, which suppress conduction and produce bidirectional block, or by type II drugs, which improve conduction and eliminate unidirectional block. Below is a list of type I and type II drugs, followed by some brief information on some of the commonly used drugs.

Type I	Type II
Quinidine	Phenytoin
Procainamide	Lidocaine
Disopyramide	
Propranolol	

When using these agents, the following points are worth noting:

1. Measure blood levels if:
   Failure to respond (on usual dosage level).
   Toxicity (on usual dosage level).
   Altered metabolism suspected.
2. Dosage schedule should not exceed half-life of the drug.
3. A loading dose before starting the maintenance dose is necessary to achieve therapeutic levels rapidly.

5

	QUINIDINE	PROCAINAMIDE	DISOPYRAMIDE	LIDOCAINE	PHENYTOIN	PROPRANOLOL	BRETYLIUM
Dosage							
IV initial	NA	100 mg IV Q 5 min to 1000 mg	NA	1-2 mg/kg (50-200 mg)*	100 mg IV Q 5 min to 1000 mg	1 mg/min IV Q 5 min to 5 mg	5 mg/kg with additional doses to 10-20 mg/kg
maintenance	NA	2-4 mg/min	NA	2-4 mg/min	NA	1-3 mg/Q4 hr	5-10 mg/kg Q6 hr
Oral loading	300 mg	0.5-1.0 grams	300 mg	NA	1000 mg in divided doses	None	NA
Total/day	1.2-3.2 gm	1-4 grams	400-800 mg	NA	300 mg	40-400 and above	NA
Schedule	Q6 hr	Q3-4 hr	Q6 hr	NA	daily	Q6 hr	Q6 hr
Half-life	6 hr	3-4 hr	6 hr	Bolus: 15-30 min Chronic: 2 hr	20-26 hr	IV: 2-3 hr Oral: 6 hr	Unknown
Therapeutic plasma levels	2-6 µg/ml	4-8 µg/ml	2-4 µg/ml	1.5-5.0 µg/ml	10-18 ng/ml	Not Established†	Not Established
Metabolism	Liver	Liver, plasma hydrolysis	Liver	Liver	Liver	Liver	Unknown
Renal excretion, unmetabolized	20-50%	50-60%	50%	<10%	<5%	<5%	Unknown
EKG Effects							
P-R	↑↓	↑↓	↑↓	↑↓	↑	↑↑	↑
Q-R-S	↑	↑	↑	↑	↑	↑	↑
Q-T	↑	↑	↑	↑↓	↓	↓	↑
Physiologic Effects							
Automaticity	↓	↓	↓	↓	↓↑	↓	→
Conduction vel.	↓	↓	↓	↑↓	↑	↓	Unknown
Effective refractory period	↑	↑	↑	↓	↓	↑	Unknown

*Pharmacokinetic considerations dictate that a second bolus be given 20 minutes after the first, so that the total loading dose falls within the recommended range.
†100-200 ng/ml is the serum level of propranolol required to produce sympathetic blockade.
NA = Not applicable.

↑ increased
↓ decreased
→ unchanged

DRUG	MAJOR ADVERSE EFFECTS	COMMENT
Quinidine	GI symptoms, cinchonism, thrombocytopenia, rashes, tachyarrhythmias, increases serum digoxin concentration	—Both IM and PO route reach peak levels at 1 to 2 hrs. —Hypoproteinemic states increase blood level —Half-life normal in dialysis patients —QRS interval correlates best with blood level —Phenobarbital and phenytoin increase metabolism and decrease serum levels of active drug —Decrease dose if QRS widens to 0.12 sec or by more than 50%
Procainamide	Lupus syndrome, rash, hypotension	—Peak levels 1 hr after oral dose —When changing from IV to oral route, give first oral dose 3 hr after discontinuing IV drug —Must decrease dosage with renal failure —80% of patients develop positive test for antinuclear antibodies (chronic use) —20 to 30% develop clinical features of lupus (chronic use) —Decrease dose if QRS widens, as with quinidine

DRUG	MAJOR ADVERSE EFFECTS	COMMENT
Disopyramide	Anticholinergic effects, hypotension, heart block, heart failure	—Must reduce dose in renal failure —Hepatic disease increases half-life —Peak levels in 2 hrs after oral dose —Urinary retention reported in 2% of patients
Lidocaine	CNS toxicity, including coma and seizures	—Decrease dose with liver disease and congestive heart failure
Phenytoin	Ataxia, nystagmus, coma, blood dyscrasias, paradoxical AV block with rapid infusion	—Neurologic effects correlate with serum levels above 20 mEq/ml —Gingival hypertrophy —Give IV dose slowly, because propylene glycol vehicle causes hypotension
Propranolol	Heart block, hypotension, heart failure, asthma	—Prolonged half-life with liver disease —Will mask signs of hypoglycemia in diabetics —May cause hypoglycemia —Rebound angina with sudden cessation of therapy
Bretylium	Hypotension, initial increase in arrhythmias	—Can be used in refractory ventricular *fibrillation* —Increases sensitivity to catecholamines (i.e., vasopressors)

References: Michaelson S. P.: Today's Clinician, September 1978, p. 39; Abramowicz M.: The Medical Letter, *20*:113, 1978; Brest A. N.: Consultant, January 1979, p. 23.

MAGNESIUM AS AN ANTIARRHYTHMIC AGENT

Magnesium deficiency may be a primary cause of serious tachyarrhythmias or contribute to digitalis induced tachyarrhythmias. Clinical states that may be associated with magnesium deficiency include:

Alcoholism
Diabetic ketoacidosis
Chronic diuretic use
Malabsorption syndromes
Malnutrition
The diuretic phase of acute tubular necrosis
Hypoparathyroidism
Primary aldosteronism
Acute pancreatitis
Therapy with cis-Platinum

The major symptoms of magnesium deficiency are neurologic and include lethargy, muscle weakness, fasciculations, tremors, positive Trousseau's sign, irritability, mental changes, convulsions, stupor, and coma. Magnesium depletion exists when the serum magnesium level falls below normal, provided the serum albumin level is also within normal limits, since about 30 per cent of magnesium is albumin-bound. Intracellular magnesium deficiency can also occur without hypomagnesemia.

Magnesium has been used successfully in hypomagnesemic patients in the treatment of both spontaneous and digitalis toxic ventricular and supraventricular tachyarrhythmias. Magnesium may also be an effective antiarrhythmic in some normomagnesemic patients and should be tried in cases refractory to other agents. The recommended schedule for magnesium therapy is: (1) 10 to 15 ml of 20 per cent magnesium sulfate IV over 60 seconds, (2) 500 ml of 2 per cent magnesium sulfate IV started simultaneously and given over six hours, and (3) subsequent doses based on status of the cardiac rhythm and level of serum magnesium.

Overdosage of magnesium can also cause significant problems, and prolonged serum levels over 5.5 mEq/liter should be avoided. The deep tendon reflexes disappear at serum levels about 6 mEq/liter, and this finding may be used to monitor continuous infusion therapy. At higher serum levels, respiratory depression, paralysis, and bradyarrhythmias may occur. The electrocardiogram does not accurately reflect serum magnesium levels.

Reference: Iseri, L. T., Freed, J., and Bures, A. R.: Am. J. Med., *58*:887, 1975.

PRIMER ON PACERS

Cardiac pacing is a common therapeutic modality for control of cardiac rate or rhythm. Pacemakers perform two basic functions: They stimulate *(drive)* the heart to contract, and they *sense* intrinsic cardiac electrical activity. The driving and sensing functions of pacers are independent of each other in that pacemakers may fail to perform one function while still adequately performing the other. Pacemakers have three main components:

1. *Pulse generator.* This provides the electrical stimulus to drive the heart and contains the sensing circuits. It is battery-powered.
2. *Transmitter wire (lead).* This carries electrical current between the pulse generator and the heart.
3. *Electrode.* This serves as the contact point with the heart for transmitting electrical stimuli and sensing intrinsic cardiac activity.

These three components can be arranged in a variety of ways. A suggested nomenclature code for cardiac pacemakers is provided in the following table. The code will help in the understanding of what each particular type of pacemaker does. As an example, a ventricular driving R-wave–triggered pacer would be labeled VVT.

There are two forms of sensing: In the inhibited mode, the pacer is turned off by intrinsic cardiac electrical activity; in the triggered mode, spontaneous cardiac activity causes the pacer to discharge its stored energy during the QRS complex. Pacers in the inhibited mode use less electrical energy than triggered pacemakers.

Nomenclature Code for Cardiac Pacemakers

1ST LETTER	2ND LETTER	3RD LETTER
(Chamber Paced)	(Chamber Sensed)	*(Mode of Response to Sensed Beat)*
V – Ventricle	V – Ventricle	I – Inhibited
A – Atrium	A – Atrium	T – Triggered
D – Both atrium and ventricle	D – Both	O – Neither
	O – Neither (i.e., doesn't sense)	

A certain minimal amount of electrical current is required for appropriate pacing function. The minimal level of current at which driving or sensing will occur is called the threshold. The threshold for both pacing and sensing should be measured at the time of insertion.

Pacemakers follow Murphy's law (anything that can go wrong will). Thus, the physician will at times be called upon to treat a malfunctioning pacemaker. The differential diagnosis of pacemaker malfunction is usually based on analysis of the electrocardiographic manifestations of pacemaker activity. The EKG manifestation of pacemaker electrical activity is a spike. The table on the opposite page summarizes the EKG pacemaker spike patterns produced by the various forms of pacemaker malfunction.

NO SPIKES	INTERMITTENT SPIKES	SPIKES WITHOUT VENTRICULAR CAPTURE (FAILURE TO DRIVE)	SPIKES WITHOUT SENSING (FAILURE TO SENSE)	SPIKES WITH CHANGING VECTOR	CHANGE IN SPIKE-TO-SPIKE INTERVAL
Normal inhibited sensing	Normal inhibited sensing	High threshold	Malposition of lead	Respiratory variation	Battery depletion
Generator malfunction	Hairline lead fracture	Malposition	Low intrinsic QRS current (i.e., not at sensing threshold)	Lead position changed	Runaway pacer
Battery failure	Changing vector of spike	Fibrosis	Generator malfunction	Break in lead insulation	T-Wave sensing
Interruption of circuit		Cardiac perforation	Pacer without sensing mode		External interference
Spike "buried" in QRS		Generator malfunction	Magnetic interference		Hysteresis
Electromagnetic interference		Battery failure			Concealed conduction of a QRS
		Spike in patient's ventricular refractory period			Faulty recording device
					Change in pacer rate (programable pacer)

Diagnosis of Pacemaker Malfunction.

Changes in the patient, such as drug reactions or electrolyte disturbances, may also affect pacemaker function and should be considered when there does not seem to be a mechanical explanation for the problem.

References: Parsonnet, V.: Primary Cardiology, January 1979, p. 60; Ryan, C., and Sudduth, B.: Practical Cardiology, April 1978, p. 142; Escher, D.: Circulation, *47*:1119, 1973.

Murphy's Law I.
If it is absolutely impossible for anything to go wrong, it will anyway. Trying to correct it will only make matters worse.

Murphy's Law II.
If anything can go wrong, it will.

Murphy's Law III.
When anything goes wrong, it does so all at once.

Murphy's Law IV.
Any error that can creep in will. It will always be in the direction that will do the most harm.

Murphy's Law V.
When left to themselves, things go from bad to worse.

Murphy's Law VI.
If two things can go wrong, the worse one will happen.

SUDDEN DEATH SYNDROME (SDS)

The sudden death syndrome usually occurs in patients with coronary artery disease. However, only a small percentage (less than 20 per cent) of patients experience an acute myocardial infarction at the time of sudden death. About half the patients with the SDS have *no* history of *symptomatic heart disease.* The cardiac dysrhythmia responsible for the SDS is ventricular fibrillation in most instances.

Since therapy to suppress premature ventricular contractions (PVCs) is difficult, often unsuccessful, and potentially dangerous, only those patients with the highest risk of experiencing ventricular fibrillation should be given antiarrhythmic agents. Cases in which antiarrhythmic agents may be useful in decreasing the frequency of PVCs and possibly reducing the incidence of the SDS include:

1. Patients experiencing ventricular fibrillation who have not suffered an acute myocardial infarction.

2. Patients with complicated PVCs (greater than 10/hour, 2 or more in a row, R on T, multifocal PVCs) within six months of an acute myocardial infarction.

3. Patients with severe symptoms related to documented arrhythmias (e.g., syncope).

4. Patients demonstrating rapid ventricular tachycardia with exercise.

5. Patients at peak exercise demonstrating both PVCs and significant ST segment depression.

6. Patients with prolonged Q-T interval and syncope.

7. Patients with angina pectoris and complicated PVCs.

Thanks to Robert Eich, M. D., for providing the organization of this material.

Murphy's Law VII.
If something goes wrong, it will be at the most inconvenient time.

Murphy's Law VIII.
Everything is always worse than you thought it was going to be.

5

CPK ISOENZYMES IN THE DIAGNOSIS OF MYOCARDIAL INFARCTION

Creatine phosphokinase (CPK) is an enzyme found primarily in muscle. There are three isoenzymes of CPK that are present in varying ratios in the different tissues of the body. The BB type is found in nervous system, smooth muscle, and the lung; the MB type is found primarily in cardiac muscle, with a small amount also present in skeletal muscle; and MM is the major isoenzyme in skeletal muscle. A small amount of MM is also present in heart muscle. Since even relatively minor skeletal muscle trauma (e.g., an intramuscular injection) can elevate the total amount of CPK, CPK isoenzyme analysis is used to improve the specificity of the test. Unfortunately, there are conditions other than myocardial infarction that can increase the amount of serum CPK MB isoenzyme. These conditions are:

Cardiac surgery
Defibrillation or cardioversion
Polymyositis-dermatomyositis
Muscular dystrophy
Rhabdomyolysis
Myopathies
    Hypothyroid
    Hypoparathyroid
    Acromegalic
Hypokalemic periodic paralysis
Postpartum

Reference: Wolf, P. L.: Practical Cardiology, January 1979, p. 126.

Murphy's Law IX.
Nothing is ever as simple as it first seems.

SYSTOLIC MURMUR AFTER MYOCARDIAL INFARCTION

The occurrence of a systolic murmur after an acute myocardial infarction is a common clinical event. Its differential diagnoses include mitral murmurs secondary to left ventricular dilatation with concomitant mitral insufficiency, papillary muscle dysfunction, or rupture and perforation of the interventricular septum. These murmurs differ in their clinical significance, course, and therapy, and therefore, a precise diagnosis is crucial. The following brief outline of their clinical presentations will allow a tentative bedside diagnosis. The ultimate distinction can be made with certainty only by angiography; however, information obtained from pulmonary artery catheterization (bedside) and echocardiography is of great help, and their contributions to diagnosis are also included.

I. Mitral murmurs
- A. Secondary to papillary muscle *dysfunction*
    1. Usually occurs within five days of infarction
    2. Dysfunction is secondary to ischemia
    3. Murmur may occur anywhere in systole; sometimes holosystolic
    4. Anterior papillary muscle dysfunction usually occurs with anterior wall infarction; posterior muscle dysfunction, with inferior wall infarction
    5. Location and radiation:
        a. Anterior leaflet affected — apex radiates to left axilla
        b. Posterior leaflet affected — apex or left sternal border radiates to base; may mimic aortic stenosis
    6. May be associated with systolic click
    7. Clinical course determined by competence of left ventricle
    8. Equal incidence of anterior, inferior infarcts
    9. S_1 increased
    10. Pulmonary edema rare
- B. Secondary to papillary muscle *rupture*
    1. Occurs in 0.9 per cent of acute myocardial infarctions
    2. Usually presents with rapid onset of pulmonary edema
    3. Posterior muscle rupture more common
    4. Usually holosytolic, low-pitched apical murmur
    5. May radiate to left axilla
    6. S_1 soft
    7. Usually no associated thrill
    8. Twice as common in inferior infarction
- C. Secondary to left ventricular dilatation
    1. Cardiomegaly present

2. Character similar to murmur of papillary muscle dysfunction

3. Resolves with improvement in left ventricular function

II. Perforation of interventricular septum
   A. Usually in first week of infarction
   B. Always in muscular septum
   C. Commonly associated with ventricular aneurysm
   D. Murmur occurs along left sternal border and may radiate to left axilla
   E. Thrill in 50 per cent of cases
   F. Interventricular conduction disturbances may occur

III. Pulmonary artery catheterization
   A. Septal rupture — O_2 saturation step-up occurs between right atrium and right ventricle
   B. Papillary muscle rupture — large "V" waves noted on pressure tracing

IV. Echocardiography data
   A. Septal rupture — right ventricular overload pattern
   B. Papillary muscle dysfunction — prolapse of leaflet into left atrium
   C. Papillary muscle rupture — flailing mitral leaflet

Reference: Dugall, C. J., Pryor, R., and Blount, S. G.: Am. Heart J., *87*:577, 1974.

Murphy's Law X.
If you tinker with something long enough, you will break it.

MORTALITY AFTER MYOCARDIAL INFARCTION

For the past 20 years the rate of first-year mortality after myocardial infarction has remained at 10 per cent despite advances in cardiac therapy. The degree of risk is predominantly a function of the amount of damaged myocardium. Other significant factors increasing the risk of mortality include:

1. An ejection fraction less than 40 per cent.
2. Presence of either AV or IV conduction disturbances.
3. Extent of underlying coronary artery disease.
4. Persistent ventricular irritability.
5. Q-T prolongation.

Murphy's Law XI.
Everything costs more than you first estimated.

AN EARLY AMBULATION PROGRAM

A major problem faces the clinician while caring for the infarction patient: How quickly can he increase his patient's level of activity to maximize rehabilitation and minimize thrombotic complications without creating undue stress on the damaged myocardium? An early ambulation program for patients with uncomplicated infarcts is provided below. Of course, these are only general guidelines and should be tailored to meet individual patient needs.

Program Guidelines

24 hrs	Out of bed to chair or commode
Day 3	Arm and leg exercises at rest
Day 4	Ambulation in room
Day 9	Ambulation in hall
Day 13	Walk down one flight of stairs
Days 14–17	Discharge from hospital
Weeks 5–6	Coitus
Weeks 9–12	Return to work
Weeks 8–12	Exercise training after treadmill test

Thanks to Dr. Murray Grossman for collection and organization of above material.

Murphy's Law XII.
It is easier to get involved in something than to get out of it.

CARDIAC PERFORMANCE STATUS

The New York Heart Association (NYHA) classification of cardiac disability may ultimately be supplanted by more sophisticated non-invasive means of evaluating cardiac performance status. However, for the nonspecialist, the NYHA classification is a widely accepted system that easily lends itself to clinical assessment.

NYHA Classification of Cardiac Disability

Class I — Patients with heart disease who have no symptoms of any sort.

Class II — Patients with heart disease who are comfortable at rest but have symptoms with ordinary activity.

Class III — Patients with heart disease who are comfortable at rest but have symptoms with less than ordinary activity.

Class IV — Patients with heart disease who have symptoms at rest.

Reference: New York Heart Association. Nomenclature and Criteria for Diagnosis of Diseases of the Heart and Blood Vessels, 6th Edition. Boston, Little, Brown & Company, 1964.

Murphy's Law XIII.
If you look for trouble, you are sure to find it.

VASODILATORS FOR HEART FAILURE

Most patients with congestive heart failure have elevation of left ventricular (LV) filling pressure and low cardiac output. An increase in systemic vascular resistance (afterload) and an increase in LV filling pressure (preload) are detrimental to the failing heart, which is unable to increase stroke volume. In the absence of a correctable cause for heart failure, digitalis, diuretics, and salt restriction are the mainstays of therapy. In severe heart failure, when conventional therapy will not suffice, vasodilators can be employed. For severe pulmonary congestion, preload reduction may be tried; with mitral or aortic regurgitation or low output states, afterload reduction may be beneficial. On a long-term basis successful therapy with vasodilators may reduce cardiomegaly, symptoms of dyspnea and orthopnea (preload), and fatigue and dizziness (afterload).

Vasodilator Drugs, Site of Action, and Hemodynamic Effects in Heart Failure

DRUG	SITE OF ACTION		HEMODYNAMIC EFFECTS				
	Arterial	Venous	Heart Rate	Arterial Pressure	Cardiac Output	Left Ventricular Filling Pressure	Systemic Vascular Resistance
Parenteral							
Sodium nitroprusside	++++	++	→	↓↓	↑↑↑	↓↓	↓↓↓
Nitroglycerin	+	+++	↓/→/↑	→↓	↑/↓	↓↓↓	↓
Phentolamine mesylate	+++	o	↑↑↑	↓↓	↑↑	↓	↓↓↓
Oral							
Nitroglycerin (sublingual, topical)	+	+++	↓/→/↑	→↓	↑/↓	↓↓↓	↓
Isosorbide dinitrate (sublingual, oral, chewable)	+	+++	→/↑	↓	→	↓↓	↓
Hydralazine	++++	o	→	→/↓	↑↑↑	↓	↓↓↓
Prazosin	++	+	→	↓	↑↑	↓↓	↓↓

↑ increase
↓ decrease
→ unchanged

SERUM DIGITALIS LEVELS-INDICATIONS AND INTERPRETATION

Several points should be kept in mind when obtaining and interpreting serum digitalis levels. Serum digitalis levels (digoxin or digitoxin) are usually obtained to verify suspected digitalis intoxication, to determine whether the patient's digitalis level is in the "therapeutic" range, or to ascertain if digitalis is being taken.

Point 1. Serum digoxin levels should be obtained *4 hours after* the previous *intravenous dose* and *8 hours after* the previous *oral dose* to ensure relative equilibrium between the serum level and the myocardial level of digoxin.

Point 2. Each laboratory should establish its own confidence limits of therapeutic digoxin levels (as well as digitoxin). As a rule of thumb, however:
— Serum dixogin level <0.5 ng/ml eliminates the possibility of digoxin toxicity — patient is underdigitalized.
— Serum digoxin levels of 0.5 to 2.5 ng/ml are optimal.
— Serum digoxin levels of 2.0 to 3.0 ng/ml overlap between optimal levels and the toxic range.
— Serum digoxin levels of >3.0 ng/ml indicate patient is overdigitalized and definitely in the toxic range.

Point 3. *High* serum digoxin levels *without toxic cardiac manifestations* may be seen in the treatment of *atrial tachyarrhythmias* and in the presence of *hyperkalemia.*

Point 4. *Low or normal* serum digoxin levels *with toxic cardiac manifestations* may be seen with *hypokalemia, hypomagnesemia, recent myocardial infarction, myxedema, hypoxia,* or *hypercalcemia.*

Point 5. Falsely low serum digoxin levels may be seen in patients receiving radioisotopes for diagnostic studies.

Point 6. Low serum digoxin levels despite adequate oral doses may be seen with *hyperthyroidism, intestinal malabsorption, rapid intestinal transit syndromes, simultaneous cholestyramine or antacids,* or *kaolin + pectin administration, abnormal digoxin metabolism.*

Point 7. Serum digitoxin levels are approximately 10 times the values for digoxin.

Point 8. Digitalis leaf, which is a mixture of many active cardiac glycosides, cannot be measured by radioimmunoassay; therefore, the adequacy of digitalization cannot be estimated from the serum digoxin level in patients receiving digitoxin or the crude leaf.

Reference: Doherty, J. E.: J.A.M.A., *239*:2594, 1978.

6
PULMONARY DISEASE

MORE ALPHABET SOUP

Because of the many initials and abbreviations now in use the jargon of respiratory care is confusing, especially to the uninitiated. The following is a listing of the currently accepted definitions for some of the more commonly discussed respiratory terms. The reader is referred to the ACCP-ATS article listed in the references for a much more extensive list of terms and symbols and a more detailed explanation of their origin.

Respiratory Physiology

General	*Gas phase*	*Blood phase*
P — Pressure	A — Alveolar	$\dot{Q}$ — Blood flow
$\overline{X}$ — A mean value	D — Dead space	Q — Blood volume
$\dot{X}$ — A time derivative	E — Expired	a — Arterial
	F — Fractional	c — Capillary
	concentration	v — Venous
	of a gas	$\overline{v}$ — Mixed venous
	I — Inspired	
	T — Tidal	
	V — Gas volume	

Measurements of Ventilation

CC	— Closing capacity	VA	— Alveolar ventilation
CV	— Closing volume	VD	— Dead space ventilation
FRC	— Functional residual capacity	$\dot{V}E$	— Minute expired volume
TV	— Tidal volume	$\dot{V}I$	— Minute inspired volume
VC	— Vital capacity	VD/VT	— Dead space/Tidal volume ratio

Measurements of Mechanics of Breathing

C	— Compliance
PAW	— Airway pressure
PIP	— Peak inspiratory pressure
R	— Resistance
W	— Work of breathing

Miscellaneous

$C(a-\overline{v})O_2$	— Arteriovenous oxygen content difference
$P(A-a)O_2$	— Alveolar–arterial oxygen pressure difference
Qsp	— Physiologic shunt flow (total venous admixture); often expressed as per cent of cardiac output (Qs/Qt)
CMV	— Controlled mechanical ventilation
CPAP	— Continuous positive airway pressure = EPAP + IPAP (see following page)
CPPB	— Continuous positive pressure breathing

CPPV   — Continuous positive pressure ventilation
EPAP   — Expiratory positive airway pressure
IAV   — Intermittent assisted ventilation
IDV   — Intermittent demand ventilation
IMV   — Intermittent mandatory ventilation
IPAP   — Inspiratory positive airway pressure
PEEP   — Positive end expiratory pressure
SIMV   — Synchronized intermittent mandatory ventilation
SPEEP   — Spontaneous positive end expiratory pressure

The system used at the University of Florida at Gainesville seems to be a precise and descriptive method of identifying the common modes of ventilation. It is presented here in the hopes that it will help you to a better understanding of the commonly used modes of ventilation and the associated airway pressure curves. As shown in Figure 6–1, an airway pressure curve can be divided into four components:

A. *Baseline,* the level from which all respiratory maneuvers are accomplished.

B. *Assist effort pressure,* the pressure the patient must reach in order to initiate a mechanical inspiration.

C. *Peak pressure,* the maximum pressure during a mechanical ventilator breath.

D. *Inspiratory effort,* the airway pressure measured during a spontaneous inspiration.

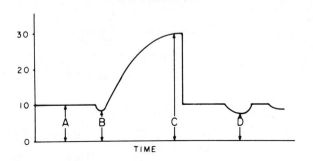

FIG. 6–1

Components of the airway pressure curve. Values on the Y axis are in cm. of water.

These phases of the airway pressure curve can be measured with an appropriate pressure gauge and should be expressed in absolute numbers, not deviations above and below the baseline.

The five commonly used modes of ventilation, their specific airway pressure curves, and the terminology that has been associated with each curve are as follows:

1. Spontaneous ventilation (*spontaneous*): The pressure differential necessary to move tidal gas is generated by the patient (Fig. 6–2).

I SPONTANEOUS VENTILATION

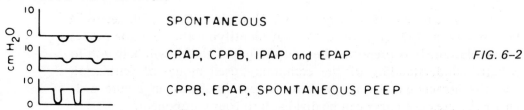

SPONTANEOUS

CPAP, CPPB, IPAP and EPAP   *FIG. 6–2*

CPPB, EPAP, SPONTANEOUS PEEP

2. Assisted ventilation (*assist*): The patients inspiratory effort signals a ventilator to deliver each mechanical ventilator breath (Fig. 6–3).

II ASSISTED VENTILATION

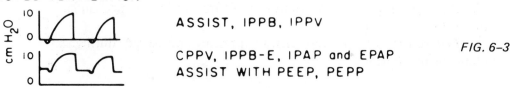

ASSIST, IPPB, IPPV

CPPV, IPPB-E, IPAP and EPAP   *FIG. 6–3*
ASSIST WITH PEEP, PEPP

3. Controlled ventilation (*CMV*): The tidal volume and rate are determined by the mechanical ventilator, so the patient cannot initiate or generate any gas flow (Fig. 6–4).

III CONTROLLED VENTILATION

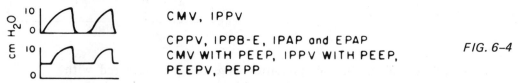

CMV, IPPV

CPPV, IPPB-E, IPAP and EPAP
CMV WITH PEEP, IPPV WITH PEEP,   *FIG. 6–4*
PEEPV, PEPP

4. Intermittent mandatory ventilation (*IMV*): The patient may breathe spontaneously between periodic tidal volumes from a mechanical ventilator (Fig. 6–5).

IV INTERMITTENT MANDATORY VENTILATION

FIG. 6–5

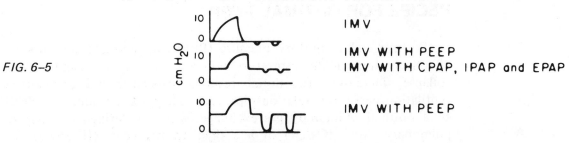

IMV

IMV WITH PEEP
IMV WITH CPAP, IPAP and EPAP

IMV WITH PEEP

5. Synchronized intermittent mandatory ventilation (*SIMV*): Same as 4, except mechanical ventilations are initiated by the patient (Fig. 6–6).

6

V SYNCHRONIZED INTERMITTENT MANDATORY VENTILATION

FIG. 6–6

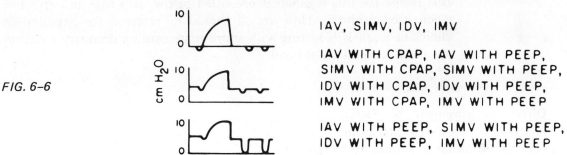

IAV, SIMV, IDV, IMV

IAV WITH CPAP, IAV WITH PEEP,
SIMV WITH CPAP, SIMV WITH PEEP,
IDV WITH CPAP, IDV WITH PEEP,
IMV WITH CPAP, IMV WITH PEEP

IAV WITH PEEP, SIMV WITH PEEP,
IDV WITH PEEP, IMV WITH PEEP

Each of these modes of ventilation can occur at ambient or elevated expiratory pressures. The ventilation data for any patient can be presented by using the appropriate abbreviation for his mode of ventilation and a set of numbers for each component of the airway pressure curve. The example in Figure 6–1 would be described as SIMV 10/8/30/7. When a numerical value is not applicable for a given measurement, a blank or an asterisk is used.

References: ACCP-ATS, Joint Committee on Pulmonary Nomenclature, Pulmonary Terms and Symbols: Chest, *67*:583, 1975; Desautels, D. A., Sanderson, R. R., and Klein, E. F.: Respiratory Care, *23*:42, 1978.

"Hypoxia not only stops the machine but wrecks the machinery."

Haldane

RECIPE FOR OPTIMAL PEEP

Positive end expiratory pressure (PEEP) in adequate amounts can effectively treat acute respiratory failure (ARF) by reversing alveolar collapse, increasing functional residual capacity, and normalizing ventilation/perfusion relationships. An adequate amount of PEEP gives optimal pulmonary gas exchange, which is defined as an intra-pulmonary shunt (Qs/Qt) of less than 15 per cent. (If you've forgotten what Qs/Qt is, see More Alphabet Soup). In some patients, cardiovascular support, volume infusions, or inotropic agents will be necessary to maintain cardiac output as PEEP is progressively increased to the level that gives optimal pulmonary function.

Although the optimal PEEP concept has been well described, the actual technique of arriving at this appropriate pressure is not as clear. One recipe for this regimen is presented below. It is safe and effective when used properly. However, it should be reserved for experienced clinicians in an ICU setting with appropriate cardiopulmonary monitoring and interventions at hand.

> Direct measurement of Qs/Qt requires a mixed venous blood gas sample obtained with a pulmonary artery catheter. An estimate of Qs/Qt can be obtained by calculating the ratio PaO_2/FIO_2. FIO_2 is expressed as a decimal. When this ratio is >300, Qs/Qt is <15%; when the ratio is <300, Qs/Qt is >15% or the $P_{\bar{v}}O_2$ is decreased.

Ingredients

1. One patient with ARF (defined as a Qs/Qt greater than 15 per cent.
2. PEEP device (several varieties available).
3. Ventilator in IMV mode.
4. Arterial line for monitoring and blood gas sampling.
5. Dash of salt (as normal saline for volume replacement).

6. Balloon-tipped, flow-directed, thermodilution pulmonary artery catheter.

7. Inotropic agents — dopamine, digoxin, calcium chloride, nitroprusside. Add according to taste.

8. Programmable calculator (very useful).

Preparation

1. Connect patient to ventilator in IMV mode (tidal volume 10 to 12 ml/kg) and to PEEP device.

2. Add PEEP in 3 to 5 cm water increments until Qs/Qt is optimal (less than 15 per cent) or cardiac output decreased. Thirty minutes after each increase in PEEP, measure blood gases and hemodynamics.

3. Stir in full hemodynamic monitoring (thermodilution catheter for measurement of cardiac output, PAo, CVP, systemic and pulmonary vascular resistance, oxygen transport, and Qs/Qt when PEEP is greater than 15 cm of water or when you are suspicious of cardiovascular compromise).

4. Adjust IMV rate independently of PEEP to minimal level necessary to maintain pH at 7.36 to 7.45 with patient's spontaneous breathing rate less than 30 per minute.

5. As oxygenation improves, decrease the FIO_2 to achieve a PaO_2 in the 80 to 100 torr range.

6. Season with cardiovascular interventions: a) Low cardiac index and low PAo — add dash of salt or packed red cells until adequate filling pressure reached. b) Low cardiac index and adequate PAo — use inotropic agent (dopamine, calcium chloride, and/or digoxin). c) Low cardiac index and high systemic vascular resistance with adequate PAo — carefully drip in nitroprusside or nitroglycerin.

7. After optimal level of PEEP is achieved, marinate at body temperature for 6 to 12 hours, then slowly remove PEEP in 3 to 5 cm increments. Monitor Qs/Qt and accept no more than a 2 to 4 per cent increase in Qs/Qt. Remember that you may have either early (within 1 hour) or late (up to 12 hours) deterioration after a decrease in PEEP. Don't hurry the batter: Too aggressive weaning from PEEP may result in return of the pulmonary pathology that often requires an even higher level of PEEP to reverse again.

8. Serve (extubate) when the patient can maintain an optimal Qs/Qt with 5 cm of PEEP (assuming all other criteria for extubation are met. See Checklist for Take-off which follows.

Early institution of this treatment, which is based on measured physiologic values rather than subjective signs and symptoms, is reported to result in mortality rates from acute respiratory failure as low as 5 per cent. Try it, you'll like it.

Reference: Gallagher, D. J., Civetta, J. M., and Kirby, R. R.: Crit. Care Med., 6:323, 1978.

CHECKLIST FOR TAKE-OFF: WEANING FROM A RESPIRATOR

Weaning a patient from mechanical ventilation is often more art than science, especially in the patient with chronic lung disease. The weaning process actually begins almost as soon as the patient is intubated and placed on mechanical ventilation. It usually flows through the following sequence:

1. Reduction of the FIO_2 to nontoxic levels (less than 60 per cent).
2. Reduction of PEEP to 3 to 5 cm H_2O. (It is the author's bias that any patient with an endotracheal tube should always be maintained on 3 to 5 cm of "physiologic PEEP" to prevent atelectasis. Exceptions are patients who already have a high FRC [functional residual capacity], (i.e., patients with acute asthma or emphysema.)
3. Removal of mechanical ventilation.
4. Removal of the endotracheal or tracheostomy tube.

The following checklist is helpful in deciding if the weaning process is complete and it is time to "pull the tube."

1. Is the primary problem resolving?
2. Is the cardiovascular system stable?
3. Is the arterial oxygenation adequate?*
   a. PaO_2 >80 torr on ≤ 40% FIO_2 and ≤3 to 5 cm PEEP.
4. Can the patient maintain an adequate alveolar ventilation without excessive work?
   a. Normal pCO_2 (40 torr) and pH (7.40) during a period of spontaneous breathing.*
   b. Respiratory rate <30/min.
   c. Minute ventilation at rest <10 liters.
5. Does the patient have enough respiratory reserve for coughing, sighing, and clearing secretions?
   a. Compliance ($C = \dfrac{\Delta\,Volume}{\Delta\,Pressure}$) >30 ml/cm H_2O.**
   b. Negative inspiratory force >−30cm H_2O.
   c. Vital capacity >15 ml/kg.
   d. Ability to double minute rate of resting ventilation voluntarily.
6. Can the patient maintain a patent airway?
   a. Is the level of consciousness adequate?
   b. Are there any mechanical factors to cause upper airway obstruction? (These often won't be apparent until the tube is removed.)

Any patient who fulfills all of these criteria should tolerate extubation without any problem. Failure to meet some or all of these criteria does not necessarily mean that the patient can not be extubated. It does mean you are going to fret a lot more if you do go ahead and pull the tube. In these marginal situations you have to weigh the risk of prolonged intubation and/or tracheostomy against the risk of recurrent respiratory failure, and then use your best clinical judgment to make the decision. After extubation the patient should be carefully observed in an ICU until it is certain that there will be no further respiratory problems. It is prudent, especially in marginal situations, to empty the stomach before extubation and keep the patient N.P.O. for a time after extubation so the risk of vomiting and aspiration will be decreased if reintubation becomes necessary.

---

*Remember that these requirements may not apply to patients with chronic lung disease. In these people the optimal arterial blood gases for weaning are the ones they have when they are doing well (which may be a PaO_2 of 45, a $PaCO_2$ of 60, and a pH of 7.38).

**To determine the compliance in practice, ΔV may be taken as the tidal volume delivered by the respirator and ΔP, the peak inspiratory pressure (PIP) minus PEEP.

6

Powner's Third Law of Critical Care Medicine:
Nothing ever happens unless you try.

SMOKE INHALATION

Smoke inhalation is a treacherous injury because the effects may not become clinically apparent until after the patient has been sent home from the emergency room. Because of the latent period that may exist between the time of the injury and the development of severe pulmonary complications, the first consideration in the management of a possible smoke inhalation victim is deciding whom to admit to the hospital. The presence of any *one* of the findings listed in the following table should be grounds for admission to the hospital for 48 hours of observation. Other patients should be observed in the emergency department for several hours before discharge. Patients who are discharged from the emergency department should be reliable and should clearly understand the necessity of immediately returning to the hospital if they develop delayed symptoms. In questionable cases it is best to be conservative and admit the patient to the hospital.

The clinical stages of inhalation injury are outlined below. In general, the more severe the injury, the sooner it will become manifest. Patients who on initial evaluation have absolutely no signs and symptoms may subsequently develop severe Stage II or Stage III injuries, so be careful.

ADMIT FOR OBSERVATION

1. Closed space fires
2. History of unconsciousness
3. Facial burns
4. Mucosal burns or singed nasal hairs
5. Wheezes, rales, rhonchi
6. Respiratory distress
7. Significant cough—especially with the production of carbonaceous material (not as useful in firefighters, who often have chronic production of carbonaceous sputum)
8. Hoarseness or dysphagia
9. Pain on deep inspiration
10. Abnormal arterial blood gases
11. Carboxyhemoglobin >10%
12. Abnormal chest x-ray
13. Acute laryngeal inflammation seen with laryngoscopy

Stage I. Acute Respiratory Distress

This occurs within the first few hours after exposure and may resemble upper airway obstruction. There often is a major bronchospastic component. The outcome is often lethal despite aggressive treatment.

Stage II. Pulmonary Edema

This develops 8 to 36 hours after injury. The onset may be insidious or acute. The syndrome may be aggravated by coexisting cardiac disease and overvigorous fluid resuscitation. During this period, upper airway edema may also occur, resulting in upper airway obstruction.

Stage III. Bacterial Pneumonia

This occurs two days to three weeks after injury. The incidence is increased by the use of prophylactic steroids or antibiotics.

Considerations in the treatment of smoke inhalation are outlined in the following table.

TREATMENT OF SMOKE INHALATION

A. All patients

1. High concentrations of humidified oxygen—to treat hypoxia and carbon monoxide poisoning

2. Vigorous pulmonary toilet
   a. Deep breathing and coughing
   b. Adequate humidification
   c. Nasotracheal suctioning and/or bronchoscopy if the patient cannot clear secretions himself

3. Careful fluid balance to avoid overhydration

B. Selected patients

1. Bronchodilators

2. Endotracheal intubation; indications:
   a. Upper airway obstruction
   b. Unmanageable secretions
   c. Severe facial or oral burns with rapidly increasing edema
   d. Need for ventilatory support
   e. Prevention of aspiration in the unconscious patients

3. Mechanical ventilation with positive end expiratory pressure (for indications see Checklist for Take-off: Weaning from Mechanical Ventilation, as the indications for ventilatory support are the reverse of the indications for weaning)

4. Selected antibiotic therapy based on blood or sputum cultures *when* and *if* pneumonia develops

C. Never indicated

1. Prophylactic antibiotics

2. Corticosteroids

3. Prophylactic tracheostomy

6

Reference: Silverman, H. M.: Smoke Inhalation. In Schwartz, G. R., et. al. (Eds.): Principles and Practice of Emergency Medicine. Philadelphia, W. B. Saunders Company, 1978, p. 837.

ADMIT THE ASTHMATIC?

A 28-year-old woman comes to the emergency room with an acute asthma attack. She is a known asthmatic taking steroids, beta-2 stimulants, and phosphodiesterase inhibitors. Do you intensify therapy and admit this patient, or do you attempt to maximize therapy in the emergency room in hopes of breaking the attack and saving an admission? With the latter course, you usually find that you tie up nursing personnnel, you occupy valuable emergency space, and you use a great deal of your time and energy only to admit an exhausted patient eight hours later. Then again, you might get lucky.

There are many factors at play in the origins and maintenance of an asthmatic attack. Some components or complications of an attack make admission obvious, whereas others may be "softer" judgment calls. Hope these hints help.

1. *Gross dehydration:* Usually the attack has been in progress for some time. There are inspissated secretions blocking the airways. It would take hours to hydrate the patient adequately in the emergency room using D5W at 250 to 500 ml an hour. Usually the patient's needs are in excess of 2500 ml. *Admit.*

2. *Dehydration with a concurrent condition that precludes rapid rehydration:* The patient may be only moderately dehydrated but have coronary artery disease or congestive heart failure, which will limit IV flow rates. *Judgment call.*

3. *Patients on steroid and bronchodilator therapy:* This is a "no win" situation. To be on this therapy in the first place is probably to be "brittle" and chronic. The patients have airways that are almost always nonresponsive or minimally responsive to additional therapy. There is frequently an underlying infection that maintains the asthma attack. *Admit.*

4. *Progression of arterial blood gases (ABGs):* The chart below shows the typical progressive deterioration of ABGs during a prolonged asthmatic attack. Stages I and II are commonly encountered. Stage III isn't just progressive hypoxemia; rather, the patient's respiratory muscles are fatigued, the airways are plugged, and the patient is dehydrated and exhausted. He is crossing the "normal values point," soon to be hypercarbic and acidemic. *Admit.*

Staging Asthma

	ARTERIAL BLOOD GASES ON ROOM AIR			
STAGE	pO_2	pCO_2	pH	COMMENTS
I	Normal	<40	>7.4	Respiratory alkalosis,
II	Mild decrease, still >65	<40	>7.4	Respiratory alkalosis, hypoxemia
III	Moderate decrease, 55–65	40	7.4	Danger! Airways are closing; exhaustion
IV	Severe, <55	>40	<7.4	Acute respiratory failure; respiratory acidosis

5. *Pulmonary infections:* If acute bronchitis with excessive secretions, pneumonitis, or lobar pneumonia is present, the odds of recurrent attacks while you are waiting for oral antibiotics to work are very high. *Admit* for IV antibiotics, continuous infusion of bronchodilators, and control of secretions.

6. *The sedated or exhausted patient: Judgment call,* depending on degree of sedation or exhaustion.

7. *Acidemic patients:* These patients are usually in acute respiratory failure, so the decision for *admission* is clear-cut. Remember that below a systemic arterial pH of 7.25, the airways are effectively resistant to cyclic AMP. Bronchodilator therapy won't work. (Suggestion: 90 to 150 ml (2 to 3 ampules) of prepackaged sodium bicarbonate (i.e., 90 to 150 mEq).

8. *Pneumothorax or pneumomediastinum:* *Obviously!*

9. *Patients with therapy-limiting cardiac conditions:* Conduction defects in the elderly, prior myocardial infarctions, ventricular aneurysms, and numerous premature ventricular contractions may severely limit asthma therapy, which is, in the main, arrhythmogenic. In addition, hypoxemia or the acidosis of an inadequately treated attack further increases the risk of cardiac arrhythmias. *Admit.*

10. *Environmental situation:* The asthmatic attack may be easy to treat, but you may return the patient right back to the same situation that triggered the attack in the first place. When the patient is comfortable enough to talk, find the precipitating event(s) (e.g., emotional trauma), and discuss factors in the physical environment (e.g., an unheated apartment, twelve cats). Then use your *judgment.*

11. *Pulmonary function tests:* Frequently, meaningful pulmonary function tests can not be obtained because of the patient's pulmonary distress. If PFTs can be obtained, please do so. Follow the FEV_1. The absolute value of the FEV_1 may not be helpful in the acute situation. If there is no change or a reduction in the FEV_1 with therapy, then *admission* is advised.

Reference: Spector, S. L.: Asthma in adults. In Conn, H. F. (Ed.): Current Therapy 1979. Philadelphia, W. B. Saunders Company, 1979, pp. 547–551.

THE MEDIASTINAL MASSES

Mediastinal masses can be a puzzling diagnostic problem for the internist. The numerous structures contained within the mediastinum may all give rise to mass lesions. In addition, a large number of congenital, developmental, and metastatic lesions may be present. The associated clinical features are usually nonspecific and add little to narrowing the differential diagnoses. Most patients are symptomatic, with either a cardiac or pulmonary complaint. Chest pain, cough, and dyspnea are the most common presenting complaints. In about 14 per cent of cases, the mass is discovered on a routine chest x-ray performed on an asymptomatic patient.

The location of the mass in the mediastinum can provide a guide for differential diagnosis. The mediastinum can be divided into four compartments. The *superior mediastinum* is the area bounded by the manubrium anteriorly and the third and fifth thoracic vertebrae posteriorly. The *anterior mediastinum* is the area anterior to the heart, from the inferior border of the superior mediastinum to the diaphragm. The *posterior mediastinum* is the area between the vertebral column and lungs that extends from the inferior border of the superior mediastinum to the diaphragm, and the *middle mediastinum* is the area bounded above by the inferior border of the superior mediastinum. It extends to the diaphragm and lies between the anterior and posterior compartments.

The normal anatomic structures found in each segment of the mediastinum are included in the following table:

SUPERIOR/ANTERIOR	MIDDLE	POSTERIOR
Thymus	Hilar regions and lymph nodes	Descending aorta
Trachea	Bifurcation of trachea	Lower portion of esophagus
Ascending aorta	Aortic arch	Part of sympathetic chain
Caval vessels	Heart and pericardium	Intercostal nerves
Phrenic, vagal, recurrent laryngeal nerves		Thoracic duct

The following chart is intended as a partial listing of the more common mediastinal masses according to site of predilection. Note that the superior mediastinum can be subdivided into anterior and posterior compartments.

Superior mediastinum	*Anterior mediastinum*
Bronchogenic cysts	Lymphadenopathy secondary to
Cystic hygroma	Hodgkin's and non-Hodgkin's
Aneurysm of ascending aorta	lymphoma
Lymphoma	TB, sarcoid
Myxoma	Teratomas
Mesothelioma	Substernal thyroid
Anterior portion: masses of	Thymoma
thymic, thyroid, or	Morgagni's hernia
parathyroid origin	Aneurysm of ascending aorta
Posterior portion: masses of	Dermoid cyst
neurogenic origin	Lymphangioma
	Sarcoma
	Parathyroid adenoma
	Mesothelioma
	Epicardial fat pad

Middle mediastinum	*Posterior mediastinum*
Hodgkin's and non-Hodgkin's	Tumors of neurogenic origin
lymphoma	Sarcoma
Primary lung malignancy	Lymphoma
Metastatic malignancy	Myxoma
Bronchogenic cysts	Enterogenous cyst
Pericardial cyst	Pancreatic pseudocyst
Hiatus hernia	Esophageal diverticulae
Lymph node involvement	Meningocoele
from various diseases (e.g.,	Thoracic duct cyst
TB, sarcoid)	Aneurysm of descending aorta
	Extramedullary hematopoiesis
	Paravertebral abscess

Approximately 18 per cent of mediastinal masses are in the superior mediastinum. Of all mediastinal tumors about 50 per cent are malignant; however, only 25 per cent of thymomas are malignant. The most common primary neoplasms and cysts of the mediastinum are in order of their frequency: neurogenic tumors, thymomas, and various cysts. The most common neurogenic tumors seen are ganglioneuromas, neurinomas, and neurofibromas. Of the cysts, the bronchogenic and dermoid types are most common.

The initial diagnostic evaluation of a mediastinal mass should include routine PA and lateral films and an overpenetrated view. A barium swallow and tomograms or the more sophisticated CT scan will also serve to delineate the mass completely. These procedures, however, will only localize the mass and will usually not yield a specific diagnosis. If a substernal thyroid is suspected, a radioiodine scan is the procedure of choice, but many substernal goiters are nonfunctional and, therefore, the procedure is helpful only if positive. If the patient has objective cardiac findings, angiography should be considered. When a histological diagnosis must be obtained, a mediastinoscopy or thoracotomy will be necessary.

References: Sabiston, D. C., and Scott, H. W.: Ann. Surg., *136*:777, 1952; Sarin, C. L., and Hohl-Oser, H. C.: Thorax, *24*:585, 1969; Friedman, H. H., and Papper, S.: Problem-Oriented Medical Diagnosis. Boston, Little, Brown & Company, 1975, pp. 168–172.

A SHORT COURSE IN THE RADIOLOGIC EXPLORATION OF THE MEDIASTINUM

The definitive detection of mediastinal disease can almost always be accomplished radiologically. Therefore the importance of reliable and thorough radiologic examination of the mediastinum cannot be overemphasized. Proper radiologic interpretation demands thorough gross anatomic, pathologic, and physiologic knowledge. This knowledge must be coupled with high quality technique and a reasoned approach to the clinical problem.

The specific nature of the disease requires pathologic and/or bacteriologic identification.

The Approach

The proper radiologic approach for evaluation of the mediastinum does not differ from an internist's approach to other clinical problems.

The following questions must be answered sequentially.

1. Is the mediastinum abnormal?
2. Where is the abnormality?
3. What is it? The answer to this question requires *your active participation* with the radiologist. Only you have access to the clinical and laboratory data that are *absolutely essential* for the best possible radiologic interpretation.

Mediastinal Road Map

Let's examine the mediastinal landmarks that help in the localization of mediastinal abnormalities.

The air-containing lungs surrounding the mediastinum provide the contrast that permits visualization of the *"rind"* of the mediastinum.

The barium-filled esophagus is used to define the *"core"* of the mediastinum. Interruption or distortion of the rind or the core or their margins signal the presence of mediastinal disease.

The important identifiable mediastinal interfaces may be divided into three groups:

Anterior (Fig. 6–7*A*, *D*, and *E*)

1. *Retrosternal stripe* (RS) (lateral view): Right lung contrasts with the retrosternal soft tissue.

2. *Parasternal stripe* (PST) (lateral view): Right or left lung contrasts with costochondral junctions and adjacent soft tissues (the internal mammary nodes).

3. *Anterior junction line* (AJL) (frontal view): This is formed by the anterior medial margins of right and left lungs meeting anteriorly.

4. *Superior paravenous stripe* (SPVS) (frontal view): Right lung contrasts with the superior vena cava.

5. *Paraarterial stripe* (PARS) (frontal view and, rarely, lateral view): Ascending aorta and its major branches contrast with the right lung. On the left, the left lung provides the contrast.

Middle (Fig. 6–7*B*, *D*, and *E*)

The projection of the azygoesophageal recess of the right lung, which takes a deep medial excursion anterior to the dorsal spine and the esophagus, provides important middle mediastinal interfaces.

1. *Paratracheal stripe* (PTS) (frontal and lateral views): The posterior and lateral stripes are seen frequently. The anterior stripe is rarely seen. The right main and intermediate bronchial wall is frequently seen.

2. *Azygos arch* (AzA) (frontal and, rarely, lateral views): The anteriorly oriented azygos arch indents the right lung from its prespinal origin to its insertion in the superior vena cava.

3. *Esophagus* (Es): Air and/or barium may be used to outline the interior of the esophagus. The lungs outline the esophageal outer surfaces, especially in emphysematous or young patients (PesS). The intimate relationships of the esophagus to the aortic arch and tracheobronchial tree are important.

4. *Heart* (frontal and lateral views): The external cardiac contours are well known to internists. The interfaces between the epicardial fat (beneath the visceral pericardium) and anterior mediastinal fat (outside the parietal pericardium), when seen, define the *pericardial stripe* (PeS). Thickening of this stripe is usually caused by pericardial fluid.

5. *Inferior paravenous stripe* (IPVS) (frontal and lateral views): The right lung contrasts with the intrathoracic inferior vena cava.

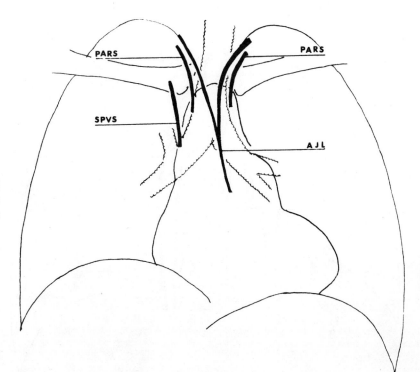

FIG. 6–7A

The anterior mediastinal interfaces, AP view. (The abbreviations for all figures are explained in the text.)

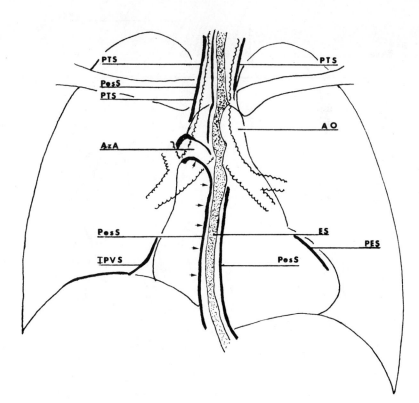

FIG. 6–7B

The middle mediastinal interfaces, AP view. The arrows point to the azygo-esophageal recess.

6

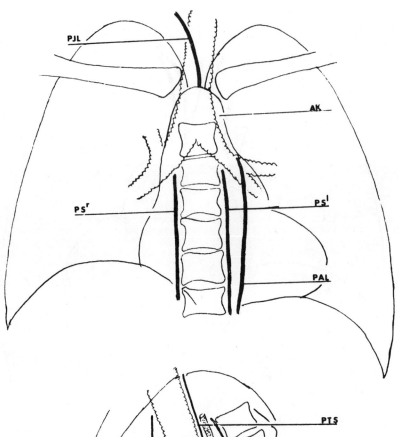

FIG. 6–7C

The posterior mediastinal interfaces, AP view.

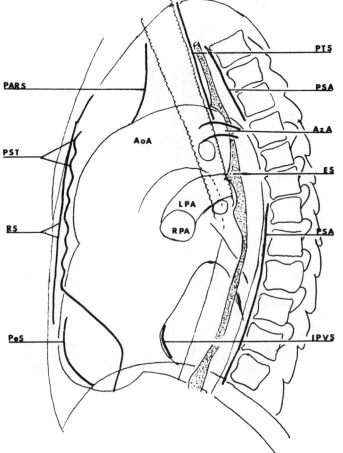

FIG. 6–7D

Lateral view of mediastinal interfaces.

ILLUSTRATION CONTINUED ON THE OPPOSITE PAGE

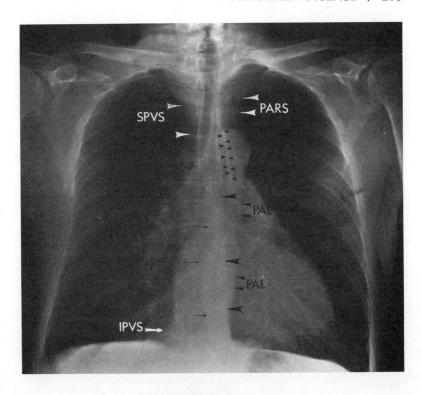

FIG. 6–7E

Posterior-anterior chest film of an emphysematous 80-year-old man.

PARS = Para-arterial stripe
PAL = Para-aortic line
SPVS = Superior paravenous stripe
IPVS = Inferior paravenous stripe
Right black arrows = Azygoesophageal recess
Multiple opposing small arrowheads = Anterior junction line
Three large arrowheads = Left paraspinal stripe

ILLUSTRATION CONTINUED ON PAGE 207

Posterior (Fig. 6–7C, D, and E)

1. *Aortic knob* (AK): This well-known shadow represents the most distal and lateral portion of the aortic arch indenting the left lung. It lies at the junction of arch and descending thoracic aorta.

2. *Paraaortic line* (PAL) (frontal view): The left lung contrasts with the descending aorta.

3. *Paraspinal stripe left lateral* (PS^L); *right lateral* (PS^R); *anterior* (PS^A): Left lung contrast produces PS^L, the most reliable and constant paraspinal stripe. The azygoesophageal recess and right lung may outline PS^R and PS^A.

4. *Posterior junction line* (PJL) (anterior view): This is formed by the meeting of the posterior medial margins of the right and left lungs behind the esophagus superiorly.

The Intrathoracic Lymph Nodes and the Clinician — Where Are They?

The following classification of intrathoracic nodal groups is designed for clinicoradiologic use. (The areas where conventional tomography (†) and computed tomography — fast scans of less than 10 secs — (*) are particularly useful are indicated.) The numbering of the nodal groups refers to Fig. 6–7*F*, *G*, and *H*.

1. Nodes of the thoracic inlet and anterior mediastinum
   A. Innominate vein angle nodes*
   B. Internal mammary nodes*
   C. Cardiophrenic angle nodes*
2. Tracheobronchial nodes
   A. Aortopulmonic window nodes
      1. Ductus nodes*
   B. Paratracheal nodes
   C. Subcarinal nodes*
3. Periesophageal nodes*
4. Posterior diaphragmatic nodes* (Fig. 6–7*J*)
5. Hilar nodes †*
   A. Inferior pulmonary ligament nodes*

What Are They?

Of course, the detection of regional adenopathy with or without a visible pulmonary lesion has strong diagnostic implications. Note once again, the radiologic method localizes but does not characterize.

The following statistical clues can help influence clinical decision making.

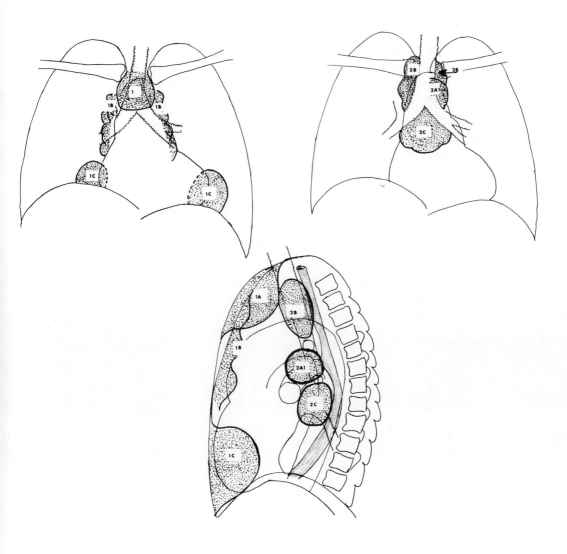

FIG. 6–7F, 6–7G, and 6–7H

The intrathoracic lymph nodes. (See p. 206 for designation of the individual nodal groups.)

6

RADIOLOGIC EXAMINATION OF MEDIASTINUM TODAY

The availability and application of fast, high-resolution CAT scanners provide exquisitely detailed images of the mediastinal anatomy. These illustrations (Fig. 6–7*I* through *K*) demonstrate the kind of information available and display the relationship of the mediastinal structures in cross-section.

The "soft tissue" and "reversal" modes of the scanner are best for imaging the mediastinum, while the "lung" mode and "bone" mode are used for analysis of the pulmonary parenchyma and the osseous thorax, respectively.

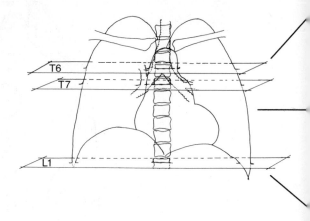

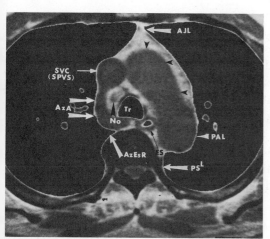

FIG. 6-7K

CT scan enlarged to emphasize mediastinal detail. (T$_6$ level)

AJL	= Anterior junction line
PAL	= Para-aortic line
PSL	= Left paraspinal stripe
Es	= Esophagus
AzEsR	= Azygo-esophageal recess
No	= Azygos node
AzA	= Azygos vein arch
SVC	= Superior vena cava
SPVC	= Superior paravenous stripe

Black arrow heads = aortic arch

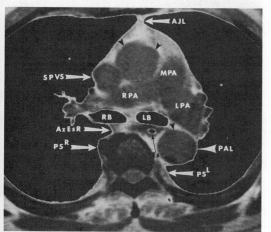

FIG. 6-7L

CT scan enlarged to emphasize mediastinal detail. (T$_7$ level)

AJL	= Anterior junction line
MPA	= Main pulmonary artery
RPA	= Right pulmonary artery
LPA	= Left pulmonary artery
PAL	= Para-aortic line
PSL	= Left paraspinal stripe
PSR	= Right paraspinal stripe (visible because of displacement by focal hypertrophic proliferative bone on right side of the body of T$_9$.)
LB	= Left main stem bronchus
RB	= Right main stem bronchus
ES	= Esophagus
AzEsR	= Azygo-esophageal recess
SPVS	= Superior paravenous stripe

Two black arrowheads = Ascending thoracic aorta
One black arrowhead = Descending thoracic aorta

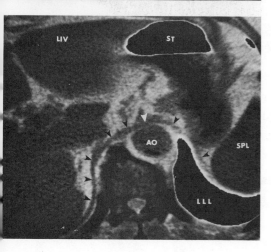

FIG. 6-7M

Enlarged CT scan taken at the level of T$_{12}$ or L. vertebral body.

ST	= Stomach
LIV	= Left lobe of liver
SPL	= Spleen
LLL	= Left lower lobe of lung
Ao	= Aorta
Arrowheads	= Diaphragm (This is the level of the diaphragmatic crura where the posterior diaphragmatic nodes lie.)

6

Sarcoidosis
(62 Patients with Sarcoidosis and Intrathoracic Adenopathy)

97% showed bilateral hilar adenopathy.

75% showed right paratracheal or aortopulmonic nodes.

20% showed subcarinal or anterior mediastinal adenopathy.

37% showed the following most common combination: aorto-pulmonic, bilateral hilar, and right paratracheal nodes.

Anterior mediastinal or subcarinal nodes are *never* seen alone (always seen in association with right paratracheal, aortopulmonic, or bilateral hilar disease).

Hodgkin's Disease (HD) vs. Non-Hodgkin's Lymphoma (NHL)
(300 Patients)

Intrathoracic disease at presentation
    HD — 67% (of 164)
    NHL — 43% (of 136)

Parenchymal lung disease present radiographically
    HD — 11.6%
    NHL — 4%

(All patients with parenchymal lung disease had intrathoracic lymphadenopathy.)

Internal mammary lymph nodes enlarged radiographically
$$\frac{HD}{NHL} = \frac{10}{1} \text{ ratio}$$

Superior mediastinal lymph nodes (anterior or tracheobronchial)
$$\frac{HD}{NHL} = \frac{2}{1} \text{ratio}$$

(Posterior mediastinal [diaphragmatic] lymph nodes and cardiophrenic angle nodes were *involved* in NHL and *not* in HD.)

Intrathoracic Lymph Node Metastases from
Extrathoracic Neoplasms
(1071 Patients)

Abnormal chest films
    15% (163 cases)

Radiographic lymphadenopathy
    2.3% (25 cases)
                Genitourinary carcinoma   12 cases
                Head and neck carcinoma   8 cases
                Breast carcinoma   3 cases
                Malignant melanoma   2 cases

Distribution of lymph nodes (25 cases)
    Right paratracheal — 15 of 25 cases
    Subcarinal and posterior mediastinal — rare

Parenchymal pulmonary disease
    10 of 25 cases

Our thanks to Alfred S. Berne, M.D., for the tour.

References: Bein, M. E., Putman, C. E., McLoud, T. C., and Mink, J. H.: Am. J. Roentgenol., *131*:409, 1978; Berne, A. S., Gerle, R. D., and Mitchell, G. E.: Semin. Roentgenol., *4*:3, 1969; Heitzman, E. R.: J. Can. Assoc. Radiol., *29*:151, 1978; Filly, R., Blank, N., and Castellino, R. A.: Radiology, *120*:277, 1976; McLoud, T. C., Kalisher, L., Stark, P., and Greene, R.: Am. J. Roentgenol., *131*:403, 1978.

THE SOLITARY PULMONARY NODULE

A logical approach to the management of the solitary pulmonary nodule will often eliminate the use of unnecessary invasive procedures. The following diagram offers a simple approach based upon whether the patient demonstrates certain symptoms. Some physicians may choose *not* to observe at several points presented in the initial portion of the diagram. The diagram merely offers a logical and reasonable approach adopted by some for evaluating the solitary pulmonary nodule. It is not meant to represent the only approach to this problem.

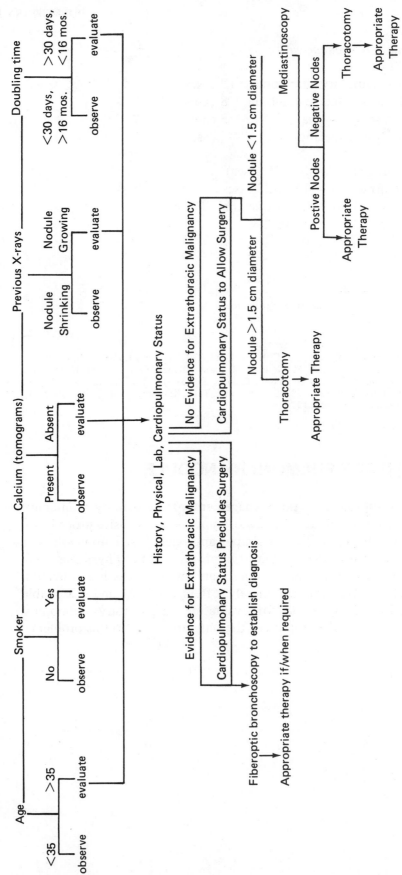

*The Solitary Pulmonary Nodule**

*The use of high resolution, "fast," computerized tomographic analysis adds an additional and probably superior dimension to radiographic analysis.

Reference: Neff, T. A.: Resident and Staff Physician, November 1978, p. 89. Reproduced by permission.

CYSTIC FIBROSIS

Das Kind stirbt bald Wieder
Dessen Stirne beim Kussen Salsig Schmiect (1857)
"The child will soon die, whose brow tastes salty when kissed"

This quotation may be the earliest reference to cystic fibrosis, which is the most frequent lethal genetic syndrome in white children. It is transmitted as an autosomal recessive trait. In recent years, more cystic fibrosis victims are living into adulthood as a result of advances in therapy, and more adults are being diagnosed as having this disorder. About one third of patients seen in cystic fibrosis centers are adults, and in 1976 approximately 2000 adult cases were recognized nationally. Most commonly, cystic fibrosis is manifest by pulmonary disease and malabsorption. Some of the clinical presentations that should suggest cystic fibrosis are listed below.

Gastrointestinal

Pancreatic insufficiency with malabsorption
Cirrhosis of the liver
Portal hypertension
Vitamin A, D, E, K deficiency
Duodenal ulcer
Rectal prolapse
Pancreatitis, acute or recurrent

Pulmonary

Chronic obstructive pulmonary disease — bronchitis or emphysema
Characteristic chest x-ray
Recurrent pulmonary infections
Bronchiectasis
Hemoptysis
Atelectasis
Staphylococcal or pseudomonas pulmonary infection
Pneumothorax
Cor pulmonale

Other

Clubbing
Diabetes mellitus
Nasal polyps
Salty taste of sweat
Hyponatremia
Hypochloremic dehydration in warm weather
Male infertility
Family history

The diagnosis is made by the sweat chloride test. Sweat testing should be performed when any of the above are present and there is no reasonable alternative explanation. The most reliable method for sweat testing is pilocarpine iontophoresis. Values of sweat chloride over 60 mEq/liter are usually diagnostic in children. In adults, values between 60 and 80 mEq/liter are less specific. A positive sweat chloride test may also be observed in untreated adrenal insufficiency, hypothyroidism, and malnutrition.

Treatment consists of vigorous attention to pulmonary toilet, early treatment of pulmonary infection (frequently staphylococcal or pseudomonas), pancreatic enzyme replacement, vitamin supplementation, and regular surveillance for complications.

Reference: Wood, R. E., Boat, T. F., and Doershuk, C. F.: Am. Rev. Respir. Dis., *113*: 833, 1976.

DRUG-INDUCED PULMONARY DISEASE

Responsibility for the prevention and early detection of drug-induced lung disease lies with the physician. Therefore a complete drug history is essential when evaluating the patient with various types of pulmonary disease. Drugs that are capable of inducing such disease are categorized below according to their clinical presentation.

Pulmonary Fibrosis

Melphalan
Nitrofurantoin
Busulfan
Cyclophosphamide
Bleomycin
Methysergide
Ganglionic blocking agents (hexamethonium, mecamylamine, pentolinium)
Pituitary snuff
Radiation
Oxygen (high FIO_2)
Mitomycin C

Pulmonary Edema

Heroin
Methadone
Propoxyphene (Darvon)
Phenylbutazone
Hydrochlorothiazide
Epinephrine
Blood (leukoagglutinins)

Hypersensitivity Pulmonary Infiltrates with Eosinophilia

Penicillin
Isoniazid
Nitrofurantoin
Sulfonamides
Aminosalicylic acid
Chlorpropamide (Diabinese)

Pulmonary Infiltrates without Eosinophilia

Narcotic analgesics
Procarbazine
Azathioprine
Methotrexate
Pituitary snuff
Radiation
Paraquat
Oxygen
Drug-induced SLE*

Mediastinal and Hilar Changes

Diphenylhydantoin (adenopathy)
Methotrexate (adenopathy)
Corticosteroids (lipomatosis)

Bronchoconstriction

Propranolol
Metoprolol
Aspirin
Pituitary snuff
Aerosolized drugs: isoproterenol, disodium cromoglycate (Cromolyn), acetylcysteine (Mucomyst)

Respiratory Muscle Paralysis

Gentamicin
Streptomycin
Kanamycin
Neomycin
Colistin
Polymyxin B
Amikacin
Tobramycin

Pleural Effusion

Nitrofurantoin
Methysergide
Drug-induced SLE*

---

*See Drug-Induced Lupus Syndrome, p. 518.

References: Rosenow, E. C.: Ann. Intern. Med., 77:977, 1972; Rosenow, E. C., Weekly Update: Pulmonary Medicine, Lesson 4. Princeton, N.J., Biomedia, Inc., 1978.

FLOW VOLUME SPIROMETRY FOR THE DIAGNOSIS OF LARGE AIRWAY OBSTRUCTION

Tracheal obstruction can be a difficult condition to diagnose. It can sometimes mimic asthma, although the patients will not respond to antiasthmatic medications. Standard spirometry, in which lung volume is plotted against time, is of no help in finding the site of airway obstruction. Flow volume spirometry, in which maximum expiratory and inspiratory flows are plotted against lung volume during maximally forced inspiration and expiration (a flow volume loop), is a sensitive test for large airway obstruction and can even identify the site of the obstruction (Fig. 6–9). A normal flow volume loop is shown in Figure 6–10. Figure 6–11 illustrates three characteristic flow volume loops produced by major airway lesions.

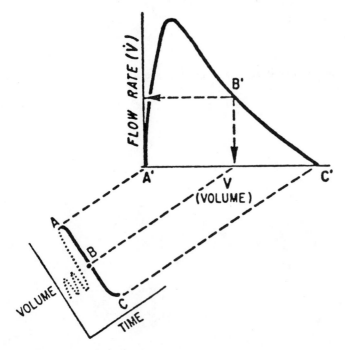

FIG. 6–9

Comparison of standard spirometry with the expiratory flow volume curve.

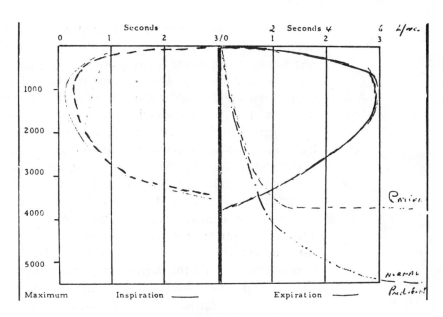

FIG. 6-10

Normal flow volume loop.

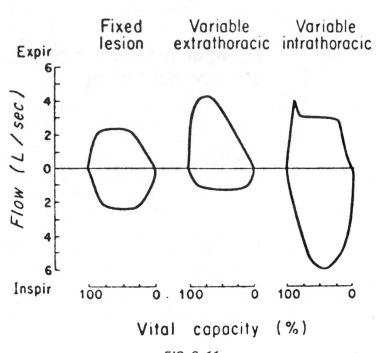

FIG. 6-11

Characteristic flow volume loops produced by major airway obstructive lesions.

Fixed lesions, usually circumferential, produce approximately equal decreases in the plateau and peak flow of both the expiratory and the inspiratory loop. Since fixed lesions have little change in diameter and are not affected by the various transmural pressure gradients, the character of the loops produced by fixed lesions is not influenced by location (i.e., intrathoracic versus extrathoracic). Variable lesions have different diameters during inspiration and expiration and thus have quite different maximal inspiratory and expiratory flows. Variable extrathoracic lesions show more distortion of inspiratory flow, whereas variable intrathoracic lesions display a distortion and reduction in expiratory flow. This difference is understandable if one considers the pressure changes that are produced by spontaneous breathing. During inspiration, intratracheal pressure is less than atmospheric, and thus the extrathoracic trachea will be smaller during inspiration because it is compressed by the surrounding atmospheric pressure. On the other hand, intrathoracic pressure is less than tracheal pressure during inspiration, so the intrathoracic trachea will be larger during inspiration and smaller during expiration.

The size of the trachea at the site of the lesion may be estimated by comparing the flow at the plateau of the patient's flow volume loop to the flows produced by breathing through tubes of known diameter.

Reference: Hyatt, R. E., and Black, L. F.: Am. Rev. Respir. Dis., *107*:191, 1973. Figure 6–11 reproduced with permission of author and publisher.

CLINICAL DIAGNOSIS OF PULMONARY EMBOLISM: MISSION IMPOSSIBLE

Several recent studies of the efficacy of thrombolytic agents in the management of pulmonary embolism have provided a large number of patients with angiographically proven pulmonary emboli for analysis. It is clear from these studies that clinical parameters are *not* reliable in the diagnosis of pulmonary embolization. There is no single sign or symptom or combination of signs and symptoms that is specific for pulmonary embolization. The table below summarizes the incidence of predisposing conditions in 167 patients while the incidence of symptoms and signs in 327 patients with significant degrees of embolization (massive = two or more lobar arteries obstructed; submassive = less than two lobar arteries obstructed) is given in the second table. Those symptoms or signs present in a high percentage of patients are so nonspecific (e.g., respiratory rate >16) they are of no diagnostic value.

Predisposing factors in 167 patients with pulmonary embolization.

Condition	% Total	Condition	% Total
Thrombophlebitis	39.5	Angina	5.4
Venous varicosity and insufficiency	15	Congestive heart failure	17.4
Peripheral arterial disease	4.8	Arrhythmia	16.2
Recent immobilization from fracture (casting)	15	Rheumatic heart disease	1.2
		Other heart disease	9.0
Bed rest	32.4	Primary pulmonary disease	7.8
Recent surgery	31.2		
Recent termination of pregnancy	1.2	Dehydration	3.6
		Diabetes mellitus	8.4
Pelvic disease	6.0	Malignancy	7.2
Obesity	30	Hemoglobinopathy	1.2
Cerebrovascular disease	6.6	Polycythemia	0
Hypertension	10.2	No predisposing etiology	6.0
Nephrotic syndrome	0.6		
Myocardial infarction	12.0		

Signs and symptoms in 327 patients with pulmonary embolization.

Symptoms and Signs	Total Series N = 327 (%)	Massive Emboli N = 197 (%)	Submassive Emboli N = 130 (%)
Symptoms			
Chest pain	88	85	82
Pleuritic	74	64	85*
Nonpleuritic	14	6	8
Dyspnea	84	85	82
Apprehension	59	65	50†
Cough	53	53	52
Hemoptysis	30	23	40*
Sweats	27	29	23
Syncope	13	20	4†
Signs			
Respirations >16/min	92	95	87
Rales	58	57	60
↑S$_2$P	53	58	45‡
Pulse >100/min	44	48	38
Temperature >37.8°C	43	43	42
Phlebitis	32	36	26
Gallop	34	39	25‡
Diaphoresis	36	42	27*
Edema	24	23	25
Murmur	23	27	16‡
Cyanosis	19	25	9†

Table continued on page 220

Symptoms and Signs	Total Series N = 327 (%)	Massive Emboli N = 197 (%)	Submassive Emboli N = 130 (%)
Predisposing condition			
Current venous disease	49	55	47
Immobilization	55	60	46 ‡
Congestive heart failure and chronic lung disease	38	36	40
Malignant neoplasm	6	8	5

NOTE: ↑S_2P = increase in the intensity of the pulmonic component of the second heart sound.
*Statistically significant (p <0.01).
†Statistically significant (p <0.001).
‡Statistically significant (p <0.05).

Reference: Bell, W. R., Simon, T. L., and DeMets, D. L.: Am. J. Med., *62*:355, 1977. Table reproduced with permission of author and publisher.

THE LUNG SCAN

Since the history and clinical examination can only suggest the diagnosis of pulmonary embolus, the physician must use further confirmatory diagnostic studies when he suspects that his patient has had an embolism. Usually radionuclide imaging of the lungs is the diagnostic modality that is chosen first. Two types of lung scan are available. The perfusion lung scan, using technetium-labeled microaggregates of albumin, outlines the distribution of pulmonary blood flow. The ventilation lung scan with radioactive xenon gas gives an idea of the distribution of ventilation throughout the lung during the "wash-in" period as the gas is inhaled and during the "wash-out" period as the gas is exhaled.

A normal perfusion lung scan performed properly with images obtained in four views (anterior, posterior, and both laterals) eliminates the possibility that the patient has had a pulmonary embolism. However, a positive perfusion lung scan — that is, a scan showing areas of lung that are not perfused — does not confirm the diagnosis of pulmonary embolism, since other pathologic conditions can also cause perfusion defects. This problem can be largely eliminated by doing both a ventilation and a perfusion scan. With pulmonary embolization, there will be a perfusion defect without any associated compromise in ventilation. The other conditions that cause perfusion defects will be associated with matching ventilation defects. The accompanying illustration (Fig. 6–12) outlines the various patterns seen with combined ventilation–perfusion lung scans. The characteristics of the isotopes are such that ventilation scanning must be done before the perfusion scan. Therefore, it is probably best to do both scans routinely when the diagnosis of pulmonary embolism is suspected.

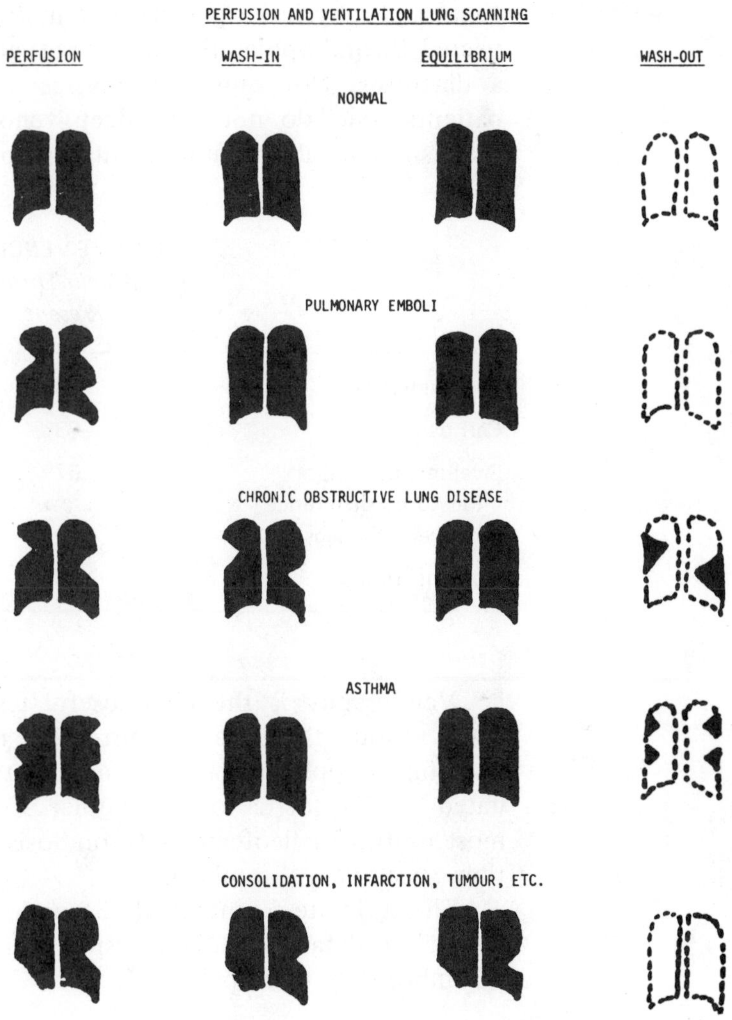

PERFUSION AND VENTILATION LUNG SCANNING

FIG. 6–12

Pulmonary angiography is the definitive diagnostic study for pulmonary embolism. This procedure should be reserved for those cases in which the diagnosis remains in doubt after lung scanning, and major therapeutic decisions must be made (e.g., anticoagulation in a patient with a history of bleeding ulcer, vena cava ligation).

Reference: Thanks to Brian Wistow, M.D., for kindly providing the illustration.

ALL THAT IS SWOLLEN AND TENDER IS NOT THROMBOSED

The diagnosis of thrombophlebitis is frequently made from clinical observations of a patient with a swollen and tender leg. It is now appreciated that symptoms and signs are not reliable for making a diagnosis of thrombophlebitis. The following table summarizes the symptoms and physical signs present in two groups of patients with suspected thrombophlebitis who subsequently had venography to establish a diagnosis. Not only are physical signs and symptoms present in patients who do not have deep venous thrombosis, but frequently these signs are absent in individuals who do have it.

	POSITIVE VENOGRAM (Deep Vein Thrombosis Present)	NEGATIVE VENOGRAM (Deep Vein Thrombosis Absent)
Leg tenderness	73%	44%
Calf pain	83%	85%
Swelling, edema, or measured difference between the legs	67%	55%
Homans' sign	50%	25%

Venography is the most useful test to establish the diagnosis of deep venous thrombosis. Currently, noninvasive tests — fibrinogen scanning, doppler ultrasound, and plethysmography — are being evaluated as diagnostic tools. Doppler studies and plethysmography are most useful for ileofemoral thrombosis but are not accurate for detection of calf vein thrombosis.

The ultimate diagnoses of 235 patients whose venograms were negative (clinical false positive) despite clinical suspicions of deep venous thrombosis are listed below.

Postphlebitic syndrome	60 patients
Congestive heart failure	56 patients
Trauma	37 patients
Malignancy causing obstruction	36 patients
Lymphangitis or cellulitis	17 patients
Arthritis or ruptured Baker's cyst	11 patients
Pregnancy	11 patients
Paralysis	7 patients

Reference: Richards, K. L., Armstrong, J. D., Tikoff, G., et al: Arch. Intern. Med., *136*:1091, 1976.

PLEURAL EFFUSIONS

Transudate vs. Exudate

The examination of pleural fluid often provides useful diagnostic information. There is an old adage in medicine that the sun should never rise or set on an undrained pleural effusion. This approach may be a bit extreme, especially when one considers the fate of many laboratory specimens obtained between sundown and sunrise. The initial examination for a pleural effusion usually consists of cultures, cytology, and a variety of laboratory determinations. Subsequent diagnostic measures and therapy often depend on whether these initial laboratory studies indicate that the fluid is a transudate or an exudate. Cell counts are not particularly useful in distinguishing transudates from exudates. Since it takes leakage of only 2 ml of normal blood into 1000 ml of pleural fluid to make a transudate bloody, the red count is of no use. A leukocyte count greater than 10,000/ml is nearly always associated with an exudative effusion. However, more than 40 per cent of exudates will have a leukocyte count of less than 2,500/ml. Thus, this measurement also seems to be of only limited use.

Simultaneous measurement of serum and pleural fluid protein and LDH can reliably distinguish transudates from exudates. The presence of any one of the following three characteristics indicates that a fluid is an exudate:

1. Ratio of pleural fluid protein to serum protein is greater than 0.5.
2. Pleural fluid LDH level is greater than 200 IU.
3. Pleural fluid LDH to serum LDH ratio is greater than 0.6.

When an exudate is found, further diagnostic studies should be undertaken to establish a definitive diagnosis. Transudates are formed when the mechanical factors influencing pleural fluid balance are altered. The list of conditions that may do this is short and consists of:

1. Congestive heart failure.
2. Cirrhosis.
3. Nephrotic syndrome.
4. Hypoproteinemia.

Tube or No Tube

Most pleural effusions accompanying acute bacterial pneumonia resolve without drainage; however, some do not. If drainage of these effusions is delayed, the patient's hospital stay may be prolonged. In addition, drainage is more complicated, since loculations will have had time to form, and the patient eventually may even require decortication.

If pleural fluid is collected anaerobically, placed on ice, and sent for pH measurement, useful information can be obtained to help determine whether a pleural effusion accompanying a bacterial pneumonia requires tube drainage. If the pleural fluid pH is greater than 7.3, spontaneous resolution is likely. When the pH is less than 7.3, or 0.15 pH units less than a simultaneously measured arterial pH in the presence of systemic acidosis, there is a high probability that tube drainage will be required. Other indications for immediate tube drainage of a parapneumonic effusion include the presence of gross pus or organisms visible on Gram stain or a fluid glucose level of less than 50 mg/100 ml. (Remember that the pleural effusions associated with rheumatoid arthritis also have a low glucose concentration.)

You may also want to consider ultrasonography when faced with a tough differential diagnostic problem that might be solved by obtaining some pleural fluid to examine. With ultrasonography, very small amounts (as little as 5 ml in some cases) of pleural fluid may be detected, localized, and aspirated.

References: Light, R. W., MacGreggor, M. I., Luchsinger, P. C., et al: Ann. Intern. Med., 77:507, 1972; Potts, D. E., Levin, D. C., and Sahn S. A.: Chest, 70:328, 1976; Gryminski, J., Krakowka, P., and Lypacewicz, G.: Chest, 70:33, 1976.

7
DRUGS

THE TOP TEN

Can you guess the ten top-selling prescription drugs of 1977? Compare your list with the list compiled below. It is worth considering the indications for each drug and to speculate why some of the drugs made it to the top ten.

1. Valium
2. Premarin
3. Ampicillin
4. Lasix
5. Tetracycline
6. Darvon Compound-65
7. Librium
8. Empirin Compound with codeine
9. V-Cillin K
10. Aldomet

Reference: Wallechinsky, D., Wallace, I., and Wallace, A.: *The Book of Lists.* New York, Bantam Books, Inc., 1978, pp. 405–406.

7

METABOLIC EFFECTS OF CERTAIN DRUGS

1. **Drugs with a high sodium content**
   Carbenicillin (4.7 mEq/gram)
   Penicillin G (1.7 mEq/million units)
   Ampicillin (3 mEq/gram)
   Cephalothin (2.5 mEq/gram)
   Kayexalate (65 mEq/16 grams)
   Fleet's Phospho-soda (24 mEq/5 ml)
   Antacids (variable amounts of sodium depending on the preparation)

2. **Drugs with a high potassium content**
   Penicillin G (1.7 mEq/million units)
   Salt substitutes

3. **Drugs with a high magnesium content**
   Antacids (absorbable)
   Laxatives

4. **Magnesium depletion**
   Diuretics

5. **Drugs with a high calcium content**
   Antacids (absorbable)

6. **Hypocalcemia**
   Anticonvulsants
   Heparin

7. **Acidosis**
   Methenamine mandelate
   Para-aminosalicylic acid
   Phenformin
   Isoniazid
   Ethanol
   Paraldehyde
   Nitrofurantoin
   Ammonium chloride
   Acetazolamide

8. **Alkalosis**
   Absorbed antacids
   Large doses of penicillin G and carbenicillin

9. **Elevation of the blood urea nitrogen**
   Tetracyclines
   Androgenic steroids
   Glucocorticoids
   Diuretics
   Hydroxyurea

10. **Fluid retention**
    Indomethacin
    Phenylbutazone
    Clofibrate
    Carbamazepine
    Vincristine

Vinblastine
Cyclophosphamide
Chlorpropamide
Thioridazine
Diazoxide
Ibuprofen

11. **Fluid depletion**
Lithium carbonate
Demeclocycline

Reference: Anderson, R. J., Gambertoglio, J. G., and Schrier, R. W.: Fate of drugs in renal failure. In Brenner, B. M., and Rector, F. C. (Eds.): The Kidney. Philadelphia, W. B. Saunders Company, 1976, p. 1917.

DRUG-INDUCED HYPERURICEMIA

The following is a partial list of drugs known to cause an elevation of the serum uric acid.

1. **Acute ethanol ingestion**

2. **Diuretics**
Thiazide diuretics
Ethacrynic acid
Furosemide
Triamterene
Mercurial diuretics
Chlorthalidone

3. **Antibiotics**
Gentamicin
Ethambutol
Pyrazinamide

4. **Antihypertensive drugs**
Diazoxide
Mecamylamine

5. **Sympathomimetic drugs**
Epinephrine
Levarterenol
Angiotensin

6. **Miscellaneous drugs**
Clofibrate
Acetazolamide

Methotrexate (when used for psoriasis)
Nicotinic acid (in large doses)
Salicylates (<4 to 5 grams/day)

Reference: Lipman, A. G.: Modern Medicine, August 1, 1976, p. 101.

ALLOPURINOL WITH 6-MERCAPTOPURINE

Patients being treated with cytotoxic drugs for malignant and non-malignant conditions (i.e., renal transplant recipients) are given allopurinol (Zyloprim) to maintain a normal serum uric acid concentration. Allopurinol competes with hypoxanthine for the enzyme xanthine oxidase and thus prevents the conversion of hypoxanthine to uric acid. By effectively inhibiting xanthine oxidase, allopurinol will also inhibit the metabolism of both azathioprine (Imuran) and 6-mercaptopurine to their inactive metabolite thiouric acid (Fig. 7–1). As a consequence, the duration of action of the active compounds will be prolonged, and the peak serum concentrations of the active parent compounds increase. The result may be severe toxicity in the form of bone marrow suppression with resulting granulocytopenia, thrombocytopenia, anemia, or any combination of the three. Thus it is recommended that the doses of both 6-mercaptopurine and azathioprine be reduced to 25

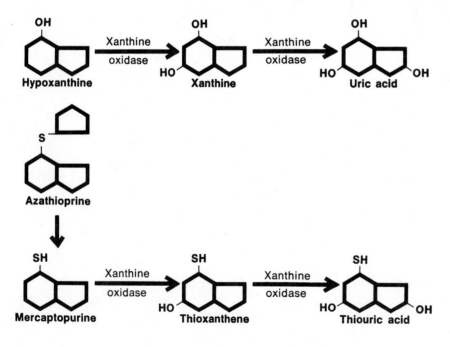

FIG. 7–1

Relation of purine metabolism (top row) to metabolism of azathioprine and mercaptopurine. Allopurinol, by competing for xanthine oxidase, inhibits both metabolic pathways.

per cent of their recommended doses when allopurinol is administered simultaneously.

Reference: Ascione, F. J.: Drug Therapy (Hospital Edition), *3*:69, 1978.

DRUGS INTERACTING WITH COUMARIN ANTICOAGULANTS

Be aware of the drugs that significantly alter the anticoagulant effect of the coumarin derivatives! The intensity of the pharmacologic effect of the coumarins is crucial, since thrombosis or disastrous bleeding may result from an alteration in therapeutic efficacy. The first two tables list drugs that have been clearly shown to interfere with the action of the coumarins in man. Other drugs that may alter the effects of the coumarin compounds based on *in vitro* and animal data or on inconclusive evidence in man are included in the other two tables.

7

	Drugs	Mechanism
	Anabolic steroids	Decrease in circulating vitamin K? Decrease in clotting-factor synthesis? Increase in clotting-factor catabolism?
	Chloral hydrate	Decrease in coumarin albumin binding
	Chloramphenicol	Inhibition of coumarin metabolism
	Clofibrate	Decrease in circulating vitamin K? Decrease in coumarin albumin binding? Inhibition of coumarin metabolism?
Drugs that potentiate coumarin action in man.	Dextrothyroxine	Decrease in circulating vitamin K? Increase in clotting-factor catabolism? Increase in coumarin receptor affinity?
	Glucagon	Decrease in clotting-factor synthesis?
	Mefenamic acid	Decrease in coumarin albumin binding
	Neomycin	Decrease in vitamin K absorption?
	Oxyphenbutazone	Decrease in coumarin albumin binding
	Phenylbutazone	Decrease in coumarin albumin binding
	Phenyramidol	Inhibition of coumarin metabolism
	Quinidine	Decrease in clotting-factor synthesis?
	Salicylate	Decrease in clotting-factor synthesis?

DRUGS	MECHANISM
Barbiturates	Acceleration of coumarin metabolism
Ethchlorvynol	Acceleration of coumarin metabolism?
Glutethimide	Acceleration of coumarin metabolism
Griseofulvin	Inhibition of coumarin absorption? Acceleration of coumarin metabolism?
Heptabarbital	Inhibition of coumarin absorption Acceleration of coumarin metabolism

Drugs that inhibit coumarin action in man.

DRUGS	MECHANISM
Acetaminophen	?
Allopurinol	Inhibition of coumarin metabolism
Diazoxide	Decrease in coumarin albumin binding
Disulfiram	?
Ethacrynic acid	Decrease in coumarin albumin binding
Mercaptopurine	Inhibition of coumarin metabolism ? Decrease in clotting-factor synthesis?
Methylphenidate	Inhibition of coumarin metabolism
Monoamine oxidase inhibitors	?
Nalidixic acid	Decrease in coumarin albumin binding
Nortriptyline	Inhibition of coumarin metabolism
Sulfinpyrazone	Decrease in coumarin albumin binding
Sulfonamides, long acting	Decrease in coumarin albumin binding
Thyroid drugs	Increase in clotting-factor catabolism

Drugs that may potentiate coumarin action in man.

DRUGS	MECHANISM
Adrenocortical steroids	Increase in clotting-factor synthesis?
Cholestyramine	Inhibition of coumarin absorption
Meprobamate	Acceleration of coumarin metabolism
Oral contraceptives	Increase in clotting-factor synthesis?

Drugs that may inhibit coumarin action in man.

Note that only drugs that directly interfere with the prothrombin-complex activity are mentioned here. Many agents may alter hemostasis by mechanisms unrelated to any direct effect on coumarin action (e.g. antiplatelet drugs, hepatotoxins), and these agents are *not* listed.

References: Koch-Weser, J., and Sellers, E. M.: New Engl. J. Med., *285*:548, 1971; Tables reproduced by permission of author and The New England Journal of Medicine. Bernstein, D.: Drug. Intell. Clin. Pharm., *8*:172, 1974.

"MINIDOSE" HEPARIN

Several large clinical studies have demonstrated the ability of low doses of subcutaneous heparin to significantly reduce the incidence of postoperative deep vein thrombosis (DVT). The amount of bleeding produced by heparin administration in these studies was not considered excessive. By reducing the incidence of DVT, it is hoped that the mortality rate of pulmonary thromboembolism will be decreased.

The following lists give the current recommendations regarding the use of "minidose" (i.e., low dose) heparin prophylaxis against DVT in surgical patients and the other clinical circumstances that warrant consideration of "minidose" heparin administration.

Minidose Heparin in Surgical Patients

1. Administer low-dose heparin to all patients who have *no* preexisting defects in their coagulation system, are *over 40*, and are to undergo major elective abdominal or thoracic surgical procedures.

2. The low-dose heparin regimen is of *limited prophylactic value* in the following:
    a. Repair of femoral fractures.
    b. Hip and knee joint reconstruction.
    c. Open prostatectomy

3. Low-dose heparin is currently *not* recommended for these operations:
    a. On the eye.
    b. On the brain.
    c. With spinal anesthesia.
    d. Transurethral prostatectomy

4. The low-dose heparin program consists of administering *5,000* USP *units* of heparin subcutaneously *two hours prior* to surgery and then *every 12 hours* while the patient is bedridden.

5. No laboratory testing is necessary to determine dosage or to establish anticoagulant effect.

Other Clinical Circumstances in Which Minidose Heparin May Be of Value

1. During hospitalization for *myocardial infarction.*
2. For control of venous thromboembolism in *pregnancy.*
3. In patients with *chronic venous insufficiency* of the lower extremities.
4. In patients with *congestive heart failure.*
5. In any *bedridden patient without* specific *contraindication* to low-dose *heparin* administration.

References: Thomas, D. P.: Semin. Hematol., *15*:1, 1978; American Heart Association, Council on Thrombosis: Circulation, *55*:423A, 1977.

THE REAL MAGIC BULLET...
GENUINE CHICKEN SOUP

Please note: All measurements are approximate. All seasonings are discretionary. Cook over heat of your choice. There are only two absolute caveats:

1. The recipe only works on Friday, and all cooking must be concluded by sundown; otherwise the magic is lost.
2. It is heretical to employ microwave ovens in the preparation of this soup.

Put one very, very, fresh whole cleaned pullet into 6 cups of water (more or less) and bring to a boil. Skim the top of the water. Add about 1 tablespoon of coarse salt (Rokeach or equivalent) and bring to a boil for about a half hour. Then simmer for 30 to 35 or 40 minutes with the pot covered.

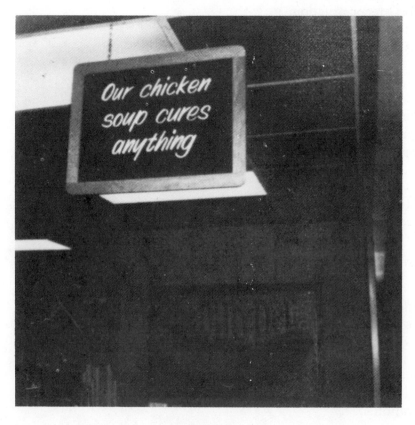

FIG. 7–2

"Our chicken soup cures anything" (photographed in the Sheraton Hotel's Dilly Deli, Toronto, October 1975).

Now add a carrot or so, an onion, a parsnip, one leek, and about one stalk of celery tied together (cotton twine only). Boil 1 hour. Add some dill, parsley, greens, a touch of pepper, and a smidge of nutmeg. Boil for about a half hour more. Remove the vegetables tied with twine, and remove the pullet (you can eat this, too).

(*Editor's note:* Best as chicken salad!)

Serve heated to a near boil for best results!

Reference: Begun, P., et al., as told to Gottlieb, D., and as transcribed by Gottlieb, C. (*Editor's note:* I never did like it! Sorry, Mom!) Fig. 7–2 reproduced with permission of author. From Mason, D.: Chest, *71*:122, 1977.

SAY CHEESE!

(Vasoactive Amines, Monoamine Oxidase Inhibitors, and Diet)

Tyramine and other amines may displace epinephrine and norepinephrine from sympathetic nerve endings and result in sympathetic discharge. As a result, hypertension, sweating, chest pain, flushing, headache, and palpitations may ensue. A number of drugs in current use are monoamine oxidase inhibitors. These drugs are listed below.

Since ingested amines are normally inactivated by monoamine oxidase in the gastrointestinal tract and liver, the simultaneous administration of these drugs and foods rich in amines may precipitate an untoward reaction. In general, the amine content of food increases with fermentation. Some foods in the fresh or unripened state contain a low amine content. The amines will increase significantly when the food ferments, ripens, or is exposed to air for a period of time. A list of foods containing high tyramine content is provided.

Should adverse reactions occur, a short-acting alpha adrenergic–blocking agent, such as phentolamine (Regitine), may be used for treatment of the hypertensive crisis in patients taking monoamine oxidase inhibitors. The use of sympathetic amines (i.e., dopa, dopamine, amphetamine) should be avoided in patients taking monoamine oxidase inhibitors.

Some Monoamine Oxidase Inhibitors

Psychiatry	*Hypertension*
Isocarboxazid (Marplan)	Pargyline (Eutonyl)
Phenelzine (Nardil)	
Tranylcypromine (Parnate)	
Iproniazid (Marsilid)	

Cancer	*Infectious Disease*
Procarbazine (Matulane)	Furazolidone (Furoxone)
	Isoniazid

Foods Containing Tyramine

> Ripened cheeses (e.g., cheddar, gruyere, Stilton, Brie, and Camembert; unripened cheeses, such as cottage cheese, cream cheese, and yogurt, contain low levels of amines until they are allowed to ferment for extended periods)
>
> Dried salted herring or vacuum packaged herring left open for two hours
>
> Fermented sausage (bologna, salami, pepperoni)
>
> Unrefrigerated chicken liver
>
> Beer (variable)
>
> Red wines
>
> Sherry
>
> Bananas (ripe)
>
> Avocados
>
> Canned figs
>
> Chocolate
>
> Fava beans

References: Horowitz, D., Lovenberg, W., Engelman, K. and Sjoerdsma, A.: J.A.M.A., *188*: 1108, 1964; Marley, E., and Blackwell, B.: Adv. Pharmacol. Chemother., *8*:185, 1970; Smith, C. K., and Durack, D. T.: Ann. Intern. Med., *88*:520, 1978.

NARCOTICS

	EQUIANALGESIC DOSE (mg)*	USUAL ADULT DOSE (mg)*	ORAL-PARENTERAL EFFICACY RATIO	AVERAGE DURATION OF ACTION (hrs)	SUGGESTED ROUTES OF ADMINISTRATION
Morphine	10	10–15	low (1/6)	4–5	IM, SC, IV, PO
Hydromorphone (Dilaudid)	1.5	1.5–2	probably low	3–4	IM, SC, IV, PO
Oxymorphone (Numorphan)	1	1–1.5	1/6	4–6	IM, SC, IV, PR
Methadone (Dolophine)	8–10	5–15	high (1/2)	4–6	IM, SC, PO
Levorphanol (Levo-Dromoran)	2	2–3	high (1/2)	4–6	IM, SC, PO
Meperidine (Demerol)	75–100	50–100	moderate (1/3–1/4)	3	IM, SC, IV, PO

*Equianalgesic dose when compared with morphine, 10 mg given subcutaneously.

Notes on narcotics:

1. All of the narcotics listed above can be given IM or SC and produce a qualitatively similar level of analgesia in equianalgesic doses.

2. With the exception of oxymorphone, all of the compounds listed are available for oral administration. When given orally they are less potent because inconstant absorption and intestinal metabolism result in lower plasma levels. Onset of action is delayed and peak levels reduced following oral administration. Methadone and levorphanol retain about 50 per cent of their potency when given orally and stand out as the preferred oral agents. Meperidine retains 1/3 its activity, while morphine and hydromorphone have the lowest oral potency.

3. Rectal administration produces a somewhat lower peak activity, with a longer duration of action than parenteral therapy. While hydromorphone and oxymorphone are available commercially for rectal administration, other narcotics may be prepared for administration by suppository. The rectal route should be considered for the therapy of chronic, severe pain.

4. In equianalgesic doses, the side effects of the various narcotics are fairly similar. Hydromorphone, methadone, and meperidine produce less sedation. Oxymorphone produces the greatest degree of respiratory depression and, with morphine, the most emesis. The least antitussive activity is seen with meperidine and hydromorphone, which are also the least constipating.

References: Catalano, R. B.: Semin. Oncology, *2*:379, 1975; Marks, R. M., and Sachar, E. J.: Ann. Intern. Med., *78*:173, 1973.

Narc — The short, colloquial, and somewhat derogatory form for the narcotics officer has an obvious derivation. The Greek root, *narke* means "numbness," and also serves as the parent of "Narcissus." Narcissus was the rather self-centered young man who spurned the advances of Echo. Poor Echo was the young lady punished for speaking too much by being permitted only to repeat the last word spoken to her. The impeded girl ultimately vanished. Only her voice remains. In the meantime, Narcissus discovered his reflection in the spring and died of exhaustion and longing while gazing at it. The flowers that bear his name are his last remains.

HYPNOTISM AND MORPHINE

Hypnos (the god of sleep) lives in the underworld realm of Hades with his brother, Thanatos (death). Both Hypnos and Thanatos are usually portrayed as winged spirits. Hypnos brings on sleep by touching the foreheads of the weary with a magic wand or by fanning them with his wings. His son, Morpheus, is the god of dreams.

METHADONE MANAGEMENT OF THE HOSPITALIZED NARCOTIC ADDICT

The Food and Drug Administration allows a physician to give methadone to a narcotic addict when the addict is admitted to the hospital for treatment of a medical condition other than addiction. An approach to the management of the hospitalized narcotic addict is given in the table on the following page.

7

Management of the Narcotic Addict

PATIENT ENROLLED IN A METHADONE MAINTENANCE PROGRAM	STREET ADDICT *(Patient stating or demonstrating addiction to narcotics but who is not enrolled in a drug abuse program)*

1. Communicate with the patient's program counselor promptly to ascertain enrollment and maintenance dose of methadone.

2. Do not try to alter the treatment for addiction in a patient enrolled in a maintenance program.

3. Administer orally once daily same dose of methadone as patient is receiving in the maintenance program.

4. At discharge, patient should return to his program.

5. If parenteral drug required, administer methadone IM or SQ in a daily dose 2/3 maintenance dose. It should be divided into 2 equal doses 12 hrs apart.

1. Support the patient's addiction to narcotics until the acute phase of the illness is over.

2. If the patient has fresh needle tracks and a positive urine test for morphine or quinine, begin methadone therapy: 10 mg orally once daily.

3. If doubt exists as to whether patient is an addict, you may decide to observe for signs of withdrawal and then administer methadone.

Sign	Initial methadone dose
Lacrimation, rhinorrhea diaphoresis, yawning, restlessness, insomnia (Grade I)	5 mg
Dilated pupils, piloerection, muscle twitching, myalgia, arthralgia, abdominal pain (Grade II)	10 mg
Tachycardia, hypertension, tachypnea, fever, anorexia, nausea, severe restlessness (Grade III)	15 mg
Diarrhea, vomiting, dehydration, hyperglycemia, hypotension, curled-up position (Grade IV)	20 mg

4. Add an additional 5 to 10 mg orally if withdrawal symptoms are not suppressed.

5. The usual stable dose in a street addict is 10 to 30 mg daily given in divided doses.

6. At discharge, the addict has 3 options:
   a. Enroll in a drug abuse program.
   b. Undergo detoxification in the hospital.
   c. Return to the street.

7. It is illegal for the hospital physician to continue to supply methadone once the treatment period is over.

Additional management points:

1. For analgesia, usual doses of hydromorphone or meperidine or morphine should be used in addition to the maintenance dose of methadone.

2. Pentazocine should *not* be used for analgesia as it may precipitate withdrawal owing to its properties as a narcotic antagonist.

3. Naloxone is the drug of choice for narcotic intoxication and/or overdose. The dose is 0.4 mg intravenously. It can be given safely every five minutes until signs of intoxication are reversed.

4. In an addict abusing multiple drugs, each withdrawal component can be treated separately—
   e.g. narcotic (methadone)
   barbiturate (phenobarbital)
   alcohol (chlordiazepoxide)

Reference: Fultz, J. M., and Senay, E. C.: Ann. Intern. Med., *82*:815, 1975.

THE HIGH COST OF A LOW URIC ACID

The benefits that result from the treatment of asymptomatic hyperuricemia have not been clearly documented. The cost of therapy with allopurinol is clear, however. It is estimated that during a 35-year course of therapy some 38,325 tablets would be ingested. At 1978 prices the cost of allopurinol is $110 per year. When the interest (at 7 per cent) that might be paid on $110 set aside each year is added to the cost of a lifetime of therapy, the total cost of therapy is almost $20,000. Not included in this estimate are physician fees and laboratory charges, transportation to the pharmacy, and the effects of inflation.

References: Liang, M., and Fries, J. F.: Ann. Intern. Med., *88*:666, 1978; Ann. Intern. Med., *89*:427, 1978.

CORTICOSTEROID PREPARATIONS

Corticosteroids are used in a myriad of conditions. *They are used in physiologic doses for replacement in adrenal insufficiency and in pharmacologic doses for their anti-inflammatory and immunosuppressive properties.*

Though the glucocorticoids may differ in anti-inflammatory potency by a factor of 25, there is no difference among them in efficacy if appropriate equivalent dosages are prescribed. In patients with hepatic disease who may be unable to adequately metabolize prednisone to its active form, prednisolone itself should be used. In the following table, the equivalent anti-inflammatory potency, biologic half-life, mineralocorticoid potency, and equivalent doses of commonly used steroid preparations are compared.

COMPOUND	EQUIVALENT DOSES (anti-inflammatory)	MINERALO-CORTICOID POTENCY	BIOLOGIC HALF-LIFE (hrs)
Cortisone	25 mg	0.8	8–12
Hydrocortisone (Cortisol)	20 mg	1.0	8–12
Prednisone	5 mg	0.8	12–36
Prednisolone	5 mg	0.8	12–36
Methyl-prednisolone	4 mg	0	12–36
Triamcinolone	4 mg	0	24–48
Dexamethasone	0.75 mg	0	24–48
Betamethasone	0.6 mg	0	—

References: Fauci, A. S., Dale, D. C., and Balow, J. E., Ann. Intern. Med., *84*:304, 1976; Axelrod, L.: Medicine, *55*:39, 1976; The Medical Letter, *17*:99, 1975; Harris, J.: Steroid Biochem., *6*:711, 1975.

STOPPING STEROIDS

The chronic administration of glucocorticoids results in suppression of the hypothalamic-pituitary-adrenal axis. In turn, adrenal suppression results in both inadequate ACTH production during stress and inadequate adrenal production of steroids consequent to adrenal atrophy. The steroid dose, frequency, route, and the duration of therapy determine the degree of adrenal suppression. Doses of less than 40 mg prednisone (or its equivalent) for less than a week or alternate-day therapy with less than 40 mg prednisone do not usually produce adrenal hypofunction following cessation of therapy. Short-term treatment with higher doses or long-term treatment with lower doses may result in pituitary-adrenal suppression. Return of normal adrenal function after long-term exogenous therapy with corticosteroids may take up to nine months after steroids are stopped.

Sudden withdrawal of prolonged or high-dose steroid therapy may produce signs and symptoms of acute adrenal insufficiency. Steroid withdrawal symptoms include fatigue, weakness, anorexia, nausea, postural hypotension and dizziness, fainting, dyspnea, and arthralgias. Hypoglycemia, hyponatremia, hyperkalemia, azotemia, and eosinophilia may also be found.

Recovery of complete hypothalamic-pituitary-adrenal function is prolonged after steroid withdrawal. During this time patients may require maintenance physiologic glucocorticoid replacement (20 to 30 mg of hydrocortisone) and supplementation during stress (e.g., illness, surgery), when the adrenal would ordinarily increase steroid output under the influence of increased ACTH. The pituitary recovers its ability to increase ACTH with stress sooner than the adrenal cortex recovers the complete ability to respond. Thus recovery of the pituitary-adrenal axis is usually complete when normal responsiveness of the adrenal to exogenous ACTH is demonstrated.

Most patients, disease activity permitting, can be slowly weaned from corticosteroids by a gradual tapering of dose and/or use of an alternate-day schedule of administration. Steroid supplementation may still be necessary in times of stress. Occasionally a patient will demonstrate profound signs and symptoms of steroid withdrawal. The following protocol has been recommended for these patients or those with severe pituitary-adrenal suppression.

1. Reduce the therapeutic doses of steroids gradually to a physiologic dose (20 mg hydrocortisone, 5 mg prednisone, 0.75 mg dexamethasone). This can be done only if the disease for which the steroid is being used is under control.

2. Begin 20 mg hydrocortisone (which is a short-acting steroid) each morning. Instruct the patient that the physiologic steroid requirement will be higher during stress.

a. Minor stress — e.g., Upper respiratory infection (URI) — 50 mg hydrocortisone in divided dosage.

b. Major infections — e.g., influenza, strep pharyngitis, otitis media, minor surgical procedures — 100 mg hydrocortisone (as 50 mg BID).

c. Major stress — e.g., pneumonia, major trauma, surgery — 200 to 250 mg hydrocortisone daily (given QID) until stress is resolved; then tapering doses back to maintenance after one week. The patient should keep a supply of parenteral dexamethasone at home, which may be used in the event of vomiting or inability to sustain oral therapy.

3. When the daily dose is 20 mg hydrocortisone, measure 8 a.m. plasma cortisol with the morning hydrocortisone dose omitted. Normal baseline 8 a.m. plasma cortisol is 5 to 25 $\mu g/100$ ml. If plasma cortisol is less than 10 $\mu g/100$ ml, then reduce the daily dose of hydrocortisone by 2.5 mg each week until the daily dose is 10 mg each morning; then measure the 8 a.m. plasma cortisol again. When the 8 a.m. plasma cortisol is greater than 10 $\mu g/100$ ml, stop maintenance hydrocortisone, since baseline pituitary-adrenal function is adequate. The patient will need supplementation for stress at this time, since adequacy of adrenal responsiveness to stress has not been tested.

4. If plasma cortisol is >10 $\mu g/100$ ml. without replacement, do an ACTH or cosyntropin stimulation test to check the responsiveness of the adrenal. Since adrenal responsiveness occurs after pituitary function has recovered, an adequate response implies that the pituitary-adrenal axis will respond normally to stress.

The following simple stimulation test is suggested:

1. Measure baseline plasma cortisol.
2. 0.25 mg synthetic ACTH (cosyntropin) is given IM.
3. Plasma cortisol is measured 30 to 60 minutes later. If plasma cortisol rises by 6 $\mu g/100$ ml and to more than 20 $\mu g/100$ ml, response to stimulation is normal and steroid supplementation for stress can be stopped. If the response is not normal, the patient should continue to receive supplementation for stress. Despite this approach, some patients may require stress supplementation at a later time or develop manifestation of chronic adrenal insufficiency. If this occurs, a more thorough evaluation of the pituitary-adrenal function is indicated (e.g., insulin tolerance test).

7

Reference: Byyny, R. L.: New Engl. J. Med., *295*:30, 1976.

WHEN YOUR PATIENT SHOULDN'T TAKE ASPIRIN

Patients often do not know when they are taking aspirin. When asked, they will answer "no" in all sincerity. Owing to the anti-platelet effect of aspirin, they are generally contraindicated in the thrombocytopenic or anticoagulated patient or in the presence of pre-existing bleeding disorders. A list of common preparations containing acetylsalicylic acid (aspirin) is provided.

Alka-Seltzer
Anacin
APC
Aspergum
Ascriptin
Bayer
BC (tablets and powder)
Bufferin
Calurin
Cope
Coricidin
Dolor

Ecotrin
Empirin Compound
Excedrin
Fiorinal
Fizrin
Measurin
Percodan
Sine-Aid
Stanback (tablets and powder)
Trigesic
Vanquish

Reference: Ted Tse, C. S.: Drug Intell. Clin. Pharm., *12*:464, 1978.

THE "PROOF" IS IN THE PUDDING

Ethyl alcohol has been included in the medical pharmacopeia for centuries. Today alcohol is frequently an ingredient in both prescribed and proprietary medications. In some, the alcoholic content can reach as high as 45 per cent (90 proof). Knowledge of the alcohol content in these preparations is essential when prescribing for the patient addicted to alcohol, for the patient taking disulfiram (Antabuse), or for the patient in whom alcohol may interfere with the desired effect of a concurrent medication. Below is a list of medications having an unusually high alcoholic content.

DRUG	PER CENT ALCOHOL
Alurate elixir	20.0
Aromatic elixir	22.0
Tincture belladonna	67.0
Benadryl elixir	14.0
Broudecon elixir	20.0
Choledyl elixir	20.0
Donnatal elixir	23.0
Elixophyllin	20.0
Nyquil Cough Syrup	25.0
Tincture paregoric	45.0
Phenobarbital elixir	14.0
Terpin Hydrate elixir	42.0
Theolixir	20.0
Mouthwashes (Scope, Listerine, Cepacol, Colgate 100, Micrin)	15.0–25.0

Reference: Patient Care, *13*:103, 1979.

7

> *Intoxicate* — The Greek word *toxon* meant "bow," and the poison used to tip the arrows was the *toxikon. Toxicum* became the Latin word for any poison. Finally, we have self-poisoning — intoxicate.

ALLERGY TO LOCAL ANESTHETICS, OR IS BITING THE BULLET EVER NECESSARY?

Many people report a history of allergy to local anesthetic agents and, as a result, have to endure minor surgical procedures without anesthetic or are subjected to an otherwise unnecessary general anesthetic. Actually, very few of the adverse reactions to local anesthetics are allergic; instead, they are due to sympathetic stimulation, vasovagal reactions, hyperventilation, or local responses to the trauma of the procedure. In addition, toxic reactions can occur if large amounts of a drug are absorbed into the circulation.

An approach to the management of local anesthetic allergy is outlined below. Since there are two unrelated classes of local anesthetic agents, you can use an agent from the other group if the available information clearly identifies a particular agent as the one producing the prior reaction. Local infiltration of 1 per cent diphenhydramine usually provides acceptable anesthesia for skin but not for dental procedures. Finally, skin testing and progressive challenge with lidocaine may be employed as outlined.

Management of Adverse Reactions to Local Anesthetic Agents

1. Use of chemically unrelated agents: Generic and proprietary names of some representative drugs:

Para-aminobenzoic acid esters:	*Miscellaneous group:*
Procaine (Novocain)	Lidocaine (Xylocaine)
Tetracaine (Pontocaine)	Mepivacaine (Carbocaine)
Butyl aminobenzoate (Benzocaine)	Dibucaine (Nupercaine)

2. Use of diphenhydramine (Benadryl) 1% (10 mg/ml).
3. Skin testing and progressive challenge with lidocaine:
   a. prick test with lidocaine 1%, diluted 1:100.
   b. prick test with lidocaine 1%, full strength.
   c. intradermal skin test with 0.02 ml lidocaine 1% diluted 1:100.
   d. intradermal skin test with 0.02 ml lidocaine 1% full strength.
   e. subcutaneous injection of 0.1 ml lidocaine 1%.
   f. subcutaneous injection of 0.5 ml lidocaine 1%.
   (Injections to be at 20 minute intervals unless the history suggests a delayed reaction; in the latter case, there should be a delay of 24 hours between steps *d* and *e*, and a similar delay after step *f* before further administration of local anesthetic.)

Reference: Nelson, H. S.: Advances in Asthma and Allergy, *3*:29, 1976. Parts reprinted with permission of the author and the publisher.

GUIDE TO SKIN TESTING FOR PENICILLIN ALLERGY

Many people think that they are allergic to penicillin, although only about 25 per cent of those claiming penicillin allergy are actually at risk of a serious immediate reaction. Since penicillin is superior to the alternative antibiotics in many clinical situations, it is often important to separate those individuals who are indeed at risk of an anaphylactic reaction from those who may be safely given penicillin. Skin testing using both penicilloyl-polylysine (PRE-PEN) and a dilute solution of penicillin G (10,000 units/ml in normal saline) is a reliable method for detection of sensitivity to "minor determinants" (antigenic sites other than the penicilloyl determinant) and to the penicilloyl moiety. These skin tests do not predict the occurrence of other penicillin reactions, such as serum sickness, drug fever, interstitial nephritis, or exfoliative dermatitis.

Since anaphylaxis does sometimes occur after intradermal skin testing, the less sensitive scratch test should be done before the intradermal injections. The scratch test is performed by placing a drop of each reagent (PRE-PEN and the dilute solution of penicillin G) on the forearm and scratching the skin through the drop with a 26-gauge needle. The scratch test is positive if there is any induration around the scratch marks persisting longer than 20 minutes. The intradermal test should not be performed if the scratch test is positive.

When the scratch test is negative, you can then perform the intradermal test with each reagent by raising in duplicate (i.e., two blebs with each reagent) a 3 mm *intradermal* bleb with 0.02 to 0.04 ml of each reagent. The test is positive when there is greater than 5 mm of induration at 20 minutes. The presence or absence of erythema is not considered when interpreting the test. If the duplicate tests for each reagent do not agree, the test for the reagent should be repeated.

If the test with *either* reagent is positive, the patient should not be given any penicillin or cephalosporin drug without prior desensitization. Concurrent antihistamine therapy may result in false negative skin tests, but moderate corticosteroid therapy will not affect the skin test response.

Reference: Adkinson, N. F.: Resident and Staff Physician, August 1977, p. 55; Penicillin Allergy, Medical Letter, *20*:13, 1978.

SENSITIVITY TO RADIOGRAPHIC CONTRAST MEDIUM

One to two per cent of patients will experience symptoms suggestive of an allergic reaction shortly after receiving an intravenous or arterial injection of radiographic contrast material. Approximately one in 50,000 patients will die following use of these agents. The mechanism of these reactions is unknown, although available data suggest that it is not immunologically mediated. Injection of a small initial test dose before giving a bolus of contrast medium has not been shown to be useful in selecting out those patients who will develop reactions. Patients with a personal history of allergy do have a greater incidence of immediate reactions than normal patients, although they do not have a higher incidence of serious and fatal reactions.

An especially difficult problem is the patient who has a history of a previous reaction to contrast medium and needs another study using such an agent. Patients who have previously had nausea and vomiting may be restudied without increased risk of an immediate generalized reaction. Patients who have had an immediate generalized reaction, such as urticaria, asthma, shock, or cardiac arrest, are at a high risk of having a recurrence. The repeat reactions are usually identical to the previously recorded reaction and not more severe. One approach to this problem is the following:

1. Prednisone, 50 mg orally every 6 hours beginning 18 hours prior to the study.
2. Diphenhydramine, 50 mg intramuscularly one hour prior to the study.

Of course the risk and potential benefits of the procedure should be clear to both physician and patient, and the potential substitution of other modalities examined, before embarking on such an undertaking.

Reference: Patterson, R., and Schatz, M.: J. Allergy Clin. Immunol., *50*:328, 1975.

DRUGS AND ACUTE INTERMITTENT PORPHYRIA

Acute intermittent porphyria has varied clinical manifestations. Painful abdominal crises, tachycardia, neurologic dysfunction (including peripheral neuropathy, seizures and coma), postural hypotension, hyponatremia, and dark urine may be present. Death may occur from an unrelenting attack. What precipitates the acute attack is not always known, but in many cases exposure to a drug is responsible. When confronted with a patient with a compatible clinical presentation after a drug exposure, you should consider porphyria. It is equally important to avoid the use of drugs that may precipitate an acute attack in the patient or family members of the patient with diagnosed porphyria. The patient should be provided with a list of drugs that are safe and unsafe for use, both for his own information and in case he requires medical care from providers who are not familiar with precipitating drugs. Drugs are listed in three categories.

1. Those that have been implicated in precipitating acute attacks of acute intermittent porphyria:

Barbiturates
Sulfonamides
Griseofulvin (Fulvicin, Grifulvin)
Chlordiazepoxide (Librium)
Meprobamate (Miltown)
Isopropylmeprobamate (Soma)
Diphenylhydantoin (Dilantin)
Methsuximide (Celontin)
Dichloralphenazone (Midrin)
Glutethimide (Doriden)
Pyrazolone compounds such as amidopyrine, anti-pyrine, isopropylantipyrine, and dipyrone
Methyprylon (Noludar)
Sulfonal
Trional
Imipramine (Tofranil)
Ergot preparations
Eucalyptol
Possibly tolbutamide (Orinase)

2. Drugs that produce significant porphyria in one or more experimental systems but have not been unequivocally implicated in producing clinical disease:

Mephenytoin (Mesantoin)
Phensuximide (Milontin)
Chloramphenicol (Chloromycetin)
2-Allyloxy-3-methylbenzamide

3. Drugs that are safe or probably safe for use in a patient with porphyria:

Morphine group
Hyoscine
Methadone
Codeine
Chloral hydrate
Meperidine (Demerol)
Penicillin (penicillin G, ampicillin, cloxacillin)
Streptomycin
Tetracyclines (chlortetracycline, oxytetracycline, tetracycline)
Chloramphenicol (Chloromycetin)
Furadantin
Mandelamine
Corticosteroids

Rauwolfia alkaloids
Guanethidine
Diphenhydramine (Benadryl)
Promethazine (Phenergan)
Promazine (Sparine)
Chlorpromazine (Thorazine)
Trifluoperazine (Stelazine)
Proclorperazine (Compazine)
Meclizine (Bonadoxin, Bonine)
Vitamin B group
Vitamin C
Digoxin
Mersalyl
Atropine
Prostigmine
Neostigmine
Tetraethylammonium bromide
Propoxyphene (Darvon)
Diazepam (Valium)

Reference: Tschudy, D. P., Valsamis, M., and Magnussen, C. R.: Ann. Intern. Med., *83*: 851, 1975.

HOW TO CONVERT

The administration of medication on the basis of body surface area rather than weight tends to reduce marked variations in dose produced by body habitus. A nomogram relating these parameters and based on the formula of DuBois and DuBois was designed by Bothby and Sandiford to facilitate the necessary calculations and has been extensively reproduced. The DuBois' formula is:

$$\text{Body surface area (square meters)} = \text{weight (kg)}^{0.425} \times \text{height (cm)}^{0.725} \times 0.007184$$

It has recently been asserted that the body surface area curve has been shifted upward in some nomograms. This results in an underestimation of the body surface area by 8 per cent. You may check the nomogram provided by applying the equation.

If you'd like to know roughly what an equivalent dose per square meter of body surface area (BSA) would be in an adult, multiply the per kg dose by 37.5. For example, a 100 kg adult being treated at 1 mg/kg is receiving approximately 37.5 mg/meter^2 BSA.

Reference: Turcotte, G.: New Engl. J. Med., *300*:1339, 1979.

THE SHOT DOCTOR (Or "Give Me a Shot, Doc")

In 1975, there were an estimated 567 million office visits to the physician in the United States. Of these, approximately 14 per cent resulted in the administration of an injection for therapeutic purposes. The drugs most frequently administered by injection in the ambulatory setting from July 1976 to June 1977 are shown in the following table.

DRUG	PER CENT OF INJECTIONS (71,329 Total Injections)
Penicillin G	17
Corticosteroids	14
Allergens	14
Insulin	7
Vitamin B_{12}	6
Estrogens	4
Local anesthetics, nonsurgical	4
Antineoplastics	3
ACTH	2
B-complex vitamins	2
Tetracyclines	2
Ampicillin	1
Progestins	1
Androgens	1

7

Administration of other antibiotics, tranquilizers, analgesics, antinauseants, diuretics, iron, antihistamines, and liver extracts account for the majority of the remaining injections.

The primary reasons for injection are the desire to have rapid, complete bioavailability of the drug administered so as to provide high blood levels promptly and to assure compliance with the therapeutic plan. Consequently, one must question the *therapeutic indications* for *injections* of many of the drugs on the list. Some do not satisfy the former rationale, because of difficulties with absorption. Although all may satisfy the latter indication, is administration of the specific drugs indicated for the problem confronting the physician?

The self-assessment quiz on the following page may help guide the discerning physician regarding the appropriateness of his injection strategies.

Is Your Shot Therapy on Target?

Try This Self-Assessment Test

1. Do you prescribe injections rather than oral medications when there's a choice?

☐ **A.** generally
☐ **B.** frequently
☐ **C.** occasionally
☐ **D.** never

2. Do you use injections for placebo effect?

☐ **A.** frequently
☐ **B.** occasionally
☐ **C.** never

3. Do you often initiate long-term injection therapy for patients?

☐ **A.** yes
☐ **B.** no

4. If a new patient wants an injection, do you acquiesce as long as its not contraindicated — even though you might consider it optional?

☐ **A.** generally
☐ **B.** frequently
☐ **C.** occasionally
☐ **D.** never

5. Do you periodically attempt to discontinue long-term injection therapy and substitute oral medication or no medication?

☐ **A.** yes
☐ **B.** no

6. Do patients often get injections from your nurse without seeing you?

☐ **A.** yes
☐ **B.** no

7. What percentage of your gross income comes from injections?

☐ **A.** under 5%
☐ **B.** 5 to 10%
☐ **C.** 11 to 15%
☐ **D.** 16 to 20%
☐ **E.** over 20%

Do You Follow These Shot Routines in Specific Situations?

8. Antibiotic injection for suspected strep throat

☐ **A.** generally
☐ **B.** sometimes
☐ **C.** rarely
☐ **D.** no

9. Antibiotic injection for probable viral URIs

☐ **A.** generally
☐ **B.** sometimes
☐ **C.** rarely
☐ **D.** no

10. Vitamins for poor nutrition

☐ **A.** generally
☐ **B.** sometimes
☐ **C.** rarely
☐ **D.** no

11. Vitamins for fatigue

☐ **A.** generally
☐ **B.** sometimes
☐ **C.** rarely
☐ **D.** no

12. Female hormones for menopausal syndrome

☐ **A.** generally
☐ **B.** sometimes
☐ **C.** rarely
☐ **D.** no

13. Male hormones for impotence

☐ **A.** generally
☐ **B.** sometimes
☐ **C.** rarely
☐ **D.** no

14. IM steroids for moderate allergic reactions (e.g., poison oak)

☐ **A.** generally
☐ **B.** sometimes
☐ **C.** rarely
☐ **D.** no

15. Intra-articular steroids for arthritis

☐ **A.** generally
☐ **B.** sometimes
☐ **C.** rarely
☐ **D.** no

16. Local steroids for bursitis

☐ **A.** generally
☐ **B.** sometimes
☐ **C.** rarely
☐ **D.** no

17. HCG for obesity

☐ **A.** generally
☐ **B.** sometimes
☐ **C.** rarely
☐ **D.** no

7

URIs indicates upper respiratory tract infection; IM, intramuscular; and HCG, chorionic gonadotrophin. Following is a scoring system for the self-assessment test; **question 1** — A, 5; B, 4; C, 2; D, 1; **question 2** — A, 5; B, 3; C, 1; **questions 3 and 6** — A, 5; B, 1; **question 4** — A, 5; B, 3; C, 2; D, 1; **question 5** — A, 2; B, 5; **question 7** — A, 1; B, 2; C, 3; D, 4; E, 5; **questions 8 through 17** — A, 5; B, 3; C, 2; D, 1. If your score is greater than 65, you may consider yourself a "shot doctor." If you scored between 65 and 30, your use of IM injections is average; a score of less than 30 is below average. Gradings are relative and represent an informal evaluation.

Reference: Alper, P. R.: Medical Economics, Aug. 5, 1974, pp. 120–126. Copyright © 1974 by Litton Industries, Inc. Published by Medical Economics Company, a Litton division, at Oradell, N.J. 07649. Reprinted by permission.

If you must use placebos, make sure that those you use really do work!

TESTING FOR FECAL BLOOD

The tests: Orthotoluidine (Occultest) is 10 times more sensitive than benzidine (Hematest) which is 100 to 1000 times more sensitive than guaiac (Hemoccult).

False positives: Because of their sensitivity, Occultest and Hematest give positive readings in patients who have meat, iron, certain bacterial flora, and vegetables with high amounts of peroxidases (e.g., turnips and horseradishes) in their stools.

False negatives: The stool guaiac may be positive with as little as 5 ml of blood of gastric origin. Since the color change in the guaiac reaction brought about by heme peroxidase is inhibited by ascorbic acid, a patient taking large doses of vitamin C may have a false negative test for fecal blood, even in the presence of significant bleeding.

Reconstitution: Untested stool that has been left on guaiac (Hemoccult) paper too long also may test negative for blood. Fortunately, it may be reconstituted with a drop of saline solution and a drop of 2 per cent acetic acid before the hydrogen peroxide is added.

Black stools: Not all black stools contain blood. Other causes include the ingestion of:

- Iron preparations
- Bismuth (Pepto-Bismol)
- Lead
- Licorice
- Charcoal, coal, dirt
- Spinach, chard, etc.

8

DUKE'S CLASSIFICATION OF COLONIC CARCINOMAS

CLASS	DESCRIPTION	APPROXIMATE PER CENT OF PATIENTS WITHOUT EVIDENT DISEASE AT 5 YEARS
A	Infiltration no deeper than the mucosa.	80
B_1	Extension into the muscularis without infiltration of the entire bowel wall. The regional lymph nodes are *negative.*	60
B_2	Extension through the entire colonic wall into the pericolic tissues. The regional lymph nodes are *negative.*	40
C_1	Infiltration of the muscularis without involvement of the entire bowel wall. The regional lymph nodes are *positive.*	15–25
C_2	Infiltration of the entire colonic wall. The regional lymph nodes are *positive.*	
D	Metastatic disease beyond the regional lymph nodes.	—

KIRKLIN MODIFICATION OF DUKES CLASSIFICATION OF COLONIC CARCINOMAS

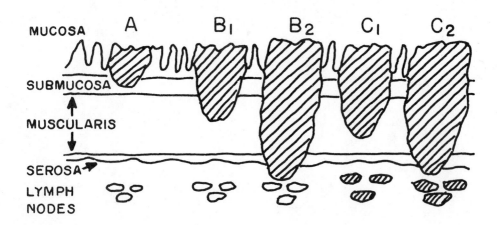

FIG. 8-1

POLYPOSIS OF THE BOWEL

	BENIGN ADENOMATOUS POLYPS	JUVENILE POLYPS	FAMILIAL POLYPOSIS OF COLON	PEUTZ-JEGHERS SYNDROME	GARDNER'S SYNDROME
Site	50% Rectosigmoid, 50% rest of colon	85% Rectosigmoid	Entire colon involved, particularly the rectum	Generalized polyposis, including stomach, but jejunum and ileum consistently involved	Throughout colon, rarely in small bowel
Age	Increases after the age of 30	First and second decade, sometimes later	Second and third decades mainly	Second and third decades, maybe later	Fourth and fifth decades
Presenting signs and symptoms	Incidental finding or bleeding	Bleeding, prolapse through rectum	Bleeding, signs and symptoms of cancer	Bleeding, intestinal obstruction	Bleeding
Pathology	True adenoma	Hamartoma	True adenoma	Hamartoma; melanin spots of lips, buccal mucosa, and digits	True adenoma; Extra-intestinal lesions, include osseous and soft-tissue tumors
Malignant potential	Relationship controversial; related to size of polyp	No	High	No	High
Treatment	Local extirpation	Local extirpation	Total colectomy	Conservative where possible	Total colectomy

8

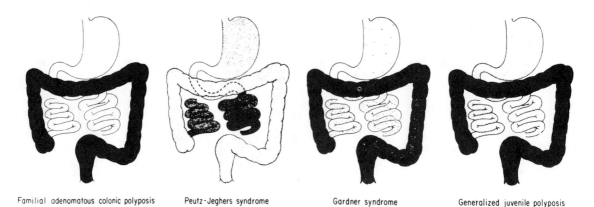

Familial adenomatous colonic polyposis   Peutz-Jeghers syndrome   Gardner syndrome   Generalized juvenile polyposis

FIG. 8-2

Localization of polyps in the polyposis syndromes. The intensity of shading reflects the frequency of anatomic involvement. (Reproduced by permission from Erbe, R.W., New Engl. J. Med., *294*: 1101, 1976.)

LAXATIVES AND CATHARTICS

Laxatives generally function by increasing intestinal peristalis or by increasing the hydration or bulk of the stool. Cathartics tend to increase intestinal peristalsis either directly or reflexively. The purpose of both groups of agents is, of course, the same. With the latter group of agents, generally a more fluid, softer stool is formed. These agents may be classified as bulk-forming laxatives, emollient laxatives, stimulant cathartics, or saline cathartics.

A. Bulk-forming Laxatives

This group includes natural and semisynthetic polysaccharides and cellulose derivatives that are hydroscopic. Consequently, they form a more or less viscous gel when mixed with intestinal contents. Fecal bulk is increased and is simultaneously kept soft and hydrated. An increase in peristalsis results from the formation of the hydroscopic mass and its mixture with indigestible alimentary residue. These agents tend to be the slowest-acting of the laxatives and cathartics. Because of their tendency to form bulk, they have been used as appetite suppressants. Adequate fluid intake should be provided to ensure passage of these agents. Rare cases of intestinal obstruction may occur when inadequate fluid is available.

1. **Psyllium (Plantago):** These agents derive from various species of plantain. Included are Metamucil and Konsyl. The usual dose of these agents is 4 to 10 grams, one to three times daily, taken in an adequate amount of fluid. Absorption of small amounts of sodium are associated with the use of these agents.

2. **Cellulose:** A variety of cellulose preparations are commercially available. They include methyl cellulose, carboxymethyl cellulose, and other hydrophilic cellulose derivatives.

3. **Bran**: Bran contains approximately 20 per cent indigestible cellulose and is a by-product of the milling of wheat. The increase in dietary fiber decreases intestinal transit time by stimulation of peristalsis, increases the weight of the feces, and acts as a stool softener. Bran is available in a variety of cereals and whole wheat flours. Roughage, or bulk, may also be obtained by the adequate use of leafy vegetables or fruits.

B. Emollient Laxatives

Emollient laxatives soften the stool, without stimulation of peristalsis. They are employed when straining at the stool should be avoided.

1. **Mineral Oil**: Mineral oil is a mixture of indigestible petroleum hydrocarbons, which are only minimally absorbed. It tends to retard gastric emptying and, as a lipid solvent, interferes with absorption of vitamins (A, D, E, and K). Consequently, mineral oil should be taken at bedtime or on an empty stomach. In addition, mineral oil has a tendency to leak from the anal sphincter, which may cause embarrassing and disconcerting side effects. The aspiration of mineral oil, which results in a lipid pneumonia, should be avoided, and the agent is probably contraindicated in those patients who have a high tendency toward aspiration.

2. **Surface-Acting Agents**: Surface-acting agents function as wetting and emulsifying agents. As a consequence, the stool is softened. The prototype surface active agent is sodium sulfosuccinate (Colace). This agent is available in a variety of formulations, including 50 and 100 mg tablets and in solution. There seems to be no serious side effects from its administration.

C. Stimulant Cathartics

It is not clear whether stimulant cathartics act by direct action on the intestinal neural plexus or smooth muscle or by the initiation of peristaltic action by intestinal mucosal irritation. Similarly, the exact role of the action of these agents in decreasing fluid and electrolyte absorption, as opposed to decreasing gastrointestinal transit time, is unclear. The use of these agents may have profound metabolic effects, which include electrolyte loss due to excessive catharsis. While they act extremely rapidly and relieve constipation quite well, they may cause abdominal cramping, excessively fluid feces, and a large amount of fecal mucus. Chronic use may result in hypokalemia, hypomagnesemia, malabsorption, gastrointestinal protein loss, and "cathartic colon."

1. **Anthraquinone Cathartics**: Included in this group are cascara sagrada, senna, and danthron. The active ingredient is an anthraquinone or anthranol derivative. These compounds may produce a brown or red discoloration of the urine and are excreted in the milk of lactating mothers. Thus, they may exert an unwanted effect in the nursing infant.

2. **Castor Oil**: Castor oil is extracted from the seeds of *Ricinus communis* and has as its major active component the triglyceride of ricinoleic acid. Ricinoleic acid, which is produced by intestinal hydrolysis, results in an active stimulation of the intestinal secretory process. The agent also produces a decreased reabsorption of water and an inhibition of the activity of intestinal circular smooth muscle. Castor oil produces a prompt, thorough evacuation of the intestinal contents, usually within three hours after its administration. The usual adult dose of castor oil is 15 to 60 ml and results in one or two large semifluid evacuations.

3. **Diphenylmethane Cathartics**: Major drugs in this group are phenolphthalein, bisacodyl, and oxyphenisatin acetate. The latency prior to evacuation is approximately six hours, since the major effects of these drugs are on the large intestine. They may be used at night to produce a laxative effect the following morning. The mechanism of action of these agents is unknown. Bisacodyl (Dulcolax) may be used both orally and by rectum. The recommended adult dosage is 10 to 15 mg orally or a 10 mg suppository.

Phenolphthalein is found in a variety of proprietary laxative preparations. About 15 per cent of a dose of 60 to 100 mg of phenolphthalein is absorbed and is subsequently conjugated to glucuronide. Excretion in the bile ultimately allows for its laxative effect. The unabsorbed dose appears in the stool, and a portion of the absorbed dose that is not detoxified appears in the urine. If alkaline, a red coloration of the excretae may result. Allergic skin reactions to phenolphthalein, including the Stevens-Johnson syndrome, have been reported. Oxyphenisatin acetate (Isocrin) is similar to bisacodyl and has no advantage over phenolphthalein. In addition, jaundice and hepatitis have been observed with bisacodyl. (Oxyphenisitin is now off the market.)

D. Saline Cathartics

The absorption of sulfate and phosphate salts of sodium and magnesium is incomplete. As a result of the osmotic effect produced in the gastrointestinal tract, these agents function as cathartics. Magnesium salts also may stimulate the release of cholecystokinin, which stimulates pancreatic and small intestine secretion and causes a decrease in absorption of fluid and sodium chloride. Consequently, the volume of gastrointestinal material is increased and the transit time decreased. Since saline cathartics are made isotonic in the stomach and duodenum, they may produce peripheral dehydration. For this reason, adequate fluid should be given with each saline cathartic. About 20 per cent of the administered dose of magnesium is absorbed and may present a problem in patients with poor renal function. A number of proprietary preparations are available, as are magnesium oxide (magnesium hydroxide) and magnesium sulfate.

The widespread and chronic use of laxatives and cathartics to insure daily bowel movement is, of course, to be decried. The side effects of excessive laxative use include crampy abdominal pain and flatulence, laxative dependence, and "cathartic colon," as well as acidosis, hypokalemia, sodium and water loss, and secondary hyperaldosteronism. Nonetheless, these agents have both an historic and a useful role in medicine. That role includes the use of emollient laxatives in painful anorectal disorders and in severe cardiovascular disease or inguinal hernia and the use of stimulant cathartics for bowel preparation prior to radiologic or endoscopic examination. A cathartic is also used in poisonings to clear the gastrointestinal tract rapidly. Similarly, cathartics may be employed to great advantage prior to the use of antihelminthic agents.

Reference: Bruckstein, A. H.: N.Y. State J. Med., *10*:78, 1978.

A RATIONAL APPROACH TO THE DIFFERENTIAL DIAGNOSIS OF DIARRHEA

The usual clinical definition of diarrhea is the passage of excessively liquid or frequent stools. Pathophysiologically, diarrhea results from either increased stool water causing excessive intraluminal volume or from abnormal gut motility. In either case there is an increase in stool bulk and volume.

The following outline categorizes diarrhea according to pathophysiologic mechanisms. Several mechanisms may play a significant role in any one disease state. However, the utility of this approach lies in its rational orientation of the differential diagnosis.

Excessive Volume

   I. Impaired absorption
      A. Malabsorption secondary to loss of normal mucosal integrity
         1. Inflammatory diseases
            a. Regional enteritis
            b. Radiation enteritis
            c. Whipple's disease
            d. Ulcerative colitis
            e. Ischemic colitis
            f. Celiac sprue
            g. Stevens-Johnson syndrome
            h. Henoch-Schönlein purpura
            i. Pseudomembranous enterocolitis
            j. Eosinophilic gastroenteritis
         2. Invasive infectious diseases
            a. Bacteria — *Shigella, Salmonella,* enteropathogenic *Escherichia coli*
            b. Viruses

   c. Protozoa — giardiasis, amebiasis
   d. Helminths — *Ascaris lumbricoides, Necator americanus, Strongyloides stercoralis*
   e. Tropical sprue
  3. Infiltrative diseases
   a. Intestinal amyloidosis .
   b. Intestinal lymphoma
   c. Intestinal scleroderma
  4. Miscellaneous
   a. Massive small bowel resection
   b. Post-gastrectomy diarrhea
   c. Carcinoma
   d. Bile salt diarrhea
   e. Steatorrhea
   f. Dermatitis herpetiformis
   g. Intestinal lymphangiectasia
 B. Maldigestion
  1. Pancreatic insufficiency
  2. Lactase deficiency
  3. Disaccharidase deficiency
  4. Other digestive enzyme deficiencies
II. Increased secretion
 A. Bacterial toxins
  1. Cholera
  2. Food poisoning — *Bacillus cereus, Clostridium welchii, Staphylococcus aureus*
  3. Enterotoxigenic *Escherichia coli*
 B. Humoral factors
  1. Non–beta islet cell tumors of pancreas
   a. Zollinger-Ellison syndrome — gastrin
   b. Vasoactive intestinal peptide (VIP) — producing tumors
   c. Other vasoactive substances
  2. Medullary carcinoma of the thyroid
 C. Miscellaneous
  1. Menetrier's disease
  2. Villous adenoma

Abnormal Gastrointestinal Motility

 I. Hypermotility with decreased transit time

A. Gastrointestinal hemorrhage
B. Post-gastrectomy with "dumping"
C. Cathartics
D. Carcinoid tumors
II. Hypomotility with intestinal stasis, bacterial overgrowth, secondary malabsorption, and maldigestion
   A. Strictures
   B. Diverticula
   C. Blind loops
   D. Scleroderma
   E. Neuromuscular disease
III. Miscellaneous
   A. Diabetic diarrhea
   B. Post-vagotomy
   C. Irritable bowel syndrome

References: Beeson, P. B., and McDermott, W. (Eds.): Textbook of Medicine, 14th Edition, Philadelphia, W. B. Saunders Company, 1975, pp. 1187–1188; Friedman, H. H., and Papper, S. (Eds.): Problem-Oriented Medical Diagnosis. Boston, Little, Brown, and Company, 1975, pp. 189–191; Phillips, S. F.: Gastroenterology, *63*:495, 1972.

What good is willpower when you've got diarrhea?   **8**

FECAL LEUKOCYTES IN DIARRHEAL ILLNESS

The diagnosis of bacterial diarrhea by clinical features is often difficult. Examination of stool for fecal leukocytes is extremely helpful in distinguishing bacterial from nonbacterial causes of diarrhea. The technique is quick and simple. A fleck of mucus or stool is placed on a clean glass slide and mixed thoroughly with two drops of Löffler's methylene blue stain. The slide is then coverslipped and examined microscopically after an interval of two to three minutes to allow proper nuclear staining. If white cells are seen under low-power scanning, a differential cell count is then made under high power. When possible, 200 cells that can be clearly identified are counted.

The presence of leukocytes is strongly associated with a bacterial cause for the diarrhea; however, fecal leukocytes do not indicate that antibiotic therapy is needed. One should also examine the stool for ova and parasites, and culture for pathogens.

DISEASE	NUMBER OF PATIENTS	NUMBER WITH FECAL LEUKOCYTES	PREDOMINANT CELL TYPE (ACUTE ILLNESS)
Shigellosis	44	44	PMN* (mean 84%)
Salmonellosis	11	9	PMN (mean 75%)
Typhoid fever	8	8	Mononuclear (mean 95%)
Invasive *E. coli* colitis	4	4	PMN (mean 85%)
Ulcerative colitis	2	2	PMN (mean 88%) and eosinophils (mean 8%)
"Allergic" diarrhea	1	1	Mononuclear (mean 95%)
Healthy controls	65	0	
Cholera	6	0	
Viral diarrhea	14	0	
Toxigenic *E. coli*	5	0	
Nonspecific diarrhea	32	3	
Giardia lamblia enteritis	2	0	
Nontyphoid salmonella carriers	2	0	
Typhoid carriers	2	0	
Shigella vaccines	15	1	

*Polymorphonuclear leukocyte.

Reference: Harris, J. C., et al.: Ann. Intern. Med., *76*:697–703, 1972. Table reproduced with permission of author and Annals of Internal Medicine.

Parasite — The wealthy of Greece and Rome were surrounded by flatterers and other groupies (how much has changed?). Their aim was to join the court and to be fed at the patron's table. Thus, the Greek *para,* "beside," and *sitos*, "food," gave rise to the Latin *parasitus* — one who eats at the side or the expense of another.

GIARDIASIS

If you've just come back from the Soviet Union, where you took a side trip to Leningrad, or been camping in the Rockies, where you got carried away with the clean taste of fresh-flowing, clear water, you may suddenly find yourself with an acute diarrheal syndrome. Suspect *Giardia lamblia.* Take comfort in the fact that you probably had a heck of a good time and now share an infestation with Leeuwenhoek of Delft. Leeuwenhoek, by the way, perfected the microscope. He also did something that you won't be able to do: He identified the parasite in his own stool during one of his diarrheal episodes and reported it in 1681!

Giardia is a ubiquitous parasite, having been found in up to 30 per cent of populations examined worldwide. Since in most studies only a single stool specimen is examined per host, these attack rates are probably underestimates. Thus it must be concluded that the majority of us harboring Giardia are at least relatively asymptomatic. Nonetheless, it now appears that giardiasis is an important cause of traveler's diarrhea.

The parasite multiplies in the duodenum and proximal small intestine following its ingestion. The pathogenesis of the diarrhea is unknown. The organism appears to be invasive with only a minimal tissue reaction. Heavy infestations appear to be the most symptomatic. There is an association with immunoglobulin deficiency states, primarily IgA and IgM deficiency. The symptoms of giardiasis may be those of an acute, chronic, or intermittent diarrheal syndrome, which may alternate with periods of constipation. Nausea, vomiting, flatulence, and colic may be additional complaints. The stools may be watery and contain mucus, but are rarely bloody. A full-blown malabsorption syndrome may be present, together with mucosal changes indicative of sprue. A protein-losing enteropathy has been reported, as has the acquired malabsorption of B_{12}, folic acid, and disaccharides. In patients with immunoglobulin disorders, serum protein electrophoresis or quantitative immunoglobulin determinations will reveal the deficiency of these proteins. Contrast radiographic studies of the small intestine are said to reveal hypersecretion, mucosal thickening, and nodular lymphatic hyperplasia.

The best way to confirm the diagnosis of giardiasis is to examine duodenal drainage. Organisms may not be present in the stool, even in patients having a choleric syndrome. Indeed, examination of the stool is positive in no more than half the cases in which the diagnosis is established by duodenal drainage. Small bowel biopsy is usually normal except for the presence of the parasite. Villous atrophy may be observed, and sprue-like changes are more common in patients with immunoglobulin deficiencies. The organism is often difficult to find on biopsy specimens, but studying the tissue with a Masson's trichrome stain helps. The parasite is usually more readily seen on touch preps made

8

by wiping a glass slide across the luminal side of the biopsy, air-drying the slide, fixing in methanol for 30 minutes, and staining with Giemsa.

Therapy with metronidazole (Flagyl) works. 250 mg are given three times a day for one week. Quinacrine (Atabrine) is only slightly less effective but causes somewhat more gastrointestinal upset. Given the usually flagrant history and symptomatology and the relative innocuousness of the therapy, a therapeutic trial may be employed, thereby circumventing a sometimes arduous and uncomfortable gastrointestinal evaluation. Structural changes in the intestine revert with adequate therapy in the vast majority of cases.

References: Brandborg, L. L.: In Sleisenger, M. H., and Fordtran, J. S. (Eds.): Gastrointestinal Disease, 2nd Edition. Philadelphia, W. B. Saunders Company, 1978, p. 1154; Wolfe, M. S.: J.A.M.A., *233*:1362, 1975.

PANCREATITIS

There are many causes of acute pancreatitis. While most cases are associated with alcoholism or cholelithiasis, a number are related to metabolic disease, drugs, trauma, infection, malignancy, vascular disease, and nutritional abnormalities. There are multiple mechanisms for the development of pancreatitis; unfortunately, most are not well understood. In alcoholism, for example, some studies have suggested that alcohol ingestion stimulates the pancreas to hypersecretion. In addition, alcohol may induce irritation, spasm, or edema of the duct papilla. Alcohol may induce atony of the sphincter, predisposing to reflux of duodenal contents into the pancreatic duct. Pancreatitis following obstruction or trauma is more easily understood. However, the manner in which pancreatitis is produced by acidosis, endotoxemia, hyperlipemia, pregnancy, or nutritional abnormalities is less clear. Hypercalcemic states appear to bring about excessive activation of trypsinogen by calcium ion or precipitate calcium in the ducts, leading to obstruction.

Etiologies of Pancreatitis

FACTOR	DESCRIPTION
Alcohol	
Cholelithiasis	
Idiopathic	
Metabolic	Uremia, acidosis, hyperlipemia (types I and V), amino-aciduria (lysine, cystine), hypercalcemic states (multiple myeloma, hyperparathyroidism, sarcoidosis, vitamin D intoxication), hemachromatosis
Drugs	Morphine, codeine, demerol, glucocorticoids, birth control pills, salicylates, salicylazosulfapyridine, azathioprine, 6-mercaptopurine, L-asparaginase, isoniazid, indomethacin, chlorothiazide, tetracycline, chlorthalidone, furosemide
Trauma	Blunt, penetrating, surgical, electrical, hypothermia
Infections	Mumps, infectious mononucleosis, viral hepatitis, Group B Coxsackie virus, scarlet fever, streptococcal food poisoning, typhoid fever, gram-negative sepsis, tuberculosis, parasitic obstruction of the sphincter of Oddi
Malignancy	Lymphoma, Hodgkin's disease, pancreatic carcinoma, any obstruction of the ducts
Vascular	Periarteritis nodosa, systemic lupus erythematosus, atheromatous emboli, atherosclerotic ischemia
Other	Perforating or penetrating peptic ulcer; nutritional: kwashiorkor, bangugu (refeeding after malnutrition); pregnancy; post-partum; hereditary pancreatitis; cystic fibrosis (obstructive); congenital stenosis of sphincter of Oddi; scorpion bite (*T. trinitatis*)

8

PROGNOSTICATING IN ACUTE PANCREATITIS

Acute pancreatitis is an illness that ranges in severity from mild abdominal discomfort to an acute fulminant process rapidly progressing to death. The 11 early objective signs listed below can be used to identify those patients who may require more vigorous therapy. Patients with less than three signs present have mild pancreatitis and a mortality rate of approximately 1 per cent. Patients with three or four positive signs have a 15 per cent rate of mortality. Patients with five or six positive signs have a 40 per cent mortality rate, and patients with seven or eight positive signs approach a 100 per cent rate of mortality.

Eleven Early Objective Signs Used to Classify the Severity of Pancreatitis

---

AT ADMISSION OR DIAGNOSIS

Age over 55
White blood cell count over 16,000/cu mm
Blood glucose over 200 mg/100 ml
Serum lactic dehydrogenase over 350 I.U./liter
Serum glutamic oxaloacetic transaminase over 250 Sigma Frankel Units/100 ml

DURING INITIAL 48 HOURS

Hematocrit falls more than 10 percentage points
Blood urea nitrogen rises more than 5 mg/100 ml
Serum calcium level below 8 mg/100 ml
Arterial PO_2 below 60 mmHg
Base deficit greater than 4 mEq/liter
Estimated fluid sequestration more than 6000 ml

References: Ranson, G. H. C., and Pasternack, B. S.: J. Surg. Res., *22*:79, 1977; Table reprinted with permission from Ranson, G. H. C., and Spencer, F. C.: Ann. Surg., *187*:565, 1978.

AGENTS AFFECTING LOWER ESOPHAGEAL SPHINCTER (LES) PRESSURE

Agents Producing Decreased LES Pressure

HORMONES
Secretin
Cholecystokinin
Glucagon
Gastric inhibitory polypeptide
Vasoactive intestinal polypeptide

NEUROTRANSMITTERS
Beta adrenergic agonist (isoproterenol)
Alpha adrenergic antagonist (phentolamine)
Dopamine
Anticholinergic (Atropine)

FOODS
Fat
Chocolate
Ethanol
Peppermint

OTHERS
Caffeine*, theophylline
Gastric acidification
Smoking
Valium
Demerol/morphine
Prostaglandins E_1, E_2, A_2
Inflammation

*Recent studies indicate that although caffeine may decrease LES pressure, the whole brew of coffee (with or without caffeine) will increase sphincter pressure.

Agents Producing Increased LES Pressure

HORMONES
Gastrin/pentagastrin
Motilin
Substance P

OTHERS
Histamine/betazole
Gastric alkalinization
Metoclopramide
Protein meal

NEUROTRANSMITTERS
Alpha adrenergic agonist
  (norepinephrine; phenylephrine)
Cholinergic
  (bethanechol; methacholine)
Anticholinesterase
  (edrophonium)

Prostaglandin $F_{2\alpha}$
Indomethacin
Coffee*
5-Hydroxytryptamine

*Recent studies indicate that although caffeine may decrease LES pressure, the whole brew of coffee (with or without caffeine) will increase sphincter pressure.

Reference: Castell, D. O.: South Med. J: *71*:26, 1978.

Nausea — The ancients, it seemed, got seasick. *Naus* meant "ship" in ancient Greece, and *nausia* was the ancient Greek *mal de mer.*

GASTROESOPHAGEAL REFLUX

Gastroesophageal reflux is a clinical syndrome caused by the passage of gastric contents into the esophagus. It is manifested by a retrosternal burning sensation traveling upward toward the mouth and is exacerbated by certain foods, the recumbent position, or bending. It is not associated with the occurrence of a hiatal hernia.

The passage of gastric contents into the esophagus is facilitated by an incompetent lower esophageal sphincter (LES). Thus, a diminished basal pressure of the LES and a failure of the LES to contract in response to elevation of either intra-abdominal pressure or gastric acid are the major abnormalities leading to LES incompetency.

The diagnosis of gastroesophageal reflux involves eliciting the patient's history. If there is question about the diagnosis, if the symptoms are severe, if the patient has not responded to the usual forms of treatment, or if there are indications that there are complications such as stricture or peptic ulceration of the esophagus, then tests to measure reflux are needed.

The management of gastroesophageal reflux should proceed by distinct steps.

Step I: *Basic maneuvers* (75 per cent of patients will respond)
    a. Eliminate coffee, alcohol, chocolate, and fatty foods from the diet.
    b. Discontinue smoking.
    c. Elevate the head of the bed with 8-inch wood blocks. Don't allow patient to assume a recumbent posture after eating.
    d. Antacids — magnesium hydroxide antacid an hour after meals and at bedtime (e.g., Mylanta II, 15 ml).
    e. Discontinue anticholinergics and beta adrenergic drugs if possible.

Step II: *Specific pharmacologic maneuvers* (15 to 20 per cent of the nonresponders to the basic maneuvers will respond to specific drug therapy)
    a. Metoclopramide hydrochloride (Maxolon), Bethanechol chloride (urecholine) — administered in adequate doses, these drugs act

to increase LES pressure.

b. Cimetidine (Tagamet) — is an H_2 antagonist and thus serves to reduce gastric acid output.

Step III: *Surgical maneuvers*

a. Surgical maneuvers are *not* aimed at repair of a hiatal hernia.

b. Surgery attempts to restore LES competence.

Reference: Cohen, S., and Snape, W. J.: Arch. Intern. Med., *138*:1398, 1978.

ANTACIDS AND UNCLE ULCER

Antacids have been one of the mainstays of therapy for peptic ulcer disease for many years. All antacids reduce gastric acidity. However, there are significant differences among the more commonly used products; these differences alter the drugs' clinical utility in certain situations.

Antacids can be divided into two basic types. The *absorbable* types include sodium bicarbonate and calcium bicarbonate (Amitone, Tetralar, and Tums). As a consequence of their absorption, alterations of the pH of the extracellular fluid may occur. Sodium bicarbonate use may result in significant systemic alkalosis and a significant sodium load (1 gram $NaHCO_3$ provides 12 mEq HCO_3^- and Na^+). In addition, the high pH to which the gastric fluid is raised may stimulate significant rebound hyperacidity. Calcium carbonate can cause hypercalcemia and hypercalciuria with its attendant risk of irreversible renal damage. Calcium-containing antacids may also stimulate acid secretion by activating gastrin release and can cause severe constipation by decreasing intestinal motility. Thus, the absorbable antacids are not recommended for chronic antacid therapy.

The *nonabsorbable* antacids are magnesium and aluminum compounds. The differences among these preparations lie in their neutralizing ability, sodium content, and effect on stool consistency. Aluminum-containing preparations (Amphojel, Basaljel, Phosphaljel, and Gelusil) tend to be constipating. The laxative preparations are those containing magnesium (Maalox, Mylanta, and Riopan in large doses).

Antacids are most effectively administered about one hour after meals, when the buffering capacity of the meal is depleted and gastric acidity is on the rise. Liquids are more efficacious than tablets, since efficacy is related to the amount of exposed surface covered.

Renal failure presents complicating circumstances for antacid therapy. A low-sodium preparation may be necessary. Titralac contains the most sodium (73.8 mg/30 ml), and Riopan the least (3.5 mg/30 ml). In renal failure, magnesium preparations should be avoided, since magnesium may be absorbed in significant amounts, and toxic levels may be reached when renal excretion is diminished. Aluminum preparations

8

that tend to bind phosphate irreversibly in the GI tract are useful in controlling the hyperphosphatemia of renal failure. Aluminum carbonate (Basaljel) is the most efficient phosphate binder.

The following table compares the more commonly used antacids. It is based on a single dose of each antacid. The standard dose is defined as the volume of antacid with the buffering capability equivalent to 30 ml of Mylanta II.

Single-Dose Comparison of Various Antacids

	CONTENTS	VOL (ml)	NA (mg)	COST (¢)
Ducon	Aluminum hydroxide Magnesium hydroxide Calcium carbonate	18	63.2	9
Mylanta II	Aluminum hydroxide Magnesium hydroxide Simethicone	30	47.9	20
Camalox	Aluminum hydroxide Magnesium hydroxide Calcium carbonate	35	17.8	16
Maalox	Magnesium hydroxide Aluminum hydroxide	48	53.8	25
Mylanta	Same as Mylanta II	52	40.6	23
WinGel	Aluminum hydroxide Magnesium hydroxide	55	13.6	22
Riopan	Aluminum hydroxide Magnesium hydroxide	56	7.9	22
Amphojel	Aluminum hydroxide	64	77.0	28
Gelusil	Aluminum hydroxide Magnesium trisilicate	93	132.7	37
Phosphaljel	Aluminum phosphate	295	767.7	118

Reference: Ippoliti, A., and Peterson, W.: Clin. Gastroenterol., *8*:53, 1979.

INTESTINAL BYPASS SURGERY FOR MORBID OBESITY: A SYSTEMIC DISEASE

Intestinal bypass surgery to achieve weight reduction in massively obese patients (defined as a body weight more than 100 pounds over ideal weight or two times ideal weight) brings about significant weight reduction in a majority of patients. The natural history of intestinal bypass surgery indicates, however, that the sequelae to the operation may induce iatrogenic, systemic disease at least as serious as the obesity.

A review of these complications may help the physician decide whether to recommend this procedure to patients.

A. *Operative mortality*
   Operative mortality has been reported to be 0 to 6.5 per cent
B. *Metabolic complications*
   Electrolyte abnormalities induced by diarrhea
       Hypokalemia, hypomagnesemia, hypocalcemia
   Hyperuricemia
   Hyperoxaluria
       Results in calcium oxalate kidney stones in 7 per cent of patients
       undergoing the operation
   Hypovitaminosis
       Decreased serum levels of vitamin E, vitamin A., folic acid, and
       vitamin D (often with elevated levels of parathyroid hormone);
       if not supplemented, vitamin B_{12} stores would become depleted
       in several years
   Hypoproteinemia
   Reduced bile salt pool leading to an increased incidence of cho-
       lelithiasis
C. *Intestinal complications*
   Intractable diarrhea
   Steatorrhea
   Gastrointestinal hemorrhage
   Bypass enteritis (increased diarrhea, abdominal pain, fever, arthritis,
       skin lesions, pneumatosis cystoides intestinales; may respond to
       antibiotics)
   Colonic pseudo-obstruction (not a mechanical obstruction)
       Paralysis of the colon at the site of drainage of the defunctional
       small bowel as well as the entire colon distal to the site of
       drainage; may respond to antibiotics aimed at colonic anaerobic
       bacteria
   Increased basal acid output.
D. *Liver disease*
   Hepatic steatosis in 15 to 25 per cent (Approximately 65 per cent
       of patients have hepatic steatosis preoperatively)
   Steatosis may proceed to fibrosis and cirrhosis in approximately
       7 per cent of patients
   Severe histopathologic changes may be present without indications
       of abnormal liver function
   Hepatic failure is the second most common cause of death after
       operative mortality
   Hepatic failure may occur as a late complication of intestinal bypass
   Re-establishing intestinal continuity restores hepatic morphology
       and function to normal if performed in time
E. *Miscellaneous complications*
   Polyarthritis (may be secondary to cryoprotein immune complex
       deposition)

Neuromyopathy (primarily proximal muscle weakness)

Alopecia (may be related to reduced Vitamin A and carotene levels)

Reanastomosis

Approximately 20 per cent of patients require reanastomosis for:

   a. Hepatic failure

   b. Worsening hepatic fibrosis

   c. Weight loss to below ideal weight

   d. Inanition

   e. Severe psychiatric problems

   f. Intractable diarrhea

   g. Disabling abdominal pain

Immunologically mediated renal disease unrelated to oxalate deposition in the kidney (progressive, may not respond to reanastomosis)

References: Halverson, J. D., Weise, L., Wazna, M. F., and Bollinger, W. F.: Am. J. Med., *64*:461, 1978; Bray, G. A., Barry, R. E., Benfield, J. R., et al.: Ann. Intern. Med., *85*:97, 1976; Drenick, E. J., Stanley, T. M., Border, W. A., et al.: Ann. Intern. Med., *89*:594, 1978.

EXTRAINTESTINAL COMPLICATIONS OF INFLAMMATORY BOWEL DISEASE

The intestinal manifestations of Crohn's colitis and ileocolitis, regional enteritis, and chronic ulcerative colitis are well known. The extraintestinal manifestations of these diseases may not be as well appreciated, but they do add considerably to the morbidity of these illnesses. An awareness of these complications may improve the care of patients with inflammatory bowel disease.

Complications that Parallel the Activity of the Inflammatory Bowel Disease

  I. Arthritis

     A. Mono-articular in large joints of lower limbs

     B. Polyarticular

     C. Spondylitis (may not coincide with the activity of the inflammatory bowel disease)

  II. Skin

     A. Erythema nodosum

     B. Pyoderma gangrenosum

  III. Mouth

     A. Aphthous stomatitis

IV. Eye
   A. Conjunctivitis
   B. Episcleritis
   C. Uveitis

Complications Related to Small Bowel Involvement with the Disease

I. Malabsorption
II. Kidney stones
   A. Oxalate
   B. Urate
III. Gallstones
IV. Genitourinary problems (other than stones)
   A. Hydronephrosis and hydroureter
   B. Enterovesical and enteroureteral fistulae
   C. Urinary tract infection

Nonspecific Complications

I. Growth retardation in children
II. Liver abnormalities
   A. Abnormal liver chemistries, especially for alkaline phosphatase
   B. Pericholangitis
   C. Chronic persistent hepatitis
   D. Chronic active hepatitis
   E. Cirrhosis
   F. Sclerosing cholangitis

Reference: Greenstein, A. J., Janowitz, H. D., and Sachar, O. B.: Medicine, 5:401, 1976.

CAUSES OF HYPERGASTRINEMIA

A. Tumorous
   Zollinger-Ellison syndrome
B. Nontumorous
   Pernicious anemia
   Chronic gastritis (atrophic)
   Massive small intestinal resection (short bowel syndrome)
   Syndrome of retained gastric antrum (hyperchlorhydria)
   Antral G-cell hyperplasia (hyperchlorhydria)
   Renal failure

DIFFERENTIATION OF HYPERCHLORHYDRIC HYPERGASTRINEMIA

TEST	SERUM GASTRIN	
	Z-E Syndrome	Nontumorous
Fasting	Often > 1 ng/ml	Usually < 1 ng/ml
Response to test meal	Slight	Pronounced increase (> 2–3 times)
Response to secretin (1–2 units/kg)	Increases 2–4 times in 10 minutes	Unchanged or decreased
Response to calcium	Pronounced, slow rise (3 hrs)	Slight change

Reference: Said, S. I., and Zfass, A. M.: Disease-A-Month, *14*:10, 1978.

PROVOCATIVE DIAGNOSTIC TESTS IN THE ZOLLINGER-ELLISON SYNDROME

The Zollinger-Ellison syndrome is characterized by peptic ulcer disease, an extremely high basal acid secretion, and fasting hypergastrinemia. In the absence of renal failure or achlorhydria, serum gastrin levels above 500 pg/ml are highly suggestive of the diagnosis of Zollinger-Ellison syndrome. About 40 per cent of patients with proven Zollinger-Ellison syndrome will have a fasting gastrin concentration of 100 to 500 pg/ml, while 10 per cent of ulcer patients without gastrinomas will have a fasting serum gastrin in that range. Since the surgical and medical approaches to the Zollinger-Ellison syndrome differ from those employed in peptic ulcer disease, the differentiation between these two syndromes is of prime importance. Three provocative tests may be employed.

1. A standard test meal
2. A bolus intravenous injection of secretin (1 to 2 units/kg).
3. An intravenous infusion of calcium gluconate (4 mg of calcium/kg/hr).

The secretin test seems to have several advantages over calcium stimulation. The test is shorter in duration, has fewer potential side effects, and results in fewer false positive and false negative results. It has been suggested that an absolute increase of 110 pg/ml in serum gastrin is preferable as a criterion for positive response to a change reflected as a per cent of the baseline levels. A negative secretin test occurs in only about 5 per cent of patients with Zollinger-Ellison syndrome. There are occasional false positive responses.

Provocation by calcium infusion should not be employed in patients with hypercalcemia. After antrectomy and Billroth II procedures, gastrin concentration does not rise following a test meal.

References: Deveney, C. W., Deveney, K. S., Jaffe, B. N., et. al.: Ann. Intern. Med., 87:660, 1977; Ippoliti, A. F.: Ann. Intern. Med., 87:787, 1977.

8

9
NUTRITION

NUTRITIONAL NEEDS

Hospitalized patients are frequently malnourished. The following table lists the recommended daily allowance of essential nutrients required for the adult to *maintain* normal nutrition. Patients who are hypermetabolic (e.g., those with trauma, fever, infection, or burns) or nutritionally depleted will need 1½ to 3 times the recommended

Recommended Daily Allowances of Essential Nutrients for Healthy Adults *

Water, *ml/calorie*	1
Energy, *kcal*	2000–2700
Protein, *gram*	46–56
Linoleic acid, *gram*	4–6
Retinol equivalents	800–1000
Vitamin D	Sunlight
Vitamin E, IU	12–15
Ascorbic acid, *mg*	45
Folic acid, *μg*	400
Niacin, *mg*	13–18
Riboflavin, *mg*	1.2–1.6
Thiamine, *mg*	1.0–1.4
Vitamin B_6, *mg*	2.0
Vitamin B_{12}, *μg*	3.0
Pantothenic acid, *mg*	5–10
Calcium, *mg*	800
Phosphorus, *mg*	800
Iodine, *μg*	100–130
Iron, *mg*	10–18
Magnesium, *mg*	300–350
Zinc, *mg*	15
Copper, *mg*	2
Potassium, *mg*	2500†
Sodium, *mg*	2500†
Chloride, *mg*	2000†
Chromium, *μg*	50–120†
Manganese, *mg*	6–8†
Molybdenum, *μg*	400†
Selenium, *μg*	50–100†

*Adapted from Food and Nutrition Board: Recommended Daily Allowances, 8th Edition. Washington, National Academy of Sciences, National Research Council, 1974. The minimum daily requirements average 0.7 times the recommended allowances.

†Recommended daily allowance not established. Values are those provided in a normal diet.

Reference: Heymsfield, S. B., Bethel, R. A., Ansley, J. D., et al.: Ann. Intern. Med., *90*:64, 1979. Table reproduced with permission of author and Annals of Internal Medicine.

daily allowances. When designing a nutrition program remember that patients who are given protein and calories without some of the other essential nutrients can develop selective nutritional deficiencies.

NUTRITIONGRAM

Malnutrition leads to depressed immunity, increased susceptibility to infection, and increased mortality in all patients, especially those who have had extensive surgical procedures or are receiving chemotherapy or radiotherapy for malignancy. The simple five-point assessment of nutritional status presented below will aid the physician in recognizing the malnourished patient so appropriate nutritional support can be provided.

How to Assess Patients by "Nutritiongram"

MEASUREMENTS		NORMALLY NOURISHED	MODERATELY MALNOURISHED	SEVERELY MALNOURISHED
Total lymphocyte count (per mm^3)		1500 or more	1000 to 1499	999 or fewer
Serum albumin (grams/dl)		3.5 or more	2.8 to 3.4	2.7 or less
Triceps skin fold (mm)	men	10 to 12.5	7.5 to 9.9	7.4 or less
	women	13.2 to 16.5	9.9 to 13.1	9.8 or less
Mid-arm circumference (cm)	men	23.4 to 29.3	17.6 to 23.3	17.5 or less
	women	22.8 to 28.5	17.1 to 22.7	17.0 or less
Delayed hypersensitivity skin tests (number of positive tests out of four)		2 or more	1	0

Column containing patient's poorest measurement determines status.

Reference: Willcutts, H. D., and Blackborn, G. L.: Medical World News, March 6, 1978, p. 16. Reproduced with permission of the authors and publisher.

TECHNIQUE FOR MEASUREMENT OF TRICEPS SKIN-FOLD THICKNESS AND MIDARM CIRCUMFERENCE

Equipment

You will need a skin-fold caliper with a standard contact surface or "pinch" area of 20 to 24 mm^2. It should read to 0.1 mm accuracy and exert a constant pressure (10 grams/mm^2) through the whole range of skin-fold thicknesses at all distances of separation of the jaws. The dial of the caliper should be reset to zero before each procedure. You will need a fiber glass or flexible steel measuring tape for measuring midarm circumference.

Technique — Skin-fold Thickness

The triceps skin-fold area will be the zone of study. For consistency, the midpoint of the left side should be studied while the arm is hanging freely.

Grasp firmly a lengthwise skin-fold and lift it up slightly between the finger and thumb of your left hand. Take care not to include the underlying muscle.

The caliper is applied 1 cm below your finger at a depth about equal to the skin-fold while the skin-fold is gently held throughout the measurement. Three measurements should be made and the results averaged.

Technique — Midarm Circumference

The middle section of the left upper arm, while hanging freely, will be used for the measurements (same as for the triceps skin-fold).

The arm circumference is measured to the nearest 0.1 cm with a flexible steel or fiber glass tape, which must be placed gently but firmly around the limb to avoid compression of the soft tissues. The overlying subcutaneous fat is measured in the triceps region with the skin-fold calipers as described above.

From these two measurements, it is possible to calculate the inner circle, which is composed principally of muscle, with a small core of bone. It is usually assumed that the bone is relatively constant in size, and the calculated value is termed the "midarm muscle circumference." The formula for the calculation of the midarm muscle circumference is:

Muscle circumference = arm circumference − skin-fold

RULE OF THUMB DETERMINATION OF IDEAL BODY WEIGHT

Females:	100 lb (45 kg) for the first 5 ft (152 cm)
	plus
	5 lb (2.2 kg) for every inch (2.54 cm) of height over 5 ft (152 cm)
Males:	110 lb (45 kg) for the first 5 ft (152 cm)
	plus
	5 lb (2.2 kg) for every 1 inch (2.54 cm) of height over 5 ft (152 cm)
Example:	female, 165 cm; 45 kg for 152 cm
	plus
	2.2 kg × 13 cm/2.54 cm = 11.4 kg
	45 kg + 11.4 kg = 56.4 kg

To adjust for frame size, 10 lb (4.5 kg) would be added in the case of a large frame or subtracted in the case of a small frame.

Reference: Krause, M. V., and Mahan, L. K.: Food, Nutrition and Diet Therapy. Philadelphia, W. B. Saunders Company, 1979, p. 31. Table reproduced with permission of publisher.

APPROACH TO NUTRITION

We would like to thank Dr. George Blackburn, Director of the Nutritional Support Service at the New England Deaconess Hospital (Boston, Mass.), for kindly allowing us to use his lucid approach to the nutritional management of the hospitalized patient.

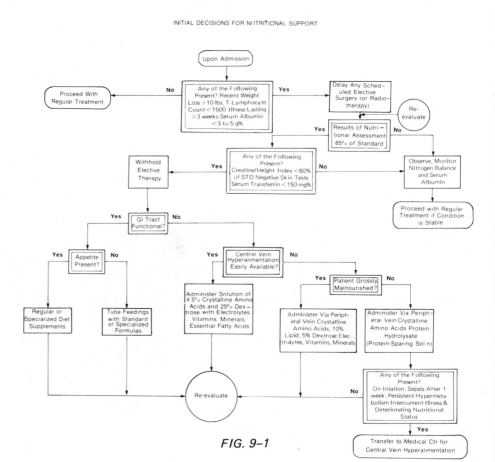

FIG. 9-1

FORMULATIONS FOR ENTERAL ALIMENTATION

The table on the opposite page summarizes the important characteristics of many of the currently available liquid formulations for enteral alimentation. There is considerable variability in both chemical composition and cost. In selecting a formulation, you need to balance the patient's particular set of problems and nutritional needs against the make-up of the available formulations and their cost. The vitamin and micronutrient profile will vary from formulation to formulation, and it is advisable to review the package inserts to see if your patient's particular situation will require any additional supplementation.

	VIVONEX	VIVONEX HN	PRECISION LR	FLEXICAL	VITAL	VIPEP	ISOCAL	OSMOLITE	SUSTACAL	ENSURE	ENSURE PLUS	MERITENE	COMPLETE B	PORTAGEN
Manufacturer	Eaton	Eaton	Doyle	Mead Johnson	Ross	Cutter	Mead Johnson	Ross	Mead Johnson	Ross	Ross	Doyle	Doyle	Mead Johnson
Calories/ml/	1	1	1	1	1	1	1	1	1	1	1	1	1	1
Protein (grams/liter)	21	42	24	19	42	25	34	37	60	37	55	55	38	35
Calories (gm nitrogen)	298	149	260	329	150	250	184	178	104	178	171	114	176	179
Protein source	L-amino acids	L-amino acids	Egg albumin	Casein Hydrolysate	Peptides Free amino acids	Peptides Amino acids	Casein soy	Casein	Milk, casein, soy	Casein, soy	Casein, soy	Milk	Beef, milk, vegetable	Casein
Fat (%)	1.3	0.33	0.7	30	9.3	22	39	38.8	20	32	32	30	36	22.7
Fat source	Safflower oil	Safflower oil	Vegetable oil	Soy oil *MCT oil	Sunflower oil	MCT Corn oil	Soy oil MCT oil	Corn oil MCT & soy oil	Soy oil	Corn oil	Corn oil	Vegetable oil	Corn oil, beef fat	MCT Corn oil
mOsm/kg	500	844	590	500	450	520	350	300	625	450	600	560	490	357
Na (mEq/liter)	37	34	36	15	17	32.6	22	23	39	31	47	40	68	27
K (mEq/liter)	30	18	27	38	30	21.8	33	23	53	33	49	43	40	40
Palatability	Poor	Poor	Poor	Poor	Good	Good	Fair	Fair	Good	Good	Good	Good	Poor	Fair
Residue	Low	Low	Low	Low	Low	Low	Medium	Medium	Medium	Medium	Medium	Medium	High	Medium
Cost/1000 KCal (1978 $)	3.33	6.67	2.40	3.00	4.43	3.96	1.59	2.00	1.44	1.21	1.51	1.77	2.37	2.43

*medium chain triglycerides

Thanks to Ms. Arlene Harris, R. D., for assembling the table.

THE PONDERAL INDEX

The ponderal index is height divided by the cube root of weight; it is a better indicator of body build and fatness than height and weight. The lower the ponderal index, the more obese the individual. There is an increased operative risk when the ponderal index falls below 11 and a dramatic decrease in life expectancy when the ponderal index is less than 11.6. The table on the opposite page of ponderal index isograms (Fig. 9–2) can be used to determine the ponderal index rapidly, even if you have forgotten how to do cube roots. Note that English, and not metric, units should be used to calculate the ponderal index.

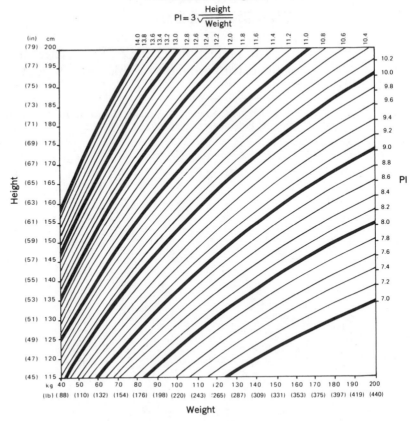

Ponderal index, quantifying obesity.

References: Selzer, C. C.: New Engl. J. Med., *274*:254, 1966; Fig. 9–2 reprinted with permission of author and publisher from Flewellen, E. H., and Bee, D. E.: J.A.M.A., *241*:884, 1979. Copyright 1979, American Medical Association.

Obesity:
A. *To live and be fat is better than not to live at all.*
B. *To live and be lean is better than to be fat.*
C. *What we eat will determine what we weigh until the second law of thermodynamics is repealed.*
D. *The only glands malfunctioning in obesity are the salivary glands.*
E. *Imprisoned in every fat man, a thin one is wildly signaling to be let out.*

CALORIC VALUE OF BEVERAGES AND SNACK FOODS

The tabulation on the opposite page should help explain why your patients (or you) have trouble losing weight!

Reference: Krause, M. V., and Mahan, L. K.: Food, Nutrition and Diet Therapy. Philadelphia, W. B. Saunders Company, 1979, p. 865.

Calorie Values of Beverages and Snack Foods

FOOD	WEIGHT (grams)	APPROXIMATE MEASURE	KCALORIES	FOOD	WEIGHT (grams)	APPROXIMATE MEASURE	KCALORIES
Beverages				Doughnut, cake type,			
Carbonated, cola type	369	1 bottle, 12 ounces	145	plain	32	1 average	125
Malted milk	235	1 regular (1 cup)	245	Doughnut, jelly	65	1 average	226
Chocolate milk				Doughnut, raised	30	1 average	120
(made with skim milk)	250	1 cup	190				
Cocoa	250	1 cup	245	Fruits			
Soda, vanilla ice cream	242	1 regular	60	Apple	150	1 medium, 2½ in. diameter	70
				Banana	100	1 medium, 6 by 1½ in.	85
Beverages, alcoholic				Grapes, European type	160	1 cup	95
Beer	360	1 bottle, 12 ounces	150	Orange	180	1 medium, 2⅝ in. diameter	65
Brandy	30	1 brandy glass	75	Pear	182	1 medium, 3 by 2½ in.	100
Gin	43	1 jigger	107			diameter	
Liqueurs (average)	20	1 cordial glass	165				
Martini		1 cocktail glass	145	Miscellaneous			
Manhattan		1 cocktail glass	165	Hamburger and bun	96	1 average	334
Rum	43	1 jigger	105	Ice cream, vanilla	62	3 ounces	95
Whiskey	43	1 jigger	107	Sherbet	96	½ cup	130
Wine, port	100	1 wine glass	160	Jams, jellies,			
Wine, sauterne	100	1 wine glass	85	marmalades, preserves	21	1 tablespoon	55
				Syrup, blended	21	1 tablespoon	60
Cake				Waffles	75	1 waffle, 4½ by 5½ by	210
Angle food	53	1 piece	135			½ inch	
Cupcake, chocolate, iced	36	1 cake, 2¾ in. diameter	130				
Fruit cake	30	1 piece, 2 by 2 by ½ in.	110	Nuts			
				Mixed, shelled	15	8 to 12	94
Candy and popcorn				Peanut butter	16	1 tablespoon	95
Butterscotch	15	3 pieces	60	Peanuts, shelled,			
Candy bar, plain	28	1 bar	145	roasted	144	1 cup	840
Caramels	28	3 medium	115				
Choc-coated peanuts	28	1 ounce	160	Pie			
Fudge	28	1 piece	115	Apple	135	4-inch sector	350
Peanut brittle	30	1 ounce	128	Cherry	135	4-inch sector	350
Popcorn with oil added	9	1 cup	40	Custard	130	4-inch sector	285
				Lemon meringue	120	4-inch sector	305
Cheese				Mince	135	4-inch sector	365
Camembert	38	1 wedge	115	Pumpkin	130	4-inch sector	275
Cheddar	28	1 ounce	115				
Cream	28	1 ounce	106	Potato chips			
Swiss (domestic)	28	1 ounce	100	Potato chips	20	10 chips, 2 inches in	115
						diameter	
Cookies				Sandwiches			
Brownies, made with				Bacon, lettuce, tomato	148	1 sandwich	282
mix	20	1 piece	85	Egg salad	138	1 sandwich	279
Cookies, plain and		1 cooky, 3 in.		Ham	81	1 sandwich	281
assorted	25	diameter	120	Liverwurst	91	1 sandwich	251
				Peanut butter	83	1 sandwich	328
Crackers							
Cheese	18	5 crackers	86	Soups, commercial canned			
Graham	14	2 medium	55	Bean with pork	250	1 cup	170
Saltines	11	4 crackers	50	Beef noodle	250	1 cup	70
Rye	26	4 crackers	85	Chicken noodle	198	1 cup	51
				Cream (mushroom)	241	1 cup	215
Desserts and doughnuts				Tomato	198	1 cup	73
Cream puff—custard				Vegetable with beef			
filling	100	1 average	233	broth	241	1 cup	80

9

VITAMIN TOXICITY

"Quackery kills a larger number of U.S. citizens each year than all the diseases it pretends to cure."

Anonymous physician (National Quarterly Review, 1861)

Megadose vitamin use is not as harmless as touted by its proponents. A partial list of the toxicities of some of the vitamins when taken in megadose quantities should help to reduce their appeal as a cure for all that ails ye. A megadose is considered to be a dose equivalent to ten times the recommended daily dietary allowance.

Vitamin C

Uricosuria and uric acid stones
Hyperuricemia and gout
Urine acidification with oxalate and cystine stone formation
Heinz-body hemolysis in G-6-P-D deficient patients
Enhanced sickling in patients with sickle disease
Rebound scurvy in people suddenly ceasing to take the drug
Inactivation of Vitamin B_{12} in food (if taken for several years, it may produce B_{12} deficiency)
A false negative urine glucose with Testape
A false positive urine glucose with Clinitest
A false negative stool for occult blood

Folic Acid

Antagonizes the anticonvulsant activity of phenytoin producing increased seizure activity.

Quack — The term for the medical charlatan who dispenses fake remedies comes from the Dutch *kwakzalver*, one who "quacks like a duck" to hawk his salves.

Vitamin A

Cirrhosis
Elevated cerebrospinal fluid pressure
Nausea, headache
Hypercalcemia
Bone pain
Premature closure of the epiphyses
Teratogenesis

Vitamin K

Water-soluble derivatives produce oxidative red blood cell hemolysis
Radiosensitization

Niacin

Flushing
Pruritus
Skin rash, pigmented hyperkeratosis
Heartburn
Nausea, vomiting
Diarrhea
Abnormal liver chemistries

Pyridoxine

Seizures
Diminished effect of L-dopa in patients with Parkinson's disease

Vitamin D

Hypercalcemia
Pseudotumor cerebri

"Vitamin B$_{17}$" (Laetrile)

Cyanide poisoning

References: Herbert, V.: Resident and Staff Physician, December 1978, p. 43; DiPalma, J. R., and Ritchie, D. M.: Ann. Rev. Pharmacol. Toxicol., *17*:133, 1977.

pH OF COMMONLY INGESTED BEVERAGES

Have you ever wondered about the acidity of things you and your patients drink? It may be desirable to avoid drinks that are extremely acidic at times. The pH values of many commonly ingested beverages are listed below.

Very Acidic (pH $\leq$ 4.5)

Orange juice	Coca Cola
Carrot juice	Yukon Club Ginger Ale
Apricot juice	Pepsi Cola
Cranberry juice	Moxie
Prune juice	Koladex
Grape juice	Beer
Apple juice	Sherry
Tea	Port
Coffee	Vermouth

Acidic (pH 5.5 to 6.0)	*Weakly acidic* (pH 6.0 to 7.0)	*Weakly alkaline* (pH $\geq$ 7.0)
Hire's Root Beer	Whiskey	Vichy water
Sparkling water	Creme de Menthe	
Rum	Gin	
	Milk	

Reference: Jarvis, D. C. Folk Medicine: A Vermont Doctor's Guide to Good Health, 9th Edition. New York Holt, Rinehart & Winston, 1959.

CAFFEINE CONTENT OF POPULAR BEVERAGES

Caffeine is a potent central nervous system stimulant. The caffeine content of a number of popular beverages is:

Beverage	*Caffeine content per 6 oz. cup*
Coffee, brewed	100 to 150 mg
Coffee, instant	60 to 80 mg
Sanka, instant	3 to 5 mg
Tea	40 to 100 mg
Cola beverages	17 to 55 mg

The ingestion of 1 gram of caffeine may produce undesired reactions, including insomnia, restlessness, excitement, delirium, ringing in the ears, tremulousness, taut muscles, tachycardia, extrasystoles, and tachypnea. Remember an "APC" (aspirin, phenacetin, and caffeine) contains 30 mg of caffeine.

Reference: The Medical Letter, *19*.65, 1977.

TEA FOR TWO

Herbal teas are made from flowers, leaves, seeds, and roots. Enthusiastic faddists may consume large quantities and may get more than they bargained for. (See table on the following page.)

> *Tea* — Tea was mentioned as long ago as 350 A.D. The Mandarin word was *ch'a,* but the sailors of the China Sea called it *t'e* or *tay* in their dialect. Tea was cultivated in Java in the seventeenth century, whence the Dutch carried it to Europe. Tea (then called tee) was first sold publicly in England in the seventeenth century.

9

TEA OR COMPONENT OF TEA BLEND*	COMMENT OR EFFECT
Aloe	Powerful cathartic
Apple, Apricot, Bitter almond	Contain a cyanogeneic glycoside; can cause cyanide poisoning
Buchu	Mild diuretic
Buckthorn	Cathartic
Burdock root	Anticholinergic
"Bush tea"	Budd-Chiari syndrome
Cassava	Cyanide poisoning
Catnip	Psychotogenic
Chamomile	Anaphylaxis, hypersensitivity reactions
Cherry, Choke cherry	Cyanide poisoning
Dandelion	Diuretic
Devil's claw root	Abortifacient
Dock root	Powerful cathartic
Ginseng	Contains estrogrens
Goldenrod	Allergic reactions
Horsetail	See *shave grass*
Hydrangea	Psychotogenic
Indian tobacco	CNS-stimulating alkaloid; can cause sweating, vomiting, paralysis, hypothermia, coma, and death
Inkberry	See *pokeweed*
Jimsonweed	Psychotogenic
Juniper	GI irritant, psychotogenic
Licorice root	Aldosterone-like syndrome
Lobelia	Psychotogenic
Mandrake root	Contains scopolamine
Marigold	Allergic reactions
Mate	Pyrrolizidine alkaloids; liver failure
Mistletoe	Gastroenteritis, vasoconstriction, shock
Nutmeg	Hallucinogenic; cramps, nausea, headaches
Peach, Pear	Cyanide poisoning
Penny royal	Induces menstruation; abortifacient; renal, liver toxicity
Plum	Cyanide poisoning
Pokeweed root	Gastroenteritis, respiratory depression, death
Quack grass	Mild diuretic
Sassafras root bark	Hepatotoxic
Senna	Cathartic
Shave grass	Nicotine and thiaminase; CNS excitation; death; beriberi
Snakeroot	Reserpine
St. John's wort	Photodermatitis, allergies
Wormwood	Psychotogenic
Yarrow	Allergic reaction

*Leaves, roots, barks, oils, flowers, seeds, and berries.
Adapted from The Medical Letter, *21*:29, 1979.

SHOWDOWN (Caloric Analysis and Sodium Content of Fast Foods)

	WEIGHT (grams)	KILOCALORIES	SODIUM (mg)
Burger Chef			
Big Chef	186	542	622
Cheeseburger	104	304	535
Double cheeseburger	145	434	691
French fries	68	187	4
Hamburger, regular	91	258	393
Mariner Platter	373	680	882
Rancher Platter	316	640	444
Shake	305	326	167
Skipper's Treat	179	604	783
Super Chef	252	600	918

(*Source:* Burger Chef Systems, Inc. Indianapolis, Ind., 1978; analyses obtained from USDA Handbook No. 8.)

	WEIGHT (grams)	KILOCALORIES	SODIUM (mg)
Burger King			
Cheeseburger	—	305	562
Hamburger	—	252	401
Whopper	—	606	909
French fries	—	214	5
Vanilla shake	—	332	159
Whaler	—	486	735
Hot dog	—	291	841

(*Source:* Chart House, Inc. Oak Brook, Ill., 1978.)

	WEIGHT (grams)	KILOCALORIES	SODIUM (mg)
Dairy Queen			
Big Brazier deluxe	213	470	920
Big Brazier regular	184	457	910
Big Brazier with cheese	213	553	1435
Brazier with cheese	121	318	865
Brazier cheese dog	113	330	—
Brazier chili dog	128	330	939
Brazier dog	99	273	868
Brazier french fries, 2.5 oz	71	200	—
Brazier french fries, 4.0 oz	113	320	—
Brazier onion rings	85	300	—
Brazier regular	106	260	576
Fish sandwich	170	400	—
Fish sandwich with cheese	177	440	—
Super Brazier	298	783	1619
Super Brazier dog	182	518	1552

9

	WEIGHT (grams)	KILOCALORIES	SODIUM (mg)
Super Brazier dog with cheese	203	593	1986
Super Brazier chili dog	210	555	1640
Kentucky Fried Chicken			
Original recipe dinner*	425	830	2285
Extra crispy dinner*	437	950	1915
Individual pieces (original recipe)			
Drumstick	54	136	—
Keel	96	283	—
Rib	82	241	—
Thigh	97	276	—
Wing	45	151	—
9 Pieces	652	1892	—

(Source: Nutritional Content of Average Serving, Heublein Food Service and Franchising Group, June 1976.)

*Dinner comprises mashed potatoes and gravy, cole slaw, roll, and three pieces of chicken, either 1) wing, rib, and thigh; 2) wing, drumstick, and thigh; or 3) wing, drumstick, and keel.

Long John Silver's			
Breaded oysters, 6 pc	—	460	—
Breaded clams, 5 oz	—	465	—
Chicken planks, 4 pc	—	458	—
Cole slaw, 4 oz	—	138	—
Corn on cob, 1 pc	—	174	—
Fish with batter, 2 pc	—	318	—
Fish with batter, 3 pc	—	477	—
Fries, 3 oz	—	275	—
Hush puppies, 3 pc	—	153	—
Ocean scallops, 6 pc	—	257	—
Peg Leg with batter, 5 pc	—	514	—
Shrimp with batter, 6 pc	—	269	—
Treasure Chest			
2 pc fish, 2 Peg Legs	—	467	—

(Source: Long John Silver's Seafood Shoppes, Jan 8, 1978; nutritional analysis information furnished in study conducted by the Department of Nutrition and Food Science, University of Kentucky.)

	WEIGHT (grams)	KILOCALORIES	SODIUM (mg)
McDonald's			
Egg McMuffin	132	352	265
English muffin, buttered	62	186	94
Hot cakes, with butter & syrup	206	472	404
Sausage (pork)	48	184	55
Scrambled eggs	77	162	167
Big Mac	187	541	215
Cheeseburger	114	306	134
Filet O Fish	131	402	158
French fries	69	211	49
Hamburger	99	257	88
Quarter Pounder	164	418	179
Quarter Pounder with cheese	193	518	257
Apple pie	91	300	23
Cherry pie	92	298	23
McDonaldland cookies	63	294	51
Chocolate shake	289	364	292
Strawberry shake	293	345	298
Vanilla shake	289	323	266

(*Source:* Nutritional analysis of food served at McDonald's restaurants, WARF Institute, Inc., Madison, Wisc., June 1977.)

9

	WEIGHT (grams)	KILOCALORIES	SODIUM (mg)
Pizza Hut *			
Thin'N Crispy			
Beef	—	490	—
Pork	—	520	—
Cheese	—	450	—
Pepperoni	—	430	—
Supreme	—	510	—
Thick'N Chewy			
Beef	—	620	—
Pork	—	640	—
Cheese	—	560	—
Pepperoni	—	560	—
Supreme	—	640	—

(*Source:* Research 900 and Pizza Hut, Inc., Wichita, Kan.)
    *Based on a serving size of one half of a 10-inch pizza (three slices).

	WEIGHT (grams)	KILOCALORIES	SODIUM (mg)
Taco Bell			
Bean burrito	166	343	173
Beef burrito	184	466	288
Beefy tostada	184	291	265
Bellbeefer	123	221	140
Bellbeefer with cheese	137	278	208
Burrito Supreme	225	457	245
Combination burrito	175	404	230
Enchirito	207	454	338
Pintos'N Cheese	158	168	210
Taco	83	186	175
Tostada	138	179	186

(*Sources:* Menu items Portions, July 1976, Taco Bell Co., San Antonio, Tex.; Adams, C. F.: Nutritive Value of American Foods in Common Units, USDA Agricultural Research Service, Agricultural Handbook No. 456, November 1975; Church, C. F., and Church, H. N.: Food Values of Portions Commonly Used, 12th Edition, Philadelphia, J. B. Lippincott Co., 1975; Valley Baptist Medical Center, Food Service Department: Descriptions of Mexican-American foods, NASCO, Fort Atkinson, Wis.)

Tantalize — For punishment for services rendered, the Greek god Tantalus was placed in water up to his chin with delicious fruits dangling about his head. Both the water and the fruits receded when he tried to reach them. Good old chairman Zeus.

10

RENAL DISEASE

ABNORMAL URINE COLOR

Urine color may be affected by disease, drugs, and other commercial chemicals or by naturally occurring substances in food. A partial list of the causes of an abnormal urine color and the colors produced is given below.

URINE COLOR	CAUSE
Colorless	Dilute urine — overhydration; diabetes mellitus, diabetes insipidus, hypercalcemia
Orange	Concentrated urine — dehydration; santonin, salicyl-azosulfapyridine (Azulfidine), phenazopyridine (Pyridium, Azo Gantrisin, Azo Gantanol), ethoxazene (Serenium)
Milky	Chyluria, pyuria
Yellow	Normal, phenacetin, quinacrine, riboflavin
Red	Hematuria, hemoglobinuria, myoglobinuria, chronic mercury poisoning, chronic lead poisoning, eosin, phenytoin (Dilantin), phenindione (Hedulin), emodin (pH > 7), anisindione (Miradon), phenolphthalein (pH ≥ 7), phenothiazines, phensuximide (Milontin), rifampin, anthracyclines (adriamycin and analogues), anthrocyanin (food pigment found in beets and blackberries)
Brown-black	Acidification of hemoglobin pigments, melanin, homogentisic acid (alcaptonuria), p-hydroxyphenyl-pyruvic acid (tyrosinosis), methyldopa (Aldomet), cascara, pyrogallol, iron sorbitol (on exposure to light), methocarbamol (Robaxin), senna, phenyl-hydrazine, rhubarb
Blue, blue-green to green	Biliverdin, indicanuria, amitriptyline, anthraquinone, arbutin, flavin derivatives, indigo blue, indigo carmine, methocarbamol, methylene blue, tetrahydro-naphthalene (a degreasing agent sold as Tetralin), thymol, phenol, resorcinol, salol, toluidine blue (Blutene), triamterene (Dyrenium, Dyazide), *Pseudomonas aeruginosa,* Clorets
Brown to red-brown	Porphyria, urobilinogen, nitrofurantoin, primaquine, chloroquine, furazolidone, metronidazole, argyrol, fava beans, aloe (seaweed)

10

IS THE KIDNEY SIZE NORMAL?

It's difficult to remember the various normal ranges for renal size, which, like the size of many other organs, varies with stature. The length of the kidney may be compared with the size of the lumbar vertebral bodies, which are almost always evaluable on the same x-ray as the kidney. The size of 3 to 3½ lumbar vertebrae is a good estimate of normal kidney size.

SODIUM, SALT, MILLIGRAMS, AND MILLIEQUIVALENTS

Each molecule of salt (NaCl) is 39.3 per cent sodium by weight. Thus, to convert *salt* in milligrams to *sodium* in mg, multiply the weight of the salt by 0.393.

To convert mg of sodium to *milliequivalents,* divide by the atomic weight of sodium, which is 23. Thus, 1 gram (1000 mg) of sodium is equal to 43.5 mEq. A teaspoon of salt contains approximately 2400 mg, or 104 mEq, of sodium.

In dietary restriction of sodium, diets considered mildly restrictive contain 2400 to 4500 mg (100 to 200 mEq) of sodium, while moderately restrictive diets contain 1000 mg (43 mEq) of sodium per day. Strict sodium restriction limits *per diem* sodium intake to less than 500 mg, or 22 mEq.

Sodium and Salt in Gram and Milliequivalent Measurements

MILLIEQUIVALENTS Na+ (Approximate)	MILLIGRAMS Na+	GRAMS SALT (Approximate)
11	250	0.6
22	500	1.3
43	1000	2.5
65	1500	3.8
87	2000	5.0
130	3000	7.6
174	4000	10.2

POTASSIUM SUPPLEMENTATION

Most patients on diuretic therapy do not develop hypokalemia, even though their total body stores of potassium may be reduced. Patients taking digitalis preparations, patients with arrhythmias, and those who develop symptomatic hypokalemia should receive potassium (K) supplementation. The usual daily intake of K is 50 to 100 mEq per day. One study reported that a K supplementation of 60 mEq daily would maintain a normal serum K in 80 per cent of patients taking hydrochlorothiazide, 50 mg BID. When the serum potassium falls below 3 mEq/ liter, approximately 200 mEq of K replacement is required to raise the serum K 1 mEq/liter. There are three basic approaches to the management of hypokalemia in patients taking diuretics:

1. Use of K-sparing drugs (spironolactone, triamterene).
2. Use of oral potassium preparations.
3. Dietary K supplementation.

Potassium preparations are one of the most widely prescribed medications, despite the fact that patient compliance may be inconstant because of poor palatability. Palatability may be improved by mixing the K with fruit juices. K supplements may produce gastrointestinal distress. Ulceration and bleeding have been reported with slow-release K tablets. In addition, the cost of 60 mEq K is between 50 and 70 cents for different K supplements. An alternative is the use of dietary supplementation. Listed below are some foods and their approximate K content.

FOODS	SERVING	APPROXIMATE mEq K
Juices		
Orange	8 oz	13
Prune	8 oz	14
Tomato	8 oz	14
Grapefruit	8 oz	10
Apple	8 oz	6
Milk	8 oz	9
Coffee, Tea	1 cup	2.5
Fruits		
Apricots (dried)	100 grams	40
Dates	1 cup	36
Raisins	1 cup	29
Peaches (dried)	100 grams	25
Cantalope	½	23
Figs (dried)	7 small	20
Banana	1 medium	16
Watermelon	½ slice	10
Meats		
Turkey	4 oz	9
Beef round	3 oz	9

10

Commercial salt substitutes can also be used for K supplementation. Most salt substitutes contain 10 to 13 mEq K per gram, or 50 to 60 mg per level teaspoon. The cost of a teaspoon of salt substitute is between 4 and 13 cents, depending on the preparation. Some clinicians have reported that dietary sources, including salt substitutes, have been used successfully to maintain normal serum potassium levels in patients requiring supplementation.

TREATMENT OF HYPERKALEMIA

Potentially lethal hyperkalemia is quickly and easily reversed. The effect of hyperkalemia on neuromuscular events is a function of both the absolute serum potassium concentration and the rate of its rise or fall. Concomitant hyponatremia or hypocalcemia will enhance the manifestations of hyperkalemia. The urgency of therapy is usually indicated by the serum potassium level and the presence of EKG changes. Note, however, that ventricular tachycardia may occur without the EKG showing the classic manifestations of hyperkalemia.

Severity	Serum concentration
Mild	less than 6.5 mEq/liter
Moderate	6.5 to 8.0 mEq/liter
Severe	greater than 8.0 mEq/liter

The therapeutic maneuvers outlined below and on the opposite page are directed at antagonizing the cellular effects of potassium, causing the potassium to shift intracellularly, or removing potassium from the body. Monitoring of the patient's EKG is essential during therapy.

THERAPY	COMMENT
1. *Calcium:* Calcium chloride 5–10 ml of 10% solution given over 2 min; repeat if necessary (IV)	—Immediately antagonizes cardiac toxicity of hyperkalemia —Should not be used if patient digitalized

2. *Sodium bicarbonate:* 45 mEq over 5 min; repeat if EKG abnormalties persist (IV)

—Causes intracellular shift of potassium
—Watch for sodium overload in patients with renal failure or congestive heart failure

3. *Glucose-insulin infusion:* 1 unit of insulin for each 2 grams glucose; add 50 ml of 50% dextrose solution to 50 ml of D5W and 12 units of insulin, and administer over 15 to 30 min (IV)

—Causes intracellular shift of potassium
—$NaHCO_3$ can be added to glucose solution to augment effect
—Requires approximately 20 min to take effect

4. *Exchange resins:* Polystyrene sulfonate (Kayexalate); *Orally:* 15–30 grams Kayexalate in 100–200 ml 20% Sorbitol solution; may repeat every 3–4 hrs up to 4–5 doses/day

—Exchange takes place in colon; therefore, reduction in potassium level may be delayed 24 hrs if given by mouth
—Sorbitol given concomitantly to avoid constipation

Rectally: 15–30 grams Kayexalate plus 50 grams Sorbitol in 200 ml of water; give as retention enema for 30–60 min; may give at hourly intervals if needed

—Single enema may reduce serum potassium concentration by 0.5–1.0 mEq/liter
—*In vivo,* approximately 1 mEq of potassium removed per gram of resin
—Hypocalcemia may result secondary to binding of calcium to resin
—15 grams of Kayexalate releases 20 mEq of sodium; use cautiously in patients with heart failure
—May produce metabolic alkalosis if given with magnesium hydroxide or calcium carbonate

5. *Dialysis*

—Both hemodialysis and peritoneal dialysis can significantly reduce serum potassium

10

Therapeutic caveats:

1. Appropriate therapy is determined by the severity of the hyperkalemia.
2. IV calcium is the only therapy that is immediately effective and that directly antagonizes the cardiotoxic effects of hyperkalemia.
3. Both sodium bicarbonate and glucose/insulin require several minutes before having significant effects on potassium concentration. The effect will persist for several hours.
4. Therapies 1 to 3 do not deplete potassium from the body and are only temporarily effective. More long-lasting therapy (therapy 4 or 5) should be instituted concomitantly. Of course, when possible, the underlying cause of the hyperkalemia should be addressed.

References: Beeson, P. B., and McDermott, W. (Eds.): Textbook of Medicine. Philadelphia, W. B. Saunders Company, 1975, p. 1588; Surawicz, B.: Am. Heart J., *73*:814, 1967; Boedecker, E. C., and Dauber, J. H. (Eds.): Manual of Medical Therapeutics. Boston, Little, Brown and Company 1974, p. 44.

DIFFERENTIAL DIAGNOSIS OF PYURIA

Although the list of causes of persistent pyuria are legion, the evaluation of this condition is relatively straightforward. One should perform a thorough external genital and rectal exam. The pelvic exam should not be deferred in the female patient. The urinary stream should be observed in males. Urine for analysis should be obtained from the beginning, middle, and end of urination. Urine collections for tuberculosis should also be obtained where indicated. An intravenous pyelogram will give the most information about upper tract disease, while a cystoscopy will detect lower tract pathology.

Differential Diagnosis of Pyuria

UPPER TRACT	BLADDER AREA	LOWER TRACT
Renal tumor	Stricture of ureteral meatus Ureterocoele; reflux	Stenosis of urethral meatus
Renal tuberculosis	Cystitis	Paraphimosis (♂)
Pyelonephritis	Congenital posterior urethral valves	Urethral stricture
Perirenal abscess	Prostatitis; prostatic abscess (♂)	Urethral diverticulum
Calyceal stone	Periprostatitis (♂)	Periurethritis; periurethral abscess
Renal pelvic stone	Seminal vesiculitis (♂)	Urethritis
Ureteropelvic junction stricture	Cowperitis (♂)	Cervicitis (♀)
Hydronephrosis	Pelvic suppuration (♂, ♀)	Foreign body in vagina (♀)
Hydroureter		Vaginitis (♀)
Periureteritis; periureteral abscess		Skenitis (♀)
Aberrant vessel (obstruction of upper ureter)		Bartholinitis (♀)
Ureteral obstruction		
Ureteral diverticulum		
Ureteral stone		
Ureteral stricture		

Reference: Roberts, J. A.: Hosp. Med., *12*:6, 1976. Table reproduced with permission of author.

HYPOURICEMIA

The clinical significance of a low serum uric acid concentration lies in its association with certain serious systemic illnesses. Hypouricemia is most often caused, however, by medications that result in an enhanced renal clearance of uric acid. Thus, a low serum uric acid concentration in a patient ill with undiagnosed systemic disease should prompt a thorough drug history and an evaluation to exclude the diseases listed below.

A. *Decreased production* (low or normal uric acid clearance)
   1. Hereditary xanthinuria
   2. Allopurinol administration
   3. Severe liver disease
B. *Increased excretion* (high uric acid clearance)
   1. Drugs (high-dose salicylates, glyceryl guaiacolate, probenecid)
   2. Radiocontrast agents
   3. Liver disease
   4. Neoplasia
      a. Hodgkin's disease
      b. Small cell carcinoma of the lung
      c. Multiple myeloma
      d. Acute myeloid leukemia
   5. Intra-abdominal abscesses
   6. Fanconi syndrome (e.g., Wilson's disease, multiple myeloma, heavy metals, outdated tetracycline)
   7. Syndrome of inappropriate secretion of anti-diuretic hormone.

10

Reference: Kelly, W. N.: Arth. Rheum., *18*(Suppl.):731, 1975.

SIMPLE APPROACH TO COMPLEX ACID-BASE DISTURBANCES, OR HOW TO EVALUATE THE PATIENT WITHOUT A NOMOGRAM

Complex or mixed acid-base disturbances result when several primary events are occurring to change the serum pH. Unless you systematically evaluate all the factors involved, you may mistake the nature of the pathophysiologic derangement and fail to initiate the appropriate corrective action. There are four primary acid-base disturbances: (a) respiratory acidosis, (b) respiratory alkalosis, (c) metabolic acidosis, and (d) metabolic alkalosis. (See table on p. 311.)

A patient may have one, two, or three of these simultaneously (one cannot have both respiratory acidosis and respiratory alkalosis), and the net result may be to give a normal or near-normal blood pH. By keeping in mind certain rules while evaluating the measured electrolytes, PCO_2 and pH, you should be able to identify the clinical problem.

Ground Rules

1. The stimulus for normal compensation in simple acid-base disturbances is the change in pH produced by the initial shift in PCO_2 or HCO_3^-.

2. Normal compensation should not "over-correct" the pH.

3. The more profound the stress of a primary acid-base disturbance, the less likely the pH is to be normal. In this setting, a normal pH indicates the presence of a mixed acid-base disturbance.

4. A pH opposite to that predicted by the initial disturbance at a time when acid-base status is stable makes the diagnosis of a mixed disturbance mandatory.

5. Acidemia begets hyperkalemia unless the patient is K^+-depleted or unless the acidemia has been caused by loss of $KHCO_3$ (diamox, diarrhea, renal tubular acidosis).

Approach

1. History and physical exam.
2. Routine check of electrolytes; note:
   a. the HCO_3^-.
   b. the anion gap.
   c. K^+.
3. Explain the pH, PCO_2, and HCO_3^-.
4. Know or look up the common causes of simple acid-base disturbances (see table on opposite page).

Common Causes of Simple Acid-Base Disturbances

METABOLIC ACIDOSIS	METABOLIC ALKALOSIS	RESPIRATORY ACIDOSIS	RESPIRATORY ALKALOSIS
I. Normal anion gap (Hyperchloremic) 1. Gastrointestinal bicarbonate loss — diarrhea, pancreatic fistula 2. Ureteroenterostomy 3. Drugs — acetazolamide, sulfamylon, cholestyramine, acidifying agents 4. Hyperalimentation 5. Renal causes — interstitial renal disease, renal tubular acidosis	1. Vomiting 2. Nasogastric suction 3. Diuretic therapy 4. Alkali therapy 5. Mineralocorticoid excess 6. K^+ depletion 7. Glucocorticoid therapy 8. IV $SO_4^=$ or $PO_4^≡$ in a Na^+-depleted patient	1. CNS depression 2. Chronic obstructive airway disease 3. Severe asthma 4. Pneumothorax 5. Abdominal distention 6. Pulmonary edema 7. Mechanical underventilation 8. Idiopathic hypoventilation 9. Neuromuscular disease	1. Salicylate toxicity 2. Hepatic failure 3. Psychogenic hyperventilation 4. Pulmonary edema 5. Asthma 6. Gram negative sepsis 7. Restrictive lung disease 8. Primary CNS disease 9. Mechanical overventilation 10. Other causes of hypoxia

II. Elevated anion gap
1. Uremia (loss of >80% renal function)
2. Ketoacidosis
3. Lactic acidosis
4. Salicylate toxicity
5. Methanol toxicity
6. Ethylene glycol toxicity
7. Paraldehyde toxicity
8. Hyperalimentation

10

Reference: McCurdy, D. K.: Chest, *62*(Suppl.):355, 1972.

GAPS—ANION AND OSMOLAR

Gross abnormalities in serum solute concentration are easily recognized. Calculations of gaps — anion and osmolar — will yield valuable clues to less obvious disturbances in acid-base and fluid homeostasis.

Anion Gap

1. To calculate the anion gap, subtract the sum of the chloride and bicarbonate concentrations from the sodium concentration (concentrations are in mEq/liter).

$$\text{Anion gap} = Na^+ - (Cl^- + HCO_3^-)$$

(Anion gap = 8 to 12 mEq/liter in the normal situation.)

2. Calculate an anion gap for every set of electrolytes obtained. This will force you to look carefully at the values and keep you from missing an important derangement when the electrolytes are not grossly abnormal.

3. Elevated anion gap
    a. Metabolic acidosis (see table, Common Causes of Simple Acid-Base Disturbances, p. 311).
    b. Therapy with certain antibiotics (e.g., carbenicillin, high dose sodium penicillin).
    c. Dehydration (if water loss exceeds electrolyte loss).
    d. Respiratory alkalosis.
    e. Chloride responsive metabolic alkalosis.

4. Low anion gap
    a. Lab error.

Bromide — A tiresome person or his trite and banal remarks. The word was created by Gelett Burgess, the perpetrator of "The Purple Cow," in the title of his book, "Are You a Bromide?" (1907). In the same edition he concocted the word "blurb," which originally referred to publisher's extravagant blurbing about the merits of their own releases.

b. Hypoalbuminemia.
c. Hyperviscosity.
d. Bromism.
e. Multiple myeloma.
f. Hypercalcemia, hypermagnesemia, lithium toxicity.

Osmolar Gap

1. Serum osmolality can be calculated from the following equation:

$$\text{Serum osmolality} = 2 \ (\text{Na}^+) + \frac{(\text{glucose})}{18} + \frac{\text{BUN}}{2.8}$$

2. The *measured* serum osmolality (280 to 300 mOsm/kg H_2O) should not exceed the *calculated* osmolality by more than 10 mOsm/kg H_2O.

3. If the *calculated* osmolality exceeds the *measured* osmolality, it is either a lab error or a mathematical error.

4. If the *measured* osmolality exceeds the *calculated* osmolality by more than 10 mOsm/kg H_2O, an abnormal osmolar gap exists:

a. If the measured osmolality is normal and the calculated osmolality is low, there is a decrease in serum water. There are no unmeasured osmols, but plasma "solids" are increased (as in hyper-triglyceridemia or hyperglobulinemia) resulting in spurious hyponatremia.

b. If the measured osmolality and the calculated osmolality are elevated, an unmeasured osmol is present in the serum (e.g., sorbitol, mannitol, glycerin, diatrizoate sodium, isoniazid, ethanol, isopropyl alcohol, methanol, acetone, ether, trichloroethanol, and other low molecular weight solutes).

10

References: Emmett, M., and Narins, R. G.: Medicine, 56:38, 1977; Smithline, N., and Gardner, K. D.: J.A.M.A., 236:1594, 1976.

RENAL TUBULAR ACIDOSIS

Your patient might have renal tubular acidosis if a hyperchloremic acidosis is observed. Many of the causes of hyperchloremic acidosis can be readily excluded.

1. Renal disease
   a. Early renal failure
   b. Renal tubular disease
      i. Proximal tubular acidosis
      ii. Distal tubular acidosis
      iii. Deficiency of titratable acid or ammonium ion excretion

2. Gastrointestinal disease
   a. Pancreatic fistula
   b. Diarrhea
3. Ureterosigmoidostomy, ureteroileostomy
4. Hyperalimentation
5. Posthypocapnea
6. Rapid IV hydration

Hypokalemia and potassium depletion may occur in both proximal and distal tubular acidosis, and the consequences of a low potassium may dominate the clinical picture. The contrasting features of the three types of overt renal tubular acidosis are presented on the opposite page. The diagnosis may be derived from the pH of the morning urine and the response to an acid and bicarbonate load. Remember the renal tubular defect in acidification may be incomplete, and its diagnosis may *require* provocation by an ammonium chloride load and an assessment of response to therapy with sodium bicarbonate. The presence of latent RTA should be suggested by a positive family history, the presence of diseases known to be associated with RTA, or unexplained nephrolithiasis.

Calcium chloride, rather than ammonium chloride, should be employed in acidification of patients with hepatic disease. Since ammonia generation by bacteria may spuriously elevate the pH of a urine specimen, make sure the samples arrive in the laboratory and are analyzed without undue delay.

The differential diagnosis of renal tubular acidosis is outlined on pages 316, 317 and 318.

Contrasting Features of Renal Tubular Acidoses

	PROXIMAL RTA	DISTAL RTA	LOW BUFFER EXCRETION
Stones or nephrocalcinosis	Rare	Common	Uncommon
Associated phosphoglycosuria	Common	Rare	Rare
Expected serum HCO_3^- (mEq/liter)	Commonly ≥15	Commonly <15	Commonly ≥15
Serum K^+	Low	Low	Normal–high
BUN	Normal initially	Normal initially	Commonly high
Urinary pH (a) Random	Inappropriately alkaline	Inappropriately alkaline	Low
(b) First morning	Commonly <6.0	Never <6.0	Commonly <6.0
(c) Post-acid load	<5.3	Never <5.3	<5.3
Tm (HCO_3^-)	Low	Normal	Mildly low
Ease of HCO_3^- replacement	Resistant (≥3–5 mEq/kg/day)	Sensitive (<2–3 mEq/kg/day)	Sensitive

10

Differential Diagnosis of Renal Tubular Acidosis

I. Bicarbonate-wasting syndrome (proximal or type II RTA)
  A. Primary
    1. Infantile
      a. Pure HCO_3^- wasting
      b. Mixed proximal defects
    2. Adult
      a. Pure HCO_3^- wasting
      b. Mixed proximal defects
  B. Secondary
    1. Disorders of *amino acid* metabolism
      a. Tyrosinemia
      b. Cystinosis
    2. Disorders of *carbohydrate* metabolism
      a. Hereditary fructose intolerance
      b. Galactosemia
      c. Glycogen storage (type I)
    3. Disorders of *protein* metabolism
      a. Myeloma
      b. Nephrotic syndrome
      c. Amyloidosis
      d. Hyperglobulinemia and malignancies
    4. Heavy metal toxicity
      a. Cadmium
      b. Lead
      c. Copper (Wilson's disease)
      d. Mercury
    5. Drugs and hormones
      a. Carbonic anhydrase inhibitors
        (1) Acetazolamide
        (2) Sulfamylon
      b. Tetracycline (outdated)
      c. 6-Mercaptopurine
      d. Hyperparathyroidism
    6. Miscellaneous
      a. Lowe's syndrome
      b. Renal transplantation

II. Distal RTA (gradient, type I)
   A. Primary
      1. Hereditary
      2. Sporadic
   B. Secondary
      1. Disorders of calcium metabolism
         a. Hyperparathyroidism
         b. Hyperthyroidism
         c. Hypervitaminosis D
      2. Disorders of protein metabolism
         a. Hyperglobulinemia
         b. Amyloidosis
      3. Disorders of sodium metabolism
         a. Edema-forming states
      4. Drugs
         a. Amphotericin B
         b. Lithium carbonate
      5. Miscellaneous
         a. Renal transplantation
         b. Medullary sponge kidney
         c. Hereditary elliptocytosis
         d. Chronic hydronephrosis
         e. Mineralocorticoid deficiency
         f. Wilson's disease
III. Low buffer excretion
   A. Phosphate depletion
   B. Failure of ammoniogenesis
      1. Azotemic hyperchloremic acidosis
      2. Gout
   C. Miscellaneous
      1. Systemic lupus erythematosus
      2. Hypoaldosteronism

10

Reference: Narins, R. G., and Goldberg, M. Renal tubular acidosis: Pathophysiology, diagnosis, and treatment. In Dowling, H. F., et al. (eds.): Disease-A-Month, *26*:23, 1977. Copyright © 1977 by Year Book Medical Publishers, Inc., Chicago. Tables and outline reproduced with permission of author and publisher.

SODIUM BICARBONATE LOADING TEST TO DISTINGUISH PROXIMAL FROM DISTAL RTA

1. Remember a first a.m. urine with a pH $<$ 5.5 effectively excludes distal RTA!
2. Give enough $NaHCO_3$ to raise the serum HCO_3^- from its usual 15 to 20 mEq/liter to 23 to 26 mEq/liter. Continue for several days.
3. Measure the serum and urine creatinine and HCO_3^-.
4. Calculate: The fraction of filtered HCO_3^- excreted = 100 $\times$ $^U HCO_3^- \times P_{Cr}/P_{HCO_3^-} \times U_{Cr}$.
5. If the fractional excretion of HCO_3^- is greater than 15 per cent, proximal RTA is present since renal disease, low buffer excretion, or distal RTA do not usually increase the fractional HCO_3^- excretion above 10 per cent.

AMMONIUM CHLORIDE LOADING TEST FOR ADEQUACY OF URINARY ACIDIFICATION

The object of the test is to establish the adequacy of the mechanisms for acidification of the urine. Ammonium chloride (0.1 mg/kg) capsules (not tablets) are taken over 45 minutes. The patient may eat and drink over the ensuing eight hours, during which hourly urine samples are collected. The dose of ammonium chloride is equivalent to about 2 mEq/kg of H^+ ion and should lower the serum HCO_3^- by 2 to 5 mEq/liter. This should be checked by a baseline venous or arterial HCO_3^- at zero time and three hours into the test. The normal kidney will respond to the systemic acidosis by lowering the urinary pH to less than 5.3. A normal response rules out distal RTA. Patients with proximal RTA and deficient buffer excretors should acidify normally. Monitoring the serum HCO_3^- or pH will exclude malabsorption of NH_4Cl as the cause of a negative test. Remember to check urinary pH promptly, and do a urine culture to rule out a urinary tract infection that will invalidate the test results.

CHANGES IN GLOMERULAR FILTRATION RATE ASSOCIATED WITH AGING

There is a 20 per cent reduction in renal mass from the fourth to the eighth decades and a loss of approximately 30 per cent of glomeruli. The creatinine clearance remains stable until age 45, at which time a decrease in creatinine clearance of 6.5 ml/min/1.73 sq m/decade occurs. The serum creatinine remains normal, as a parallel reduction in muscle mass reduces the amount of creatinine available for excretion. Therefore, the serum creatinine cannot be used as an accurate guide to renal function in the elderly patient. This fact assumes clinical importance when potentially dangerous drugs that are excreted primarily by the kidney, such as the aminoglycoside antibiotics and digoxin, are used. The creatinine clearance becomes a more accurate assessment of renal function in the elderly and should be employed, rather than the serum creatinine, to determine appropriate drug dosages.

Reference: Rowe, J. W.: Resident and Staff Physician, *24*:49, 1978.

URINARY DIAGNOSTIC PROFILE

Oliguria is a common clinical problem. After you have ruled out an obstructive basis for the oliguria (remember that an obstruction in the circuit can occur at any site from the entry of the tube into the urimeter to the renal pelvis), the major differential is between renal hypoperfusion and an intrinsic renal disease, such as acute tubular necrosis. It is useful to be able to identify those patients with renal hypoperfusion, because appropriate intervention may prevent acute renal injury. In most instances, it is possible to distinguish renal hypoperfusion from acute tubular necrosis with a battery of urinary chemical indices. To construct a urinary diagnostic profile, you need to measure urine sodium, osmolality, creatinine, and urea, and plasma creatinine, sodium, and urea.

The table below summarizes the characteristic indices obtained in patients with prerenal azotemia and acute oliguric renal failure (acute tubular necrosis, or ATN). A few patients with oliguric and most patients with nonoliguric renal failure exhibit values between those of patients with prerenal azotemia and oliguric acute renal failure. These indices are not helpful in the diagnosis of acute glomerular lesions or obstructive uropathy, but careful clinical evaluation and examination of the urine sediment will usually distinguish these disorders.

10

INDEX	UNITS/FORMULA	PRERENAL	RENAL
Urine osmolality	mOsm/kg H_2O	> 500	< 350
Urine sodium	mEq/liter	< 20	> 40
Urine/plasma urea nitrogen	—	> 8	< 3
Urine/plasma creatinine	—	> 40	< 20
Renal failure index	$U_{Na}/U/P_{CR}$	< 1	> 1
Fractional excretion of filtered sodium	$\dfrac{U/P_{Na}}{U/P_{CR}} \times 100$	< 1	> 1

Reference: Miller, T. R., Anderson, R. J., Linas, S. L., et al.: Ann. Intern. Med., *89*:47, 1978.

MYOGLOBINURIA IN THE ABSENCE OF OBVIOUS CRUSH INJURY

The release of myoglobin into the plasma and myoglobinuria occur when there is muscle injury. It is becoming increasingly apparent that many circumstances besides crush injury may lead to liberation of sufficient quantities of myoglobulin to produce myoglobinuria. The combination of myoglobinuria and dehydration are associated with a form of acute renal failure in which hyperkalemia and hypocalcemia occur very rapidly. These electrolyte disturbances may in turn lead to severe cardiac rhythm disturbances. Thus, recognition of the syndrome of nontraumatic myoglobinuria becomes clinically important if one is to prevent or treat the exaggerated metabolic consequences of this particular type of acute renal failure. The triad of orthotoluidine-positive urine, pigmented granular casts in the urine sediment, and a very high serum creatine phosphokinase level in association with one of the conditions listed below strongly suggests the presence of myoglobinuria.

Non-Traumatic Myoglobinuria

I. Hereditary
   A. McArdle's disease (phosphorylase deficiency)
   B. Carnitine palmityl transferase deficiency
   C. Malignant hyperthermia following anesthetics and succinylcholine
II. Grand mal seizures
   A. From any cause (e.g., idiopathic epilepsy, meningitis, cerebral metastases, alcohol withdrawal)
   B. Electric shock therapy
III. Prolonged coma
   A. Compression by body in prolonged coma
IV. Infection
   A. Viral illness in the absence of fever
V. Strenuous exercise
VI. Heat stroke
VII. Electrical injuries
VIII. Chronic hypokalemia
IX. Ischemia
   A. Arterial occlusion of extremity
   B. Carbon monoxide poisoning
X. Toxins
   A. Alcohol
   B. Malayan sea snake bite poison
   C. Heroin (without coma)

References: Grossman, R., Hamilton, R., Morse, B., et al.: N. Engl. J. Med., *291*:807, 1974; Rowland, L., and Penn, A.: Med. Clin. North Am., *56*:1233, 1972.

RENAL DISEASE ASSOCIATED WITH ANALGESIC USE

One of the most common causes of chronic end-stage renal disease is chronic analgesic ingestion! In the United States, analgesic nephropathy has been implicated in 5 per cent of patients with chronic renal failure. Data from other parts of the world indicate that analgesic-associated renal failure occurs with a frequency ranging from 11 to 22 per cent in patients with chronic renal failure.

Most patients with this syndrome have ingested aspirin and phenacetin-containing compounds. Data exist to suggest that the combination of the two drugs are more nephrotoxic than if either is taken alone.

The initial lesions involve the renal papillae and ultimately lead to medullary interstitial scarring and the changes of chronic interstitial nephritis of the renal cortex.

Thus, the urine findings and the natural history of the disease are those of chronic interstitial nephritis with minimal proteinuria (less than 1 gram/day), the absence of red cell casts, the presence of pyuria, and occasionally the presence of papillary necrosis. The patients are usually asymptomatic until azotemia supervenes. Hypertension occurs in 50 to 70 per cent of patients and may be present prior to the development of azotemia. The earliest functional problem is a renal concentrating defect, with isosthenuria (constant specific gravity) or hyposthenuria (urine constantly hypotonic to plasma) resistant to vasopressin. Hyperchloremic metabolic acidosis and a sodium losing tendency may also develop.

The syndrome occurs most often in middle-aged women taking analgesics for recurrent headaches and backaches. The threshold dose for the development of nephrotoxicity is unknown. Stopping the drugs leads to stabilization or improvement in the azotemia in the majority of patients. Thus, a history of chronic headache or backache in a patient should prompt an inquiry into the patient's use of analgesic drugs, as analgesic nephropathy is one of the few chronic renal diseases that is both preventable and partially reversible.

10

Reference: Goldberg, M., and Murray, T. G.: N. Engl. J. Med., *299*:716, 1978.

THE UREMIC SYNDROME

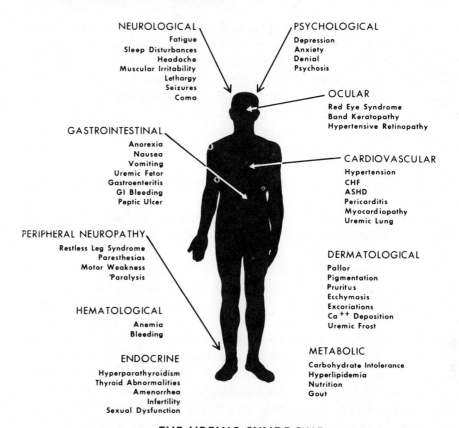

NEUROLOGICAL
Fatigue
Sleep Disturbances
Headache
Muscular Irritability
Lethargy
Seizures
Coma

PSYCHOLOGICAL
Depression
Anxiety
Denial
Psychosis

OCULAR
Red Eye Syndrome
Band Keratopathy
Hypertensive Retinopathy

GASTROINTESTINAL
Anorexia
Nausea
Vomiting
Uremic Fetor
Gastroenteritis
GI Bleeding
Peptic Ulcer

CARDIOVASCULAR
Hypertension
CHF
ASHD
Pericarditis
Myocardiopathy
Uremic Lung

PERIPHERAL NEUROPATHY
Restless Leg Syndrome
Paresthesias
Motor Weakness
Paralysis

DERMATOLOGICAL
Pallor
Pigmentation
Pruritus
Ecchymosis
Excoriations
Ca^{++} Deposition
Uremic Frost

HEMATOLOGICAL
Anemia
Bleeding

ENDOCRINE
Hyperparathyroidism
Thyroid Abnormalities
Amenorrhea
Infertility
Sexual Dysfunction

METABOLIC
Carbohydrate Intolerance
Hyperlipidemia
Nutrition
Gout

THE UREMIC SYNDROME

Schematic representation of symptoms and abnormalities of the uremic state.

FIG. 10–1

Reference: Schoenfield, P. Y., and Humphreys, M. H.: A general description of the uremic state. In Brenner, B. M., and Rector, F. C. (Eds.): The Kidney. Philadelphia, W. B. Saunders Company, 1972, p. 1432. Figure reproduced with permission of author and publisher.

SOME DRUGS EXCRETED PRIMARILY BY THE KIDNEY

Barbital	Methotrexate
Carbenicillin	Methyldopa
Chlorpropamide	Neomycin
Colistin	Phenformin
Cycloserine	Phenobarbital
Digoxin	Quaternary ammonium anticholinergics
Ethambutol	Sulfinpyrazone
5-Fluorocytosine	Tetracycline
Gentamicin	Tobramycin
Kanamycin	Vancomycin

Reference: Reidenberg, M. M.: Am. J. Med., *62*:482, 1977.

CARDIAC GLYCOSIDES IN PATIENTS WITH RENAL INSUFFICIENCY

Digoxin

The usual loading doses (i.e., 0.75 to 1.25 mg) are given, but maintenance doses are modified. One suggested schedule is:

Creatinine clearance (ml/min)	Average dose (mg)
0	0.125 given 3 to 5 times a week
25	0.20 daily
50	0.25 daily
75	0.30 daily
100	0.35 daily

If a patient with renal insufficiency requires dialysis, maintain a K^+ concentration of 3.0 to 3.5 mEq/liter in the dialysis bath to prevent sudden decreases in serum K^+ concentration during dialysis. No supplemental dose is required after dialysis.

Digitoxin

The usual loading dose (i.e., 0.8 to 1.4 mg) is administered, and the maintenance dose should be modified in either of two ways:

a. $D = 7.7 + (0.035 \times C_{CR})$
    D = daily maintenance dose expressed as *per cent* of *loading dose*
    C_{CR} = creatinine clearance in ml/min
    e.g., loading dose = 1.2 mg
    $\qquad C_{CR} = 10$ ml/min
    $\qquad D = 7.7 + (0.035 \times 10)$
    $\qquad D = 7.7 + 0.35$
    $\qquad D = 8.05\%$
    $\qquad (0.080) \times (1.2) = 0.1$ mg daily dose

b. Give a maintenance dose equal to $^2/_3$ to $^3/_4$ the usual maintenance dose of patients with normal renal function, e.g., 0.1 mg given five days a week.
    No supplemental dose is required after dialysis.

Reference: Cheigh, J. S.: Am. J. Med., *62*:555, 1977.

DRUG OVERDOSE/TOXICITY MOST RESPONSIVE TO DIALYSIS

Aminoglycosides
Barbiturates
Bromide
Phenytoin
Ethchlorvynol
Glutethimide
Lithium
Methaqualone
Meprobamate
Methyprylon
Salicylates
Thiocyanate

Reference: Maher, J. F.: Am. J. Med., *62*:475, 1977.

ANTIMICROBIAL AGENTS NOT REQUIRING DOSE MODIFICATION IN PATIENTS WITH RENAL INSUFFICIENCY

Certain penicillins (oxacillin, cloxacillin, dicloxacillin, nafcillin)
Clindamycin
Chloramphenicol
Doxycycline
Erythromycin
Ethionamide
Pyrimethamine
Rifampin

Reference: Anderson, R. J., Gambertoglio, J. G., and Schrier, R. W. Fate of drugs in renal failure. In Brenner, B. M., and Rector, F. C., (Eds.): The Kidney. Philadelphia, W. B. Saunders Company, 1976, p. 1917.

SOME DRUGS REQUIRING SUPPLEMENTAL DOSES AFTER DIALYSIS

Aminoglycosides

Gentamicin
Tobramycin
Kanamycin
Streptomycin

Cephalosporins

    Cephalothin
    Cephalexin
    Cephapirin
    Cephazolin

Penicillins

    Penicillin
    Ampicillin
    Carbenicillin

Other Antimicrobials

    Sulfonamides
    Chloramphenicol
    Trimethoprim
    Cycloserine
    Ethambutol
    5-Fluorocytosine

Other Drugs

    Aminophylline
    Methyldopa
    Procainamide
    Methotrexate
    5-Fluorouracil
    Cyclophosphamide

10

Reference: Maher, J. F.: Am. J. Med., *62*:475, 1977.

DRUGS IN THE PATIENT WITH RENAL INSUFFICIENCY

The vast number of drugs makes it impossible to list the recommended dose adjustments for patients with renal insufficiency. The following reference list, however, will provide ready access to the desired information.

1. Bennett, W. M., Singer, I., Golper, T., et. al.: Ann. Intern. Med., *86*:754, 1977. (An updated list will be published in 1980.)
2. Anderson, R. J., Gambertoglio, J. G., and Schrier, R. W.: Fate of drugs in renal failure. In Brenner, B. M., and Rector, F. C., (Eds.): The Kidney. Philadelphia, W. B. Saunders Company, 1976, pp. 1911–1948.
3. Bennett, W. M., Singer, I., and Coggins, C. J.: J.A.M.A. *230*:1544, 1974.
4. Cheigh, J. S.: Am. J. Med., *62*:555, 1977.

PERITONEAL DIALYSIS

The peritoneum is an inert, semipermeable membrane with a surface area approximately equal to that of the glomerular capillaries. Thus it lends itself to the exchange of solutes and fluids with 20 per cent of the efficiency of hemodialysis.

Peritoneal dialysis is most often employed in patients with acute oliguric renal failure, azotemia, hyperkalemia, or fluid overload or in patients with a drug intoxication if hemodialysis is unavailable. Consequently, the physician may have to institute peritoneal dialysis away from a referral center. An outline of some of the features of peritoneal dialysis may prove helpful (see pp. 328 and 329).

(For the composition of various dialysis solutions, see table on opposite page.)

Composition of Dialysis Solutions

PER CENT DEXTROSE	OSMOLALITY (mOsm/kg water)	Na⁺ (mEq/liter)	Cl⁻ (mEq/liter)	Ca⁺⁺ (mEq/liter)	Mg⁺⁺ (mEq/liter)	ACETATE OR LACTATE (mEq/liter)
1.5	372–375	140–142	101–102	3.5–4.0	1.0–1.5	33–45
3.0	435	132	102	3.0	1.0	33
4.25	526	140	101	4.0	1.5	45
7.0	677–686	140–146	101–102	3.5–4.0	1.5	45

Notes:
1. Under most circumstances, 7 per cent dextrose solutions should not be used unless one is treating severe pulmonary edema in a patient with renal failure.
2. Commercial dialysates contain no K⁺. Potassium is added to the dialysis fluid as needed.

10

A. Contraindications
1. *Absolute:* A patent opening between the peritoneal cavity and the pleural space.
2. *Relative:*
   a. Recent severe abdominal trauma.
   b. Previous abdominal surgery with adhesions.
   c. Recent abdominal surgery requiring insertion of a prosthetic device.
   d. Peritonitis.

B. Rate of solute clearance
1. *Equilibration time:* The longer the fluid remains in the abdomen, the greater the amount of solute removed.
2. *Rate of dialysate flow:* The greater the rate of dialysate flow, the greater the clearance. The usual rates of flow are 2.5 to 3.3 liters/hr.
3. *Temperature:* Heating the dialysis fluid to 37°C increases urea clearance.
4. *Dialysis fluid:* The use of more hypertonic fluid increases urea clearance.

C. Relative rates of clearance of solutes
1. Urea $> K^+ > CL^- > Na^+ >$ creatinine $>$ phosphate $>$ uric acid $> HCO_3^- > Ca^{++} > Mg^{++}$.
2. Maximum urea clearance is 15 to 30 ml/min.
3. Maximum creatinine clearance is 10 to 15 ml/min.

D. Complications
1. *Minor:* Abdominal pain, bleeding or leakage around the cannula; subcutaneous dissection of fluid.
2. *Major:* Peritonitis (5 to 10 per cent), bladder perforation, bowel perforation, loss of cannula into peritoneum, atelectasis, pleural effusion, pneumonia.
3. *Metabolic:* Volume depletion with hypotension and worsening oliguria, fluid overload with pulmonary edema, hyperglycemia, occasionally hyperglycemic hyperosmolar nonketotic coma, hypocalcemia, lactic acidosis in patients with liver disease, hypernatremia, metabolic alkalosis, protein and amino acid loss (20 to 60 grams protein/48 hr of dialysis; 5 to 10 grams essential amino acid loss/48 hr of dialysis).

E. Management of Peritoneal Dialysis

Once the cannula is in position, the routine dialysis orders should include:

1. Specify the *type* of *dialysis fluid* to be used and warm to 37°C (e.g., 1.5 per cent dextrose).
2. Specify the *exchange times* for each 2-liter run (e.g., *inflow time* – 15 minutes; *dwell time* – 20–25 minutes; *outflow time* – 20 minutes).
3. Add 500 U heparin to every other exchange.
4. Check vital signs hourly.
5. Culture the dialysate twice daily.
6. Determine levels of serum electrolytes, glucose, creatinine and BUN every 12 hours.
7. Add KCl to the dialysis fluid as needed after the first 24 hours.
8. Order insulin as needed.
9. Weigh the patient daily.
10. Record accurate total intakes and outputs.
11. Write orders for intravenous fluid replacement as required.

To reduce the likelihood of peritonitis, the dialysis should not be maintained for longer than 36 to 48 hours. Intraperitoneal antibiotics should not be instilled prophylactically. If peritonitis develops, the patient is treated with systemic (as opposed to intraperitoneal) parenteral antibiotics.

The organisms usually involved in peritoneal dialysis peritonitis are *Staphylococcus aureus* and the gram negative aerobic bacilli.

References: Table adapted from Gault, M. H., Ferguson, E. L., Sidhu, J. S., and Corbin, R. P.: Ann. Intern. Med., *75*:253, 1971; Miller, R. B., and Tassistro, C. R.: N. Engl. J. Med., *281*:945, 1969; Dunea, G.: Med. Clin. North Am., *55*:155, 1971.

10

KIDNEY STONES

Kidney stones account for approximately 200,000 hospitalizations per year plus untold emergency room visits. The types of renal stones are shown in Fig. 10–2. Calcium oxalate and calcium oxalate–calcium phosphate (hydroxyapatite) stones account for 66 to 75 per cent of kidney stones. Magnesium ammonium phosphate (struvite) accounts for 15 per cent, uric acid stones for 10 per cent, and cystine stones 1 per cent of all renal stones. Pure calcium phosphate (apatite) stones account for a very small per cent of all kidney stones and tend to be found in urine that is persistently alkaline, as in distal renal tubular acidosis.

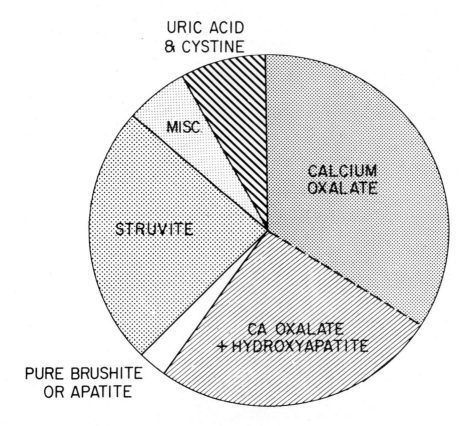

Types of Renal Calculi.

FIG. 10–2

Calculate — In ancient Rome, *calculi* meant "little stones." These stones were used as a primitive calculator and were the forerunners of calculus.

Evaluation

A logical approach to the patient with nephrolithiasis involves defining the pathogenetic mechanism(s), reducing the concentration of stone constituents in the urine, and reducing the risk factors predisposing to stone formation. The risk factors for calcium stone formation include:

1. *Dehydration:* Leads to a concentrated urine and promotes saturation of the urine with stone constituents.
2. *Diet:* Attention should be paid to the calcium, oxalate, and purine intake.
3. *Family history:* 25 per cent of people with recurrent calcium stones have a close relative with a history of kidney stones.
4. *Hypercalciuria:* Enhanced calcium excretion is found in patients with recurrent calcium oxalate stones.
5. *Hyperoxaluria:* A minority of patients with calcium oxalate stones have high normal or high oxalate excretion (normal oxalate excretion is 15 to 60 mg/day). Only a few clinical syndromes demonstrate marked increases in oxalate excretion. (See Hyperoxaluria, p. 333.)
6. *Hyperuricosuria:* Hyperuricosuria is associated with a propensity to form calcium oxalate stones.
7. *Medications:* Vitamins A and D are associated with hypercalcemia, hypercalciuria, and nephrolithiasis. Vitamin C is metabolized to oxalate, leading to hyperoxaluria. Acetazolamide causes a persistently alkaline urine, which leads to pure calcium phosphate stone formation.
8. *Urine pH:* Acid urine promotes uric acid and cystine stone formation. Alkaline urine promotes pure calcium phosphate stone formation. Variations in urine pH in the physiologic range have little influence on the solubility of calcium oxalate.

10

Evaluation of the patient with a *first* episode of kidney stones should include a urinalysis and the following tests: urine pH, urine culture if pyuria is present, serum calcium, 24-hour urine for calcium with the patient on at least a 1000 mg elemental calcium diet, serum uric acid, and 24-hour urine uric acid.

If the patient has a history suggestive of recurrent episodes of renal stones, a more comprehensive evaluation should be undertaken. Again the patient should be consuming at least a 1000 mg elemental calcium diet.

Metabolic Evaluation for Recurrent Kidney Stones

TEST	DAY			
	1	*2*	*3*	*4*
serum calcium	+	+	+	+
serum electrolytes	+	–	–	–
serum uric acid	+	+	+	+
serum creatinine	+	+	+	+
24-hour urinary uric acid excretion	+	–	–	+
24-hour urinary calcium excretion	–	+	+	–
24-hour urinary creatinine excretion	+	+	+	+
urine cystine screen	+	–	–	–
fresh urine pH	+	–	–	–
urinalysis	+	–	–	–
urine culture	+	–	–	–

+ means the test *is* performed.
– means the test is *not* performed.

Additional evaluation is required if any of the data generated above suggest hypercalciuria, hyperuricosuria, renal tubular acidosis, oxaluria, cystinuria, or infection.

Management

The long term management of patients with nephrolithiasis consists of eliminating any underlying pathogenetic mechanism (e.g., primary hyperparathyroidism) and reducing the risk factors:

A. Hypercalciuric states
1. Idiopathic hypercalciuria
   a. *Absorptive:* No truly effective therapy exists.
   b. *Renal:* Thiazide diuretics.
2. Distal renal tubular acidosis (complete): Systemic alkalinization. (See Renal Tubular Acidosis, p. 313.)
3. Hypercalcemic states causing hypercalciuria: Correct the condition causing the hypercalcemia (e.g., primary hyperparathyroidism, vitamin D intoxication, thyrotoxicosis).
4. Maintain a high fluid intake, especially at night.

B. Hyperuricosuria
1. Give allopurinol.
2. Alkalinize the urine.
3. Maintain a high fluid intake especially at night.
C. Hyperoxaluria
1. Treat the condition causing the hyperoxaluria or reduce the intestinal absorption of oxalate (see Hyperoxaluria, below).
D. Magnesium ammonium phosphate stones
1. These stones form in persistently alkaline urine caused by recurrent urinary tract infection by urea-splitting organisms.
2. The therapy is aimed at acidifying the urine and eradicating any infection.
3. Maintaining a high fluid intake is important.
E. Cystine stones
1. Cystinuria is an autosomal recessive trait characterized by an impairment of cystine, arginine, lysine, and ornithine transport by the mucosal cells of the kidney and small intestine.
2. Cystine is the least soluble naturally occurring amino acid and precipitates in an acid urine, producing radiopaque stones.
3. D-penicillamine may be used to dissolve cystine stones and prevent formation of new stones.
4. Alkalinize the urine to a pH of greater than 7.5.
5. Maintain a high fluid intake, especially at night.

References: Williams, H. E.: N. Engl. J. Med., *290*:33, 1974; Broadus, A. E., and Thier, S. O.: N. Engl. J. Med., *300*:839, 1979; Coe, F. L.: The clinical and laboratory assessment of the patient with renal disease. In Brenner, B. M., and Rector, F. C. (Eds.): The Kidney. Philadelphia, W. B. Saunders Company, 1976, p. 801. Fig. 10–2 reproduced with permission of author and the New England Journal of Medicine, *290*:33, 1974.

10

HYPEROXALURIA

Oxalate is a component of the majority of kidney stones. In most patients with calcium oxalate stones, oxalate excretion is within the normal range of 15 to 60 mg/24 hours. There are, however, a few clinical conditions in which urinary oxalate excretion is increased, resulting in a marked tendency to form calcium oxalate stone.

A. *Increased Intake of Oxalate or its Precursors*
1. spinach (and spinach family), rhubarb, parsley, pepper, cocoa, tea, vitamin C
(all must be ingested in large amounts)
2. ethylene glycol poisoning
3. methoxyflurane anesthesia

B. *Increased Absorption of Dietary Oxalate*
1. jejunoileal bypass, ileal resection, Crohn's disease
2. intestinal bacterial overgrowth syndromes
3. any intestinal condition associated with fat malabsorption, e.g., chronic pancreatic and biliary tract disease
C. *Increased Endogenous Production of Oxalate*
1. pyridoxine deficiency
2. primary hyperoxaluria Type I and Type II

References: Williams, H. E.: N. Engl. J. Med., *290*:33, 1974; Broadus, A. E., and Thier, S. O.: N. Engl. J. Med., *300*:839, 1979.

11
ENDOCRINOLOGY

DIABETES MELLITUS—WHO HAS IT?

To be sure, a diagnosis of diabetes mellitus demands the demonstration of hyperglycemia. What samples to obtain, when to do a glucose tolerance test (GTT), and how to interpret the GTT are areas upon which there is little agreement. As an aid in the evaluation of a patient suspected of having diabetes, the following guidelines should be useful. If plasma is used instead of whole blood for the glucose determinations, add 15 per cent to the glucose value measured in whole blood (i.e., plasma glucose = whole blood glucose × 1.15).

a. Any fasting blood glucose concentration > 110 mg/100 ml is suspect.

b. A random blood glucose concentration > 125 mg/100 ml is suspect.

c. A 2-hour postprandial blood glucose concentration > 160 mg/100 ml is suspect.

If several specimens repeatedly demonstrate one of the above abnormalities, then no further diagnostic study is required. However, if reasonable doubts about the diagnosis exists, and the blood glucose falls below these levels, an oral GTT should be performed.

Oral GTT

1. The patient should consume at least 200 grams of carbohydrate per day for three days prior to the test.

2. Perform after an overnight fast.

3. Administer 100 grams of flavored glucose in a 25 per cent solution *chilled* to minimize nausea and vomiting.

4. Venous blood is drawn prior to administration of glucose and at hourly intervals for three hours.

5. Draw blood at hourly intervals for five hours if reactive hypoglycemia is suspected.

6. A sample of blood is not drawn 30 minutes after administration of the glucose unless intestinal malabsorption is suspected.

11

Many interpretations of the oral GTT have been made. The first table offers three different published criteria for an abnormal oral GTT arranged by the stringency of the criteria for making a diagnosis of diabetes mellitus. The second table lists the criteria for interpretation of the oral GTT in pregnancy.

Abnormal Oral GTT

WHOLE BLOOD GLUCOSE (mg/100 ml)

	Most Sensitive– Least Selective	Middle Ground	Most Selective– Least Sensitive
Fasting	110 (125)	110 (125)	125 (140)
1 hour	160 (185)	170 (195)	225 (260)
1½ hours	145 (165)	—	—
2 hours	120 (140)	120 (140)	200 (230)
3 hours	—	110 (125)	—

The numbers in parentheses are the *plasma* glucose concentrations. Add 10 mg/100 ml per decade for patients over 50 for all glucose values.

Maximal Normal Values for the Oral GTT in Pregnancy

WHOLE BLOOD GLUCOSE (mg/100 ml)

Fasting	90 (104)
1 hour	165 (190)
2 hours	145 (167)
3 hours	125 (145)

The numbers in parentheses are the *plasma* glucose concentrations.

Reference: Whitehouse, F. W.: Med. Clin. North Am., *62*:627, 1978.

INSULIN C-PEPTIDE

Insulin consists of a pair of polypeptide chains, designated the A and B chains, joined by disulfide linkages. Endogenous insulin is synthesized as a larger molecule called proinsulin. The C terminal portion of the B chain is initially connected to the N terminus of the A chain by a connecting polypeptide, which, depending on the species, is 30 to 35 amino acids in length. Transformation of proinsulin by cleavage of the connecting peptide occurs in the Golgi apparatus and is completed in the secretory granules of the pancreatic beta cells. In humans, the connecting peptide, or "C-peptide," consists of 31 amino acids of known sequence and is released into the circulation along with insulin. Its presence may be assessed by radioimmunoassay and constitutes a marker for endogenous insulin release. Although the C-peptide assay is quite new, a number of applications have been found for it.

Hypoglycemic States

1. Diagnosis of insulinoma or beta cell hyperplasia in insulin-requiring diabetics (increased).

2. Diagnosis of insulinoma by suppression test employing exogenous insulin-induced hypoglycemia (not suppressed in insulinoma).

3. Diagnosis of surreptitious injection of insulin (low). (See Malingering, Chapter 1.)

Euglycemic States

1. Diagnosis of remission phase or recovery from diabetes (normal).

Hyperglycemic States

1. Evaluation of completeness of pancreatectomy (absent with complete extirpation).

2. Distinction of the truly "brittle" diabetic (complete loss of beta cell function) from poor diabetic control due to exogenous insulin deficiency.

Reference: Horowitz, D. L., Kuzuya, H., and Rubenstein, M. B.: New Engl. J. Med., *295*:207, 1976.

11

HEMOGLOBIN AIc AND DIABETES MELLITUS

In the normal red cell, glucose reacts irreversibly in a nonenzymatic fashion with the β chains of hemoglobin A ($\alpha_2\beta_2$) to form a glycosylated variant known as hemoglobin AIc. Hemoglobin AIc is formed continuously throughout the life span of the red cell.

In nondiabetic patients, hemoglobin AIc constitutes approximately 3 to 4 per cent of the total hemoglobin. In diabetic subjects, the levels of hemoglobin AIc appear to reflect the degree of control of the diabetic state. Since the binding of glucose to hemoglobin A is irreversible, and binding occurs through the life span of the red cell (120 ± 20 days), the percentage of AIc present reflects an average of the blood glucose concentrations for two to three months prior to the determination. Thus, it is hoped that AIc measurements will allow the clinician to regulate the diabetic state of patients with greater precision. In addition, AIc determinations may be used to screen patients for unsuspected diabetes. Finally, by providing a sensitive index of diabetic control AIc determinations may also aid in answering the question of whether the vascular complications of diabetes mellitus are related to the degree of control of the blood sugar.

Reference: Bunn, H. F.: Resident and Staff Physician. December, 1978, p. 53.

WHEN THE INSULIN REQUIREMENTS DECREASE

Hypoglycemia occurring in the insulin-dependent diabetic patient may cause serious morbidity and demands immediate investigation by the clinician. Simply decreasing the insulin dose is inadequate therapy, as many of the conditions listed on the opposite page will require further therapeutic intervention.

Conditions Associated with a Decreasing Insulin Requirement

CONDITION	COMMENT
1. Exercise	—Facilitates glucose movement into muscle —Facilitates absorption of insulin from injection site
2. Institution of good control	—So-called "honeymoon period" —Occurs more frequently in juvenile onset type —May be related to restoration of ability to secrete insulin or induction of insulin receptors by insulin administration
3. Spontaneous remission of immunogenic insulin resistance	
4. Uremia	—Decrease in hepatic glucose production —Increased half-life of plasma insulin
5. Endocrine deficiency states: hypopituitarism, hypoadrenalism, hypothyroidism	—These deficiency states occur with increased frequency in the insulin-dependent diabetic
6. Autonomic neuropathy	—Secondary to partial deficiency of catecholamines and glucagon release —May be induced by beta blockers
7. Insulinoma	—Very rare —A positive tolbutamide tolerance test or measurable levels of C-peptide support the diagnosis
8. Surreptitious insulin administration	—Diagnosis made by demonstrating high serum insulin levels and no measurable C-peptide —C-peptide secreted with endogenous insulin only; does not occur in commercial insulin preparations

11

INSULIN AND ORAL HYPOGLYCEMIC AGENTS

Insulin is the therapy of choice for all juvenile onset diabetics and is also frequently used in the adult onset or non-ketotic–prone diabetic. A variety of oral hypoglycemic agents may be used in the latter group. The currently recommended oral agents are sulfonylureas. It should be noted that phenformin has been removed from the market, as its use was associated with a significant incidence of severe and often fatal lactic acidosis.

The following tables outline some characteristics of the insulins and oral hypoglycemic agents.

Varieties of Insulin

TYPE OF INSULIN*	ACTION	PROTEIN	PEAK ACTION (hrs)	DURATION (hrs)
Regular	Rapid	None	1–2	5–6
Semilente	Rapid	None	1–2	12–16
Globin	Intermediate	Globin	2–4	18–24
NPH	Intermediate	Protamine	2–8	24–28
Lente	Intermediate	None	2–8	24–28
PZI	Long-acting	Protamine	8–12	36
Ultralente	Long-acting	None	8–14	36

*All commercially available insulins are now U-100.

Oral Hypoglycemics

AGENT	AVAILABLE FORM (mg)	APPROXIMATE POTENCY RATIO	DURATION OF ACTIVITY (hrs)	AVERAGE DOSE (mg)
Tolbutamide (Orinase)	500	1	6–12	500–3000 (usually divided)
Acetohexamide (Dymelor)	250 500	2.5 —	12–14	125–1000 (single or divided)
Tolazamide (Tolinase)	100 250 500	5 — —	approx. 24	100–1000 (single, may be divided)
Chlorpropamide (Diabinese)	100 250	5 —	up to 60	100–500 (usually single)

Reference: Thorn, W. G., Adams, R. D., and Braunwald, E. (Eds.): Harrison's Principles of Internal Medicine, 8th Edition. New York, McGraw-Hill Book Company, 1977, pp. 574–575.

TEACHING PROGRAM FOR THE DIABETIC PATIENT

Effective management of the patient with diabetes mellitus requires the patient's active participation. An adequate understanding of the disease will help assure this. The following outline might serve as a syllabus around which the physician can organize a teaching program for the patient with diabetes mellitus.

Thanks to Crouse-Irving Memorial Hospital, Syracuse, N.Y., for organization of this material.

Outline of the Program

    I. Importance of patient education in diabetes
        A. Prevention of complications
        B. Insight as to controlling own problems
        C. Recognition of early warning signs to seek medical help
   II. Explanation of diabetic pathophysiology
  III. General management principles
        A. Diet
        B. Medication
        C. Exercise
  IV. Urine testing
        A. Physiologic significance
        B. Blood test vs. urine tests
        C. Sugar
            1. Types of testing and equipment
            2. Technique
            3. Appropriate testing times
        D. Acetone
            1. Types of testing and equipment
            2. Technique
            3. Appropriate testing times
        E. Signs of trouble in urine: When to seek medical advice
    V. Medications
        A. Oral agents vs. insulin
        B. Oral hypoglycemic agents
            1. Type
            2. Dosage
        C. Insulin
            1. Type, strength, dosage
            2. Types, brands available
            3. Preparation and administration techniques
  VI. Diet: Individual dietary instruction by dietician
 VII. Hyperglycemia
        A. Causes
        B. Symptoms
        C. Treatment
        D. Prevention

11

VIII. Hypoglycemia
    A. Causes
    B. Symptoms
    C. Treatment
    D. Prevention
IX. What to do when "sick"
    A. Medication
    B. Diet
    C. Medical attention
X. Preventing long-term complications
    A. Importance of keeping diabetes under control *every day*
    B. How to accomplish this
        1. Urine testing
        2. Following prescribed diabetic program
        3. Medical follow-up
    C. Consequences of uncontrolled diabetes
XI. Personal hygiene
    A. Importance
    B. Decreased circulation
    C. Skin
    D. Feet
    E. Eyes
    F. Teeth
XII. Identification
    A. Diabetic I.D. card
    B. Medic alert tag
XIII. Traveling with diabetes
XIV. Miscellaneous
    A. Publications
    B. Associations and organizations
    C. Community resources for diabetics

FASTING HYPOGLYCEMIA

A. *Glucose underproduction*
1. Hepatic
   a. Fulminant hepatitis
   b. Severe passive congestion
   c. Malnutrition
   d. Hepatotoxins (e.g., phosphorus, chloroform)
   e. Galactosemia (following foods containing galactose)
   f. Hereditary fructose intolerance (following food containing fructose)
   g. Glucose-6-phosphatase deficiency (type I) (associated with hypertriglyceridemia, hyperlactatemia, and hyperuricemia)
   h. Debrancher enzyme deficiency (type III)
   i. Phosphorylase deficiency (type VI) (cholesterol and lactate elevated, liver enlarged, growth retarded)
2. Adrenal insufficiency
   a. Primary adrenal insuffiency
   b. Secondary to decreased pituitary ACTH
   c. Adrenogenital syndrome
   d. Adrenocortical carcinoma
3. Pituitary insufficiency
4. Disturbances of the fasting equilibrium
   a. Alcoholic hypoglycemia
   b. Exogenous insulin or hypoglycemic agents
   c. Ackee fruit ingestion (the ripe fruit contains hypoglycine, an amino acid that interferes with metabolism of long-chain fatty acids)
B. *Glucose overutilization or loss*
1. Insulinoma
2. Extensive neoplastic disease
3. Lactation
4. Exercise
5. Renal glycosuria

11

HYPOPHOSPHATEMIA

Be sure to measure phosphorus in the diabetic with ketoacidosis and in the alcoholic.

Phosphorus is the major intracellular anion. Eighty per cent of the body's phosphorus (total is approximately 712 grams, or 23,000 mmoles) is in bone, 9 per cent is in skeletal muscle, and the rest is in red cells and viscera. The serum level does not accurately reflect total body levels, and phosphate depletion may exist in the presence of a normal serum phosphate. Total body phosphorus deficiency is rare, but moderate hypophosphatemia (1 to 2.5 mg/100 ml) is common. Hypophosphatemia can be produced by:

1. *Inadequate intake:* Starvation, hyperalimentation without phosphorus administration, excessive use of phosphate-binding antacids (e.g., Amphogel).
2. *Factors that produce phosphaturia:* Volume expansion, metabolic acidosis, vitamin D deficiency, hypomagnesemia, increased parathyroid hormone levels.
3. *Transport of phosphorus into cells with glucose:* Glucose administration, fructose administration, insulin administration, and respiratory alkalosis.

The main clinical conditions in which severe hypophosphatemia (less than 1 mg/100 ml) occurs are alcohol withdrawal, diabetes mellitus with ketoacidosis, hyperalimentation, refeeding after starvation, and severe respiratory alkalosis. About 50 per cent of hospitalized alcoholics have hypophosphatemia. The mechanism may be related to any or all of the following: poor intake, vomiting, diarrhea, an effect of ethanol itself, magnesium deficiency, hypocalcemia, and ketoacidosis. Hypophosphatemia is usually most pronounced on the second to fourth day of hospitalization (probably because of refeeding) and may be manifest by myopathy and central nervous system dysfunction; the latter may complicate the alcohol withdrawal state.

In diabetic ketoacidosis the serum phosphorus is usually normal or elevated on admission, although there is phosphate depletion (approximately 400 mmoles) due to the phosphaturia that occurs as a result of the acidosis. As insulin is administered, phosphorus moves intracelluarly, causing a decrease in serum phosphorus. In some cases, hypophosphatemic ketoacidotic patients in coma awake following phosphate administration.

When severe hypophosphatemia occurs, significant effects on bodily functions may be present, including:

1. Red cell dysfunction.
   a. Extreme hypophosphatemia may cause hemolysis.
   b. Lower levels of erythrocyte 2,3 DPG will lower the P50 (oxygen tension at which hemoglobin is 50 per cent saturated), thereby impairing O_2 delivery to tissues.
2. Leukocyte dysfunction: impaired chemotaxis, phagocytosis, and bacteriocidal activity.
3. Platelet dysfunction.
4. Central nervous system dysfunction: metabolic encephalopathy, weakness, paresthesias, seizures, and coma.
5. Rhabdomyolysis, with elevated CPK values and myopathy.

Phosphate may be repleted in the following ways:

1. Milk: contains 1 gram (33 mmoles) of phosphorus and calcium per quart (skim milk).

2. $NaH_2PO_4 \cdot Na_2HPO_4$: contains 1.63 mmoles/ml. This can be given orally as a dose of 15 to 30 ml three times a day.

3. $KH_2PO_4 \cdot K_2HPO_4$: for intravenous use, 2 mmoles of phosphorus per milliliter. This can be alternated with KCl in ketoacidosis to correct potassium and phosphate deficiency (see below).

You must check the label of each solution for mmoles of phosphorus present, since the amount of available phosphorus is dependent on the pH of the preparation used. Treatment should be directed at raising the serum phosphorus to greater than 1 mg/100 ml, since the complications of hypophosphatemia occur when the serum phosphorus is below that level. Daily requirements of phosphate intake for patients receiving parenteral nutrition are 12 to 15 mmoles/day. For patients with phosphate depletion, a much higher intake (up to 400 mmoles) may be required to replete stores.

Reference: Knochel, J. P.: Arch. Intern. Med., *137*:203, 1977.

PARENTERAL PHOSPHATE ADMINISTRATION

Phosphate should be prescribed in terms of *millimoles* of *phosphate* or *milligrams* of *elemental phosphorus* and not milliequivalents, when it is used to correct hypophosphatemia. In the hypophosphatemic patient, neither the size of the body deficit nor the response of the serum phosphorus to therapy can be predicted. Therefore, the effect of replacement on serum phosphorus levels should be monitored carefully. Some rough guidelines to use when administering parenteral phosphorus are provided below. Keep in mind 1 *mmole* of *phosphate* = 31 *mg* of *elemental phosphorus.*

1. In severe hypophosphatemia (serum phosphate concentrations of < 0.32 mmole/liter or < 1 mg/100 ml), parenteral preparations are preferred, as oral preparations may cause diarrhea and make intestinal absorption unreliable.

2. The initial dose should be between 0.08 mmole *phosphate*/kg body weight and 0.16 mmole *phosphate*/kg body weight (or 2.5 mg phosphorus/kg body weight and 5 mg phosphorus/kg body weight).

3. The initial dose should be administered intravenously over six hours. Subsequent doses are determined by the level of serum phosphorus.

11

4. Initial doses may be 25 to 50 per cent higher if the patient is symptomatic; lower if he is hypercalcemic.

5. To minimize risks, no dose should exceed 0.24 mmole phosphate/kg body weight (7.5 mg phosphorus/kg body weight).

6. *Calcium*-containing salts should *not* be administered through the same intravenous tubing as the phosphate. They may precipitate!

7. *Oral* phosphate should be administered to correct hypophosphatemia if the serum phosphate concentration is greater than 0.32 mmole/liter or 1 mg/100 ml.

8. Hazards of parenteral phosphate administration include:
   a. Profound hypocalcemia
   b. Metastatic calcification.
   c. Hypotension unrelated to dehydration.
   d. Dehydration from osmotic diuresis caused by hypertonic phosphate solutions.
   e. Hyperphosphatemia, which can accelerate deterioration of renal function in chronic renal failure.

The table on the opposite page lists some of the various commercially available phosphorus preparations.

Examples of Therapeutic Phosphorus Preparations

PREPARATIONS	COMPOSITION	pH	mOsm/kg/H_2O	PHOSPHATE (mmole/ml)	PHOSPHORUS (mg/ml)	SODIUM (mEq/ml)	POTASSIUM (mEq/ml)
Oral							
Whole cow's milk	...	...	288	0.029	0.9	0.025	0.035
Neutra-phos	Na_2HPO_4, NaH_2PO_4, K_2HPO_4, KH_2PO_4	7.3	...	0.107	3.33	0.095	0.095
Phospho-soda	180 mg $Na_2HPO_4 \cdot 7H_2O$ + 480 mg $NaH_2PO_4 \cdot H_2O$/ml	4.8	8240	4.150	128.65	4.822	0
Acid Na phosphate	136 mg $Na_2HPO_4 \cdot 7H_2O$ + 58.8 mg H_3PO_4 (NF 85%)/ml	4.9	1740	1.018	35.54	1.015	0
Neutral Na phosphate	145 mg $Na_2HPO_4 \cdot 7H_2O$ + 18.2 mg $NaH_2PO_4 \cdot H_2O$/ml	7.0	1390	0.673	20.86	1.214	0
Parenteral							
Neutral Na phosphate	10.07 mg Na_2HPO_4 + 2.66 mg $NaH_2PO_4 \cdot H_2O$/ml	7.35	202	0.090	2.80	0.161	0
Neutral Na, K phosphate	11.5 mg Na_2HPO_4 + 2.58 mg KH_2PO_4/ml	7.4	223	0.100	3.10	0.162	0.019
Na phosphate	142 mg Na_2HPO_4 + 276 mg $NaH_2PO_4 \cdot H_2O$/ml	5.7	5580	3.000	93.00	4.000	0
K phosphate	236 mg K_2HPO_4 + 224 mg KH_2PO_4/ml	6.6	5840	3.003	93.11	0	4.360

References: Knochel, J. P.: Arch. Intern. Med., *137*:203, 1977; Lentz, R. D., Brown, D. M., and Kjellstrant, C. M.: Ann. Intern. Med., *89*:941, 1978. Table reproduced with permission of author and Annals of Internal Medicine.

11

CALCIUM SUPPLEMENTATION

Some factors influencing calcium absorption and excretion may produce conditions that necessitate calcium supplementation.

1. *Formation of poorly absorbable calcium complexes in the upper gastrointestinal tract.* Included are phytates, oxalates, phosphates, and excessive amounts of fatty acids, which may be found in malabsorptive states. An alkaline intestinal pH decreases the ionization of calcium and thus its absorption (achlorhydria, gastric resection).

2. *Vitamin D.* Vitamin D deficiency may result from poor dietary intake, lack of actinic exposure, or malabsorption (sprue syndrome, chronic diarrhea or, rarely, the excessive use of nonabsorbable materials that dissolve fat-soluble vitamins, e.g., mineral oil). Vitamin D is activated first by the liver to 25-hydroxy–vitamin D and then by the kidney to the more active metabolite 1,25-dihydroxy–vitamin D. Kidney activation is enhanced by increased levels of parathyroid hormone. Patients with chronic renal disease may have an increased renal calcium loss and may not be able to activate vitamin D adequately.

3. *Glucocorticoids.* Calcium metabolism is affected at three sites. GI absorption of calcium is inhibited by glucocorticoids, renal excretion is enhanced, and bone formation is decreased.

4. *Hypoparathyroidism.* A negative calcium balance is found in hypoparathyroidism. A decrease in intestinal absorption of calcium and a decrease in renal activation of vitamin D are observed. An increase in renal excretion of calcium is a consequence of a decrease in tubular reabsorption of phosphate.

5. *Anticonvulsant drugs.* Long-term administration of phenytoin and phenobarbital will induce activity in the hepatic microsomal enzymes responsible for the inactivation of active 25-hydroxy–vitamin D. Less hydroxy–D is available for renal conversion to 1,25-dihydroxy–vitamin D and consequently for facilitation of intestinal calcium transport.

6. *Diuretics.* Diuretics such as furosemide increase calcium excretion. Thiazides and chlorthalidone conversely produce hypocalciuria, presumably as a result of a preservation of the mechanism for proximal reabsorption of calcium.

7. *Phosphate depletion.* Phosphate depletion may result in osteomalacia. This may be seen in patients taking large quantities of phosphate-binding antacids, in patients undergoing hemodialysis with low-phosphate solutions, and in patients maintained on low-phosphate parenteral nutrition.

8. *Acidosis.* Urinary calcium loss is influenced by the plasma ionized calcium, which is increased in acidosis.

9. *Immobilization.* Prolonged immobilization results in an increase in bone reabsorption and calcium excretion.

Calcium Requirements

Suggested daily dietary requirements of calcium are:

800 mg	Children (1 to 10 years old)
1200 mg	Adolescents
800–1000 mg	Adults
1200–1300 mg	Pregnant and lactating women
360 mg	Infants younger than 6 months
540 mg	Infants 6 to 12 months

Treatment with Calcium Salts

The treatment of calcium depletion syndromes should be aimed at correcting the underlying cause when possible. Calcium supplements administered for inappropriate indications may result in hypercalcemia or extraskeletal precipitation of calcium and phosphate.

Oral calcium therapy may be indicated as part of the overall therapy of osteoporosis, osteomalacia, chronic hypoparathyroidism, rickets, latent tetany, or hypocalcemia due to the administration of anticonvulsant drugs. Calcium supplementation is often indicated for pregnant, lactating, and postmenopausal women.

Several calcium salts are available for oral administration. The advantages offered by each salt are as follows (see table on p. 353):

1. Phosphate salts may be of some advantage in patients who require phosphorus as well as calcium. They should not, however, be used in patients with hypocalcemia accompanied by hyperphosphatemia (e.g., as in renal hyperparathyroidism). Phosphate salts have, to a large extent, been replaced by more soluble calcium salts, which are absorbed more readily.

2. Calcium carbonate is a calcium supplement that has also been given to patients with renal disease and hyperphosphatemia. It is used to bind phosphate in the intestine to reduce serum phosphate levels. Calcium carbonate is also an antacid found in many proprietary antacid preparations.

3. Significant differences exist among the various calcium salts. They are the amount of elemental calcium supplied by the salt, its solubility (therefore, absorption), and the amount of drug per tablet.

4. Calcium chloride has been associated with severe gastrointestinal irritation and is therefore not often used as a calcium supplement.

5. One of the difficulties of oral calcium therapy is compliance. Each dose may require several tablets, some of which are distasteful and must be chewed. If tolerated, salts containing a high percentage of available calcium may be used to overcome this problem.

11

Toxicity

The toxicities of oral calcium supplementation administered in usual doses are minimal and usually consist of GI upset or constipation.

Hypercalcemia is rarely produced when the drug is administered for appropriate indications and in usual supplemental doses. Symptoms of hypercalcemia include anorexia, nausea, vomiting, constipation, abdominal pain, dryness of mouth, thirst and polyuria, and muscle weakness. The most serious problem associated with hypercalcemia may be the result of the precipitation of calcium in vital organs and tissues and CNS effects such as depression, drowsiness, and disorientation.

Dosage

The dosage of the oral calcium supplements depends on the requirements of the individual patient. (See section on requirements, p. 351.) Calcium requirements can be estimated by clinical assessment and plasma calcium determination.

The average oral dosage of elemental calcium for prevention of hypocalcemia in adults is approximately 1 gram per day. The usual oral dose for the treatment of calcium depletion is 1 to 2 grams or more per day. Plasma and urinary calcium determinations may be used as guides to providing adequate dosage without inducing hypercalcemia.

In children, the usual supplemental daily dosage of elemental calcium is 45 to 65 mg per kilogram.

Oral calcium supplements are usually administered in three to four doses daily. It has been recommended that oral calcium be administered an hour before or 1 to 1½ hours after meals. This schedule avoids the formation of insoluble salts with foodstuffs and thereby assures maximal absorption.

Oral Calcium Preparations

CALCIUM SALT	AVAILABLE CALCIUM	FORMULATIONS	MILLIGRAMS OF CALCIUM PER DOSE
Calcium chloride	27%	No commercial preparation (solutions can be prepared)	(Very irritating to GI tract)
Calcium gluconate	9%	Tabs 325 mg 500 mg 650 mg 1000 mg	29 mg 45 mg 58 mg 90 mg
Calcium lactate	13%	Tabs 325 mg 650 mg	42 mg 84 mg
Calcium carbonate	40%	Tabs 650 mg 1300 mg	260 mg 500 mg (Os-Cal-500)
Calcium glubionate	6%	Syrup 1.8 grams/5 ml	115 mg (Neocalglucon Syrup)
Dibasic calcium phosphate	29.5%	Tabs 500 mg	147 mg (poor solubility)
Tribasic calcium phosphate	38.7%	No commercial preparation	

Adapted from material prepared by J. F. DeGrazio, R.Ph.

11

ADRENAL FUNCTION TESTING WITHOUT TEARS

Serum Cortisol

Serum cortisol should be measured by the specific and sensitive radioimmunoassay. Samples are obtained at 8:00 a.m. (normal: 10 to 25 µg/dl) and 4:00 p.m. (normal: 5 to 10 µg/dl), so both the diurnal variation and the absolute values are examined.

1. *Normal values* — represent fairly good evidence for normal ACTH secretion but do not exclude partial adrenal insufficiency.
2. *Loss of diurnal variation* — typical of adrenal hyperfunction, particularly when coupled with elevated p.m. values.
3. *Low values* — imply adrenal hypofunction or exogenous adrenal suppression secondary to corticosteroid administration.
4. *Elevated values* — suggests adrenal hyperfunction or exogenous corticosteroid administration. Estrogens and oral contraceptives increase the concentration of corticosteroid-binding globulin in the serum. Elevated serum cortisol in the absence of hypercorticism may result.

Plasma ACTH

Plasma ACTH may be determined by radioiomunoassay and is helpful in differentiating between pituitary and end-organ failure in hypoadrenalism and between a pituitary abnormality and an adrenal tumor or hyperplasia in cases of adrenal hypersecretion.

1. *Elevated values* — suggests pituitary tumor (hyperadrenalism) or adrenal failure (hypoadrenalism). Ectopic ACTH–producing tumor.
2. *Low values* — suggests adrenal tumor (hyperadrenalism) or pituitary failure (hypoadrenalism).

Dexamethasone Suppression Tests

Dexamethasone in low doses inhibits pituitary secretion of ACTH. The procedures suggested have fewer false negatives than the overnight dexamethasone suppression test, which is often employed for screening.

1. *Low dose* — 0.5 mg of dexamethasone is given every 6 hours for 48 hours. Urinary 17-hydroxycorticoids are measured during the second 24-hour period. Normal excretion is less than 4 mg/24 hrs (or 2 mg/gram creatinine). Inadequate suppression indicates presumptive hypercorticism.

2. *High dose* — 2.0 mg of dexamethasone are given every 6 hours for 48 hours. Urinary 17-hydroxycorticosteroids are measured during the second 24 hours. Partial suppression to less than half the basal value indicates pituitary-dependent Cushing's disease (ACTH-secreting adenoma). Partial suppression, but to more than half the basal value, indicates autonomously secreting adrenal tumor.

Cosyntropin Stimulation Test

Use of this synthetic peptide with ACTH activity has replaced ACTH stimulation in assessing adrenal function. 250 μg of cosyntropin is given IV each 12 hours for 24 hours. A more rapid method is provided in the following essay.

1. *Pituitary ACTH deficiency* — A twofold or threefold increase in cortisol is seen within 8 hours, with normal values obtained by 24 hours.

2. *Hypoadrenalism* — no response or blunted response.

Metyrapone Stimulation

Metyrapone blocks adrenal hydroxylation just prior to production of cortisol with accumulation of 11-deoxycortisol; a loss of the feedback inhibition of ACTH normally produced by cortisol results.

A basal 24-hour urine is collected for 17-hydroxycorticosteroids. On the day of testing, an 8:00 a.m. serum sample for cortisol and 11-deoxycortisol is obtained. 750 mg of metyrapone is then administered each 4 hours for 6 doses. At 8:00 a.m. the following day (4 hours after the last dose), blood is again drawn for cortisol and 11-deoxycortisol testing, and a 24-hour urine collection is begun for 17-hydroxycorticosteroids. In patients who have been on long-term replacement therapy, two days of cosyntropin stimulation and three days of rest may be employed prior to metyrapone testing. Since this provocative test may occasionally induce an adrenal crisis, the patient should be hospitalized and observed closely throughout for signs of postural hypotension, nausea, vomiting, tachycardia, or excessive sweating.

1. *Normal* — rise in urine 17-hydroxycorticoids to at least twice basal levels (or a rise of 8 to 10 mg/24 hrs).

2. *Pituitary hyperadrenalism* — increase of greater than 50 per cent in 17-hydroxycorticosteroids.

3. *Adrenal tumor or ectopic ACTH* — no response.

11

INTERPRETATION OF DYNAMIC TESTING IN PATIENTS WITH CUSHING'S SYNDROME

TEST	RESULT	BEST WORKING DIAGNOSIS
17-hydroxycorticoid response to high-dose dexamethasone	>50% decrease	Pituitary dependent Cushing's disease
	<50% decrease	Adrenal tumor or ectopic ACTH syndrome
17-hydroxycorticoid response to metyrapone	Increase	Pituitary dependent Cushing's disease
	No increase	Adrenal tumor or ectopic ACTH syndrome
Plasma ACTH	Increased	Pituitary dependent Cushing's disease
	Marked increase	Ectopic ACTH syndrome
	Decreased	Adrenal tumor

Reference: Neelon, F. A., and Sydnor, C. F.: Disease-A-Month, January 1978.

BILATERAL ADRENAL HEMORRHAGE IN THE ADULT

Bilateral adrenal hemorrhage was found in 1.1 per cent of 2000 consecutive autopsies performed at the Baltimore City Hospitals between 1966 and 1974. Signs and symptoms of adrenal insufficiency were rarely recognized antemortem, as they tended to occur in clinical circumstances not usually associated with Addison's disease.

The factors implicated most frequently in the finding of bilateral adrenal hemorrhage at postmortem were:

a. *Serious systemic illness* — most often infection, severe cardiac disease, or burns. Undoubtedly, these illnesses represent marked physiologic stress with resultant increased endogenous ACTH stimulation of the adrenal glands. This may be the final common pathway predisposing to adrenal hemorrhage in patients not receiving anticoagulants.

b. *Anticoagulation.* A third of the patients with adrenal hemorrhage reported in the literature were receiving anticoagulant therapy at the time. The hemorrhage tended to occur in the second or third week of anticoagulant therapy.

The most frequent clinical findings in patients later shown to have bilateral adrenal hemorrhage were:

1. Hypotension (74 per cent)
2. Fever (59 per cent)
3. Abdominal pain (56 per cent)
4. Nausea/vomiting (46 per cent)

Thus, in patients ill with systemic disease, *especially those receiving anticoagulants* (heparin or coumadin), unexplained clinical deterioration necessitates consideration of adrenal insufficiency secondary to bilateral adrenal hemorrhage. Intramuscular or intravenous injection of 250 μg (25 units) of α1-24 corticotropin (cosyntropin), with measurements of plasma cortisol prior to injection and 30 and 60 minutes after injection, will allow the clinician to establish the diagnosis.

Reference: Xarli, V., Steele, A., Davis, P. J., et al.: Medicine, *57*:211, 1978.

CLINICAL INDICATIONS FOR PITUITARY FUNCTION EVALUATION

Evaluation of pituitary function is expensive, tedious, and time consuming. The following list may help you decide when to undertake such tests.

A. *Syndromes that may require total assessment of pituitary hormone reserve.*
    1. Visual loss, suggesting a lesion of the optic chiasm, or demonstrated lesion of the chiasm (used to establish diagnosis, assess functional loss, plan replacement therapy, or evaluate the response to therapy).
    2. Pituitary tumor.
    3. Perisellar tumor.
    4. Diabetes insipidus.
    5. Established abnormality or pituitary malfunction.
    6. Following pituitary or hypothalamic surgery or trauma (two to three months post-op).
B. *Syndromes that may require evaluation of specific hormone reserve for either loss of function or possible hyperpituitarism.* (Demonstrations of the lack of a trophic hormone should probably precede total pituitary evaluation. Alternatively, demonstration of end-organ failure

(i.e., cosyntropin stimulation) may circumvent the need for an evaluation of pituitary function.

    1. Hypothyroidism.
    2. Amenorrhea (including premature menopause).
    3. Impotence or loss of libido (with low serum testosterone).
    4. Hypoadrenalism.
    5. Growth failure.
    6. Delayed pubescence.

C. *Syndromes requiring testing for specific hormone hypersecretion.* If testing is positive, total evaluation should be carried out.

    1. Cushing's syndrome.
    2. Nonpuerperal galactorrhea (particularly with amenorrhea).
    3. Acromegaly and gigantism.

BRIEF EVALUATION OF PITUITARY FUNCTION

When time is severely limited, the following schedule for evaluation of pituitary function may be appropriate. Since the insulin induced hypoglycemia should produce symptoms (glucose <40 mg/dl) if cortisol and prolactin responses are to be optimally evoked, the attendance of a physician is required. The usual insulin dose is 0.1 U/kg. Since patients with decreased or absent pituitary function may be unduly sensitive to insulin, small (0.05 U/kg) doses of crystalline insulin are employed if hypopituitarism is a strong possibility. Insulin-hypoglycemic provocation should not be attempted in patients whose basal morning serum cortisol is less than 5 μg/dl.

Day 1
    12:00 midnight: Begin overnight fast.
Day 2
    7:30 a.m.:   Insert indwelling intravenous line.
    8:00 a.m.:   Test blood for thyroxine index, TSH, estradiol or testosterone, LH, FSH, prolactin, growth hormone, cortisol, osmolality, and glucose.
                   Test urine for osmolality.
    8:05 a.m.:   Give intravenous insulin.
    8:20 a.m.:   Test blood for glucose, growth hormone, and prolactin.
    8:35 a.m.:   Test blood for glucose, growth hormone, prolactin, and cortisol.
    8:50 a.m.:   Test blood for glucose, growth hormone, prolactin, and cortisol.
    9:05 a.m.:   Test blood for glucose, growth hormone, prolactin, and cortisol.

9:35 a.m.:   Test blood for glucose, growth hormone, and prolactin.

12:00 noon: TRH stimulation test of TSH and prolactin (optional).

Reference: Suggested by Neelon, F. A., and Sydnor, C. F.: Disease-A-Month, January, 1978.

GROWTH HORMONE

A number of factors have been reported to effect growth hormone secretion. Consideration of these situations should be given in all evaluation of growth hormone testing.

Static Tests

The growth hormone level after a fast is normally so low that static tests of growth hormone are usually not performed. While fasting growth hormone is usually elevated in acromegaly, it should not be used as the only basis for diagnosis.

Suppressive Tests

Glucose suppression test: Hyperglycemia suppresses growth hormone in healthy persons. The glucose suppression test is performed by the oral administration of 100 grams of glucose. Serum samples for growth hormone are obtained prior to glucose and then hourly for three hours. In healthy individuals, growth hormone falls to less than 2 ng/ml during the test. In patients with acromegaly, growth hormone levels usually exceed 5 ng/ml throughout. At times, a paradoxical rise of hormone levels may occur.

Provocative Tests

These are useful in the evaluation of growth failure or fasting hypoglycemia as well as in complete delineation of the hypothalamic pituitary axis in the adult.

Exercise test: Growth hormone levels are compared after a half hour of rest to those obtained after 15 minutes of brisk walking and 5 minutes of running upstairs. A normal response is a level of greater than 6 ng/ml after exercise. The test is not completely reliable, as "normal" levels are not attained by 20 per cent of children and a greater percentage of adults. A normal response, however, excludes growth hormone deficiency. The use of beta adrenergic blockade with propranolol

11

(20 to 40 mg orally) before exercising enhances growth hormone release. The normal response exceeds 7 ng/ml, and the abnormal is less than 4 ng/ml.

L-Dopa: Five hundred mg of L-Dopa are given to the rested, fasting subject, and growth hormone levels are measured at 30, 60, 90, and 120 minutes thereafter. Normal responses lie between 6 and 10 ng/ml. Values decrease below baseline in patients with acromegaly. Most recently, enhancement of the test by beta-adrenergic blockade has been employed.

Insulin hypoglycemia: Provocation of growth hormone response is most reliably done by the induction of hypoglycemia. A fall of at least 50 per cent in the initial blood glucose level is required in a fasted patient for appropriate evocation of growth hormone. Depending on the index of suspicion of hypopituitarism, from 0.05 to 0.2 U/kg crystalline insulin is administered as an IV bolus. Serum glucose and growth hormone levels are measured initially and each 15 minutes for 1½ hours. The test is terminated by glucose injection or feeding. Growth hormone should reach concentrations above 10 ng/ml and rise quickly once hypoglycemia is attained. The growth hormone response is augmented by propranolol. Prolactin and ACTH levels may be assessed during the same test period. Clearly, the patient must be closely monitored during the examination, with a 50 per cent glucose solution immediately available.

Reference: Neelon, F. A., and Sydnor, C. F.: Disease-A-Month, January 1978.

SIADH

The syndrome of inappropriate ADH (SIADH) secretion is increasingly being recognized as a cause of hyponatremia. By definition in SIADH, release of ADH occurs without the appropriate trigger of plasma osmolality and/or hypovolemia. Hyponatremia secondary to inappropriate water retention results when urine osmolality is inappropriately elevated above plasma osmolality.

The criteria for the diagnosis of SIADH are:

1. Normal renal, thyroid, and adrenal function.
2. Grossly normal total body sodium (no edema or hypovolemia).
3. Inappropriately concentrated urine.
4. Hypotonic plasma.
5. Urinary sodium concentration during volume expansion greater than 30 mEq/liter.

6. Correction of hyponatremia by water restriction alone.
7. Absence of diuretics.

To establish a definitive diagnosis, follow this procedure for a water load test:

1. Omit breakfast (no smoking prior to or during test).
2. Weigh patient (kg).
3. Draw blood for plasma osmolality and ADH (heparinized blood).
4. Have patient empty bladder, and record time. Save urine.
5. Give oral water load of 20 ml/kg of body weight over 15 to 20 min, and record time.
6. Keep patient recumbent throughout test except when voiding.
7. Collect urine at hourly intervals for five hours starting at the time water load is begun. Record times.
8. Draw blood for plasma osmolality and ADH at 1½ to 2 hr intervals after start of water load. Record times.

Prior to water loading assure yourself that the patient's sodium is at a safe level (generally above 125 mEq/liter) and that the patient is asymptomatic from hyponatremia. Excretion of more than 80 per cent of the water load by the fifth hour and a fall in the urinary osmolality to less than 100 milliosmoles per kilogram, constitute a normal water load test. In patients with SIADH, less than 40 per cent of the water load is excreted in five hours, and the urine is not diluted to hypotonic levels. To prevent water intoxication, no further free water should be given to the patient suspected of SIADH until the serum sodium returns to pretest values.

The causes of SIADH are listed under the following general headings:

Drugs	*Malignancy*
Chlorpropamide	Small cell carcinoma of the lung
Clofibrate	Carcinoma of the duodenum
Carbamazepine	Carcinoma of the pancreas
Vincristine	Thymoma
Vinblastine	Hodgkin's and non-Hodgkin's lymphoma
Cyclophosphamide	
Barbiturates	
Narcotics	
Tricyclic antidepressants	
Thiazides	
General anesthesia	
Oxytocin	

11

Pulmonary disease	*Neurologic disturbances*
Pneumonia	Pain
Lung abscess	Physical or emotional stress
Tuberculosis	Skull fracture
Any inflammatory pulmonary process	Subdural hematoma
	Subarachnoid hemorrhage
	CVA
Miscellaneous	Meningitis
	SLE
Acute intermittent porphyria	Guillain-Barré syndrome
Hypothyroidism	Encephalitis
Positive pressure ventilation	

The therapy for SIADH is aimed at increasing the serum sodium concentration. In mild cases, simple water restriction will suffice. When hyponatremia is life-threatening, administration of 3 per cent or 5 per cent saline will correct the low serum sodium more quickly. If volume overload is a consideration (congestive heart failure), simultaneous administration of furosemide will have an additional therapeutic effect.

References: Wintrobe, M. M., et al.: Harrison's Principles of Internal Medicine, 7th Edition, New York, McGraw-Hill Book Company, 1974, pp. 487–500.

THYROID FUNCTION TESTS

Here is a brief guide to the measurement of thyroid function.

Causes for Increase or Decrease in Thyroid-Binding Proteins

PROTEIN	INCREASE	DECREASE
Thyroid-binding globulin	Estrogens, including oral contraceptives	Androgens, including anabolic steroids
	Pregnancy	Active acromegaly
	Newborn infant (due to maternal estrogen)	
	Hepatic disease* Acute intermittent porphyria	Hepatic disease* Acute illness or surgical stress† Exogenous steroids
		Nephrotic syndrome
	Perphenazine (Trilafon)	Phenytoin (Dilantin)‡
	Hypothyroidism	Hyperthyroidism
	Hereditary	Hereditary
Thyroid-binding prealbumin	Androgens, including anabolic steroids	Acute illness or surgical stress
	Exogenous steroids	Nephrotic syndrome
	Hepatic disease	Salicylates‡
		Hyperthyroidism

*May cause either increase or decrease in TBG.
†May be due to inhibitor of T4 binding.
‡May be due to competition for T4-binding sites.

11

Thyroxine (T4) by Radioimmunoassay (RIA)

Commonly, serum T4 (RIA) is used to screen for thyroid dysfunction or to monitor hyperthyroid patients when there are no abnormalities of thyroid-binding proteins. If the thyroid-binding proteins are increased or decreased, there is an increased or decreased level of T4. In these circumstances serum T4 (RIA) is not an accurate estimate of thyroid function (see table on thyroid-binding protein).

Triiodothyronine (T3) by RIA

T3 is the major active thyroid hormone. In most clinical situations T4 (RIA) correlates well with T3 (RIA). However, early in the course of thyrotoxicosis the T3 (RIA) may be elevated before a rise in T4 (RIA) is seen. In T3-thyrotoxicosis (which affects less than 5 per cent of hyperthyroid patients) the T3 (RIA) is elevated but the T4 (RIA) remains normal. In patients who are very ill (including those with cirrhosis, renal failure, and malnutrition), the T3 (RIA) is characteristically low, the T4 (RIA) is normal, the free thyroxine values are borderline high or elevated, the TSH levels are normal, and the patient is clinically euthyroid ("sick euthyroid"). Occasionally, patients with reduced thyroid reserve and those on an iodine-deficient diet may have normal T3 (RIA) levels and low T4 (RIA) hormone levels despite being clinically euthyroid.

Free Thyroxine (FT4)

As previously noted, the T4 measured by the RIA method is affected not only by thyroid function but also by the level of thyroid-binding proteins. On the other hand, the free thyroxine is unaffected by changes in thyroid-binding proteins. When there are alterations of thyroid-binding proteins, the level of FT4 is more closely correlated with the true hormonal status of the patient. The FT4 is technically more difficult to measure and more expensive than the T4 (RIA).

Thyroid-Stimulating Hormone (TSH) by RIA

Patients with primary hypothyroidism have elevations of the pituitary hormone TSH. Conversely, in patients with hypothyroidism due to pituitary or hypothalamic disease, TSH is not elevated.

The TSH is an excellent measure of adequate exogenous thyroid replacement in patients with primary hypothyroidism. The TSH will drop to a normal range when a patient is hormonally euthyroid and remain elevated when the thyroid dose is inadequate. Since TSH levels are undetectable or normal in hyperthyroid and euthyroid patients, there is little rationale for measuring TSH levels in these settings.

Thyroid-Releasing Hormone (TRH)

TRH is composed of only three amino acids and probably is the trophic hormone responsible for TSH release. It is found in highest concentrations in the hypothalamus.

To test TSH response, one vial (400 μg) of TRH is given by intravenous bolus, and the TSH response measured. Patients with a normal pituitary axis will respond to the stimulus with at least a twofold increase in TSH. A peak response occurs in 30 minutes, with return to normal in two hours. During the two hours of testing, there is no significant change in the T4 (RIA). Patients with primary hypothyroidism (thyroid failure) exhibit an exaggerated and prolonged TSH response. Little or no response is observed in hyperthyroidism. TRH is a most valuable aid in the diagnosis of hypothyroidism in patients who have a normal or slightly elevated levels of TSH but are not yet clinically hypothyroid. TRH testing is also of value in the distinguishing patients with secondary (pituitary hypothyroidism) from those with hypothalamic hypothyroidism. Patients with secondary hypothyroidism will not respond to a TRH infusion, while those with a hypothalamic disorder will have a TSH response.

Basal Metabolic Rate (BMR)

This is the most direct measure of metabolic activity, but the wide range of normal values and the changes in BMR caused by nonthyroidal factors make this determination of limited diagnostic value.

Protein-Bound Iodine (PBI)

This test measures all the iodine that is bound to protein (mainly thyroid hormone) in the serum and thus precipitable by protein-denaturing agents. However, if large quantities of iodine or any of the roentgenographic contrast media that contain iodine are present, the level is falsely elevated. Thyroid-formed iodoproteins other than thyroxine are also precipitated and may be grossly elevated in subacute thyroiditis.

11

Butanol Extractable Iodine (BEI)

Butanol extractable iodine excludes iodoproteins. If the PBI exceeds the BEI by 20 per cent, abnormal amounts of iodoproteins are present. This situation is most commonly seen in subacute thyroiditis.

SITUATION	TESTS
Standard screen	T4 (RIA); may also use T3 (RIA)
Screen in patients with altered binding proteins	FT4
Suspected thyrotoxicosis	T4 (RIA), T3 (RIA); may also need FT4
Suspected hypothyroidism	T4 (RIA), FT4, TSH
Hypothyroidism with normal or slightly elevated TSH	TRH; prolonged, exaggerated TSH response in primary hypothyroidism
Hypothyroidism with low TSH	TRH: secondary pituitary hypothyroidism has no response; hypothyroidism from hypothalamic failure shows marked response
Hypothyroidism on replacement therapy	TSH (T4 falsely elevated if patient on Synthroid; T3 falsely elevated if Cytomel is used)

If hypothyroidism or hyperthyroidism is suspected, T4 (RIA) may be used for a screen, except in those patients who may have changes in the thyroid hormone–binding proteins (see the table above). (In these patients the free thyroxine measure is an appropriate screening test.) TSH should be measured in all patients with hypothyroidism to delineate primary from secondary hypothyroidism. If the diagnosis of hypothyroidism is strongly suspected but not yet obvious, the TRH stimulation test would be appropriate.

GYNECOMASTIA

Gynecomastia (it may be unilateral) occurs in association with the following:

Normal puberty
Gonadotropin secreting neoplasms
    testes, lung, adrenal, liver
Estrogen-secreting tumors
    adrenal, testes
Pituitary tumors associated with increased serum prolactin
    (may or may not have galactorrhea)
Liver disease
Hyperparathyroidism
Chronic renal failure with hemodialysis
Drugs
    Estrogens
    Testosterone

Chorionic gonadotropin
Phenothiazines
Meprobamate
Hydroxyzine
Reserpine
Spironolactone
Marijuana
Digitalis(?) (may be related to the presence of congestive heart
    failure and diminished hepatic blood flow)
Hyperthyroidism
Hypothyroidism
Refeeding gynecomastia
    Recovery from malnutrition
Hypogonadotrophic hypogonadism
    Klinefelter's syndrome
    Reifenstein's syndrome

Evaluation

Serum HCG, serum estradiol, serum prolactin
Skull x-rays, chest x-ray, computerized tomography (head)
Buccal smear if Klinefelter's syndrome is suspected
Drug history
Biopsy if carcinoma is suspected

Reference: Paulsen, C. A.: The testes. In Williams, R. H. (Ed.): Textbook of Endocrinology. Philadelphia, W. B. Saunders Company, 1974, pp. 360, 361.

Amazon — The word is derived from *a,* "without," and *mazon,* "breast." Supposedly, this condition arose from a practice of these legendary female warriors designed to facilitate the drawing of the bow-string.

11

CESSATION OF MENSES

Menstruation is dependent upon normal genital anatomy and a balanced cyclical interaction between hypothalamic-pituitary and ovarian hormones. A multitude of factors affecting either the stimulus-feedback system or the quantity of hypothalamic-pituitary-ovarian hormones can lead to irregular menses or complete cessation of menstruation. The internist should be acquainted with the causes of secondary amenorrhea, as some of them may have significant medical implications (e.g., pituitary tumor), while others may require only reassurance of the patient (i.e., functional amenorrhea).

Diagnostic intervention is usually warranted after four to six menstrual periods are missed. *Pregnancy is the most common cause* of secondary amenorrhea and should be ruled out before further investigations are initiated.

The following is a list of the etiologies:

1. *Pregnancy*
2. *Ovarian disease*
   Normal menopause
   Acquired lesions—infection, oophoritis, tumor (may be hormone-producing)
   Premature menopause (usually defined as occurring before the age of 40)
   Polycystic ovaries
3. *Hypothalamic-pituitary disease*
   Tumors—nonsecretory or secretory (acromegaly, galactorrhea, Cushing's disease)
   Infiltrative disease (sarcoid, histocytosis)
   Prolactin secretion in absence of tumor — idiopathic or drug-induced (phenothiazines)
   Postpubertal hypogonadotrophic hypogonadism
   Empty sella syndrome
4. *Adrenal disease*
   Cushing's syndrome — adenoma, carcinoma
   Adrenal tumors with virilization
   Addison's disease
5. *Drug-induced*
   Contraceptives
   Spironolactone
6. *Chronic systemic disease*
   Malignancy
   Collagen-vascular disease
   Anemia
   Chronic active hepatitis
   Chronic infection
7. *Anorexia nervosa*
8. *Massive obesity*
9. *Anatomic lesions of genitals*
   Asherman's syndrome — scarring of cervical os
10. *Functional amenorrhea*
    Secondary to emotional trauma

11. *Idiopathic*
12. *Acute systemic disease*
    Acute infection

The evaluation of the patient with secondary amenorrhea begins with a detailed and complete history and physical examination. Careful pelvic examination will help determine the size of the uterus and ovaries and detect any mass lesions or signs of infection. Where indicated, laboratory evaluation can be directed at the specific disease suggested by the history and physical examination (e.g., thyroid disease).

The following approach is designed to uncover abnormalities as they might exist in the controlling endocrine organs. A complete gynecologic evaluation may include laparoscopy, laparotomy, or endometrial biopsy. Remember, pregnancy and menopause are the most common etiologies!

1. *Progesterone challenge* (Provera, 10 mg a day orally for 5 days)
   A. Positive test: Withdrawal bleeding; anovulatory cycle and at least minimal function of ovary, pituitary, and the hypothalamus established. Indicates previous endometrial stimulation by estrogens.
   B. Negative test: No withdrawal bleeding. Go to step 2.
2. *Estrogen challenge* (Premarin, 1.25 mg a day orally for 21 days)
   A. Positive test: Withdrawal bleeding; normal uterine response to estrogen prime established. Go to step 3.
   B. Negative test: No withdrawal bleeding; target organ or out-flow tract failure.
3. *Gonadotropin (FSH, LH) and prolactin levels*
   A. To distinguish end-organ (ovarian) failure (high levels) from hypothalamic-pituitary failure (low levels).
   B. To rule out prolactinoma (hyperprolactinemia, amenorrhea-galactorrhea syndrome).
   C. *Pituitary-hypothalamic failure or hyperprolactinemia:* x-rays of sella turcica and/or computerized tomography, pituitary evaluation (see Pituitary Function Testing, p. 357).
4. *Therapy* (What does the patient want?)
   A. Watchful waiting.
   B. Treatment of anovulation (clomiphene citrate [Clomid]).
   C. Therapy of any underlying associated disorder.
   D. Symptomatic therapy of secondary amenorrhea (progesterone, progesterone/estrogen).

11

Reference: Speroff, L., Glass, R. H., and Kase, N. G.: Clinical Gynecologic Endocrinology and Infertility. Baltimore, The Williams and Wilkins Company, 1973, p. 75.

HAIRY MARY, OR THE HIRSUTE FEMALE

You may be confronted by the female patient who has developed the very disturbing sign of hirsutism, or evidence for virilization such as acne, temporal baldness, deepening of the voice, increased muscle mass, amenorrhea, and clitoral enlargement. The differential diagnosis involves ovarian or adrenal pathology. The evaluation depends upon the fact that adrenal tumors secrete weak androgens that must be produced in large amounts to cause virilization. Thus, the urinary 17-ketosteroids are markedly elevated in adrenal causes. The ovarian tumors, however, secrete the potent androgen testosterone and are, therefore, characterized by normal or modest elevations of the 17-ketosteroids. On the opposite page is a flow chart for the evaluation of androgen excess in the female.

Virile — From the Latin *vir,* meaning "man." *Virtus,* from which "virtue" is derived, having the traits of a man. All the progeny of *vir,* including "virtuoso," have strongly positive connotations.

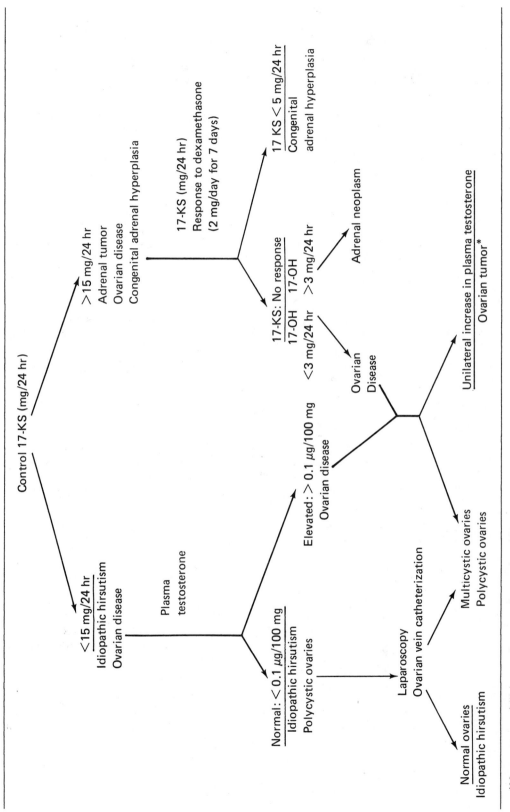

*Most common virilizing ovarian tumor is an arrhenoblastoma

Reference: Thorn, W. G., Adams, R. D., and Braunwald, E. (Eds.): Harrison's Principles of Internal Medicine, 8th Edition, New York, McGraw-Hill Book Company, 1979, p. 545. (Reproduced by permission.)

12

HEMATOLOGY/ ONCOLOGY

APPROACH TO ANEMIA

History, Physical Exam, CBC, Reticulocyte Count, Peripheral Smear Examination, and Red Cell Indices As Guides to Diagnosis

MICROCYTIC HYPOCHROMIC (MCV<$82\mu^3$)

Iron deficiency anemia
Lead poisoning
Thalassemia syndromes
Sideroblastic anemia
Severe protein deficiency
(Anemia of chronic disease)

NORMOCYTIC (MCV 82 to $98\mu^3$)

Elevated reticulocyte count
  Hemorrhage
  Hemolysis
  Unstable hemoglobins
  Red cell enzyme deficiencies

Normal reticulocyte count
  Early iron deficiency anemia
  Anemia of chronic disease

Low reticulocyte count
  Aplastic anemia
  Pure red cell aplasia
  Endocrine disease
  Renal disease
  Infection: viral, bacterial, fungal
  Acute leukemia, lymphoma, multiple myeloma, myelofibrosis
  Splenomegaly ("hypersplenism")
  Toxic agents: radiation, cancer chemotherapy, lead, carbon tetrachloride

MACROCYTIC (MCV>$98\mu^3$)

Nonmegaloblastic bone marrow
  Reticulocytosis
  Liver disease (in absence of folate deficiency)
  Hypothyroidism

Megaloblastic bone marrow
  Folic acid deficiency
  Vitamin B_{12} deficiency
  Vitamin C deficiency (scurvy)
  Erythroleukemia
  Cancer chemotherapy
  Pyridoxine responsive megaloblastic anemia
  Refractory sideroblastic anemia
  Hereditary orotic aciduria

12

NORMAL HEMOGLOBIN AND HEMATOCRIT VALUES IN ADULTS

MEAN AND RANGE (± 2 S.E.)

	Adult male	Adult female	
Hemoglobin	15 grams/100 ml (13–17)	13.5 grams/100 ml (11.5–15.5)	(Finch[1])
	15.5 grams/100 ml (13.3–17.7)	13.7 grams/100 ml (11.7–15.7)	(Williams[2])
	15.5 grams/100 ml (13.5–17.5)	13.5 grams/100 ml (11.5–15.5)	(S.U.H.[3])
Hematocrit	47% (41–53)	41% (35–47)	(Finch)
	46% (39.8–52.2)	40.9% (34.9–46.9)	(Williams)
	47% (43–51)	40.5% (36–45)	(S.U.H.)

[1] Data from Hillman, R. S., and Finch, C. A.: Red Cell Manual, 4th Edition. Philadelphia, F. A. Davis Company, 1974.

[2] Data from Williams, W. J., et al.: Hematology, 2nd Edition. New York, McGraw-Hill Book Company, 1977.

[3] Data from clinical pathology laboratory, State University Hospital, Upstate Medical Center, Syracuse, N. Y.

MCVMCHMCHC: SOME USES

Automated electronic counters are employed in virtually all clinical laboratories to determine blood counts. The counters measure red and white blood cell counts by registering the interruption of charge produced when a nonconducting particle passes through a voltage gate. Since the magnitude of the electrical interference is proportional to cell size, an accurate assessment of the mean corpuscular volume (MCV) is also made electronically. Hemoglobin level is determined colorimetrically, and values for hematocrit, mean corpuscular hemoglobin (MCH), and mean corpuscular hemoglobin concentration (MCHC) are computed. The normal adult values employed at our medical center are:

$$MCV = \frac{Hct}{RBC} = \frac{80-96}{\mu^3(fl)} \qquad MCH = \frac{Hb}{RBC} = \frac{27-33}{\mu\mu g(pg)} \qquad MCHC = \frac{Hb}{Hct} = 32-36\%$$

Alterations in MCH and MCHC

These indices have added little to what may be determined from the MCV, since the hemoglobin falls as the MCH falls. A *high* MCHC means that hemoglobin is packed in the red cell with a minimum of excess membrane. Spherocytosis, whether hereditary in origin or caused by immune or microangiopathic hemolysis, is almost always the explanation for an elevation in the MCHC.

A. *The low MCV:* The three major clinical conditions associated with a red cell with a low MCV are:

1. Iron deficiency: The earliest change in iron deficiency is a fall in bone marrow iron and serum ferritin. A fall in serum iron and a rise in free erythrocyte protoporphyrin (FEP) then follow. The MCV drops just prior to the fall in hemoglobin.

2. Thalassemia minor: The MCV may be employed as a screening test in thalassemia minor. The MCV is usually between 60 and 65 fl in β-thal and somewhat higher in α-thal. In thalassemia major, the macrocytosis tends to raise the otherwise low MCV.

3. Lead poisoning: Microcytosis is seen in lead poisoning less often than is a rise in RBC FEP. The FEP tends to be higher in lead poisoning per degree of anemia than in iron deficiency.

Iron Deficiency or Thalassemia Trait?

It's possible to make a presumptive diagnosis of iron deficiency or thalassemia trait in over 90 per cent of cases based on the data obtained on the CBC. These formulas are useful in the stable, uncomplicated patient. Hemolysis, brisk reticulocytosis, active bleeding, or secondary polycythemia makes them less reliable.

$$\textit{Mentzer formula} = \frac{MCV}{RBC}$$

Values greater than 14 are seen in iron deficiency, while values less than 12 indicate thalassemia.

$$\textit{Discriminate function} = MCV - RBC - (5 \times Hb) - 3.4$$

Positive values for the discriminate function suggest iron deficiency, while negative values are found in thalassemia.

12

B. *The normocytic anemia:* Think of recent blood loss, the anemia of chronic disease, hemolysis, or bone marrow failure.

C. *The high MCV:*
1. Nutritional megaloblastic anemias (B_{12} or folate): The LDH is almost always elevated!
2. Reticulocytosis: The reticulocyte is a large cell.
3. Antineoplastic therapy: Interference with cell division produces a large RBC.
4. Liver disease: An increase in membrane lipid increases the size of the membrane.
5. Hypothyroidism.
6. Down's syndrome.
7. Drugs: They can interfere with folate metabolism by a variety of mechanisms. Check for alcohol, birth control pills, phenytoin, triamterene, sulfa and similar drugs.
8. Miscellaneous: "Preleukemia."

MCHC IN HEREDITARY SPHEROCYTOSIS

The following chart (Fig. 12–1) shows the mean corpuscular hemoglobin concentration (MCHC) in patients with hereditary spherocytosis and in their relatives.

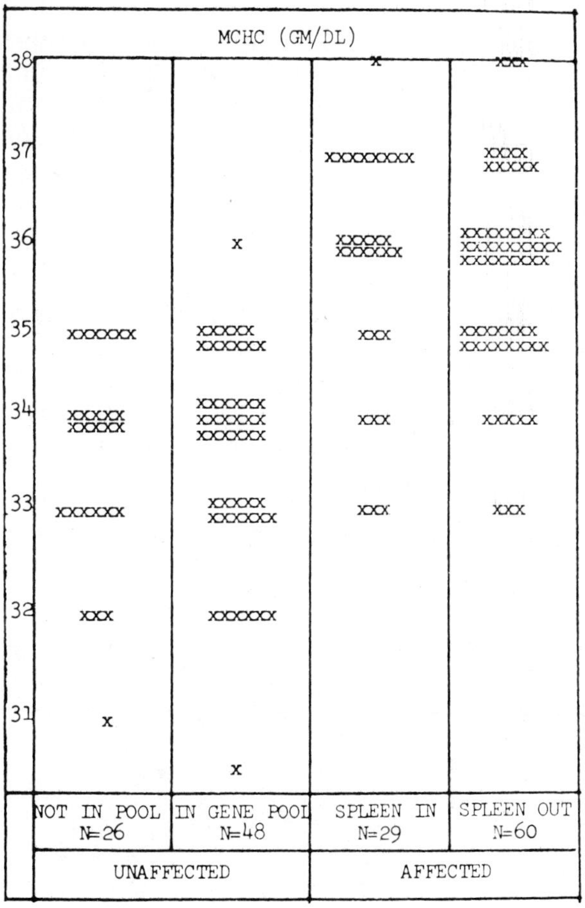

FIG. 12–1

The MCHC in patients with hereditary spherocytosis and their relations.

MCHC (GM/DL)	NOT IN POOL N=26	IN GENE POOL N=48	SPLEEN IN N=29	SPLEEN OUT N=60
38			x	xxx
37			xxxxxxxx	xxxx / xxxxx
36		x	xxxxx / xxxxxx	xxxxxxxx / xxxxxxxxx / xxxxxxxx
35	xxxxxx	xxxxx / xxxxx	xxx	xxxxxxx / xxxxxxxxx
34	xxxxx / xxxxx	xxxxxx / xxxxxx / xxxxxx	xxx	xxxxx
33	xxxxxx	xxxxx / xxxxx	xxx	xxx
32	xxx	xxxxxx		
31	x			
		x		
	UNAFFECTED		AFFECTED	

Reference: Schilling, R. F.: Hereditary spherocytosis. Semin. Hematol., *13*:169, 1975. Figure reproduced with permission of author and Grune & Stratton, Inc.

12

ANEMIA OF CHRONIC DISEASE

The anemia of chronic disease is usually a mild, normocytic, normochromic anemia seen with infection, inflammatory disease, and malignancy. For a variety of reasons, iron, stored in the reticuloendothelial system, fails to recirculate (via transferrin) to the developing erythrocyte. Thus, in the maturing red cell, the anemia of chronic disease represents a "relative" iron-deficient state.

The table on the opposite page compares the anemia of chronic disease with true iron deficiency anemia and the anemia of recent GI bleeding and highlights some of the more salient features of each.

Iron "Deficient" Erythropoiesis

	ANEMIA OF CHRONIC DISEASE	TRUE IRON DEFICIENCY	RECENT BLEEDING
Peripheral smear	Normal to slightly microcytic	Normal or hypochromic microcytic	Normal or shift macrocytes
Reticulocyte count	Normal or decreased	Normal or decreased	Increased
Serum Fe	$\leqslant 30\ \mu g/100\ ml$	$< 50\ \mu g/100\ ml$	$> 45\ \mu g/100\ ml$
TIBC*	150–300 $\mu g/100\ ml$	350–500 $\mu g/100\ ml$	300–400 $\mu g/100\ ml$
Per cent saturation	10–20	1–15	15–35
Ferritin	Normal to increased	Decreased	Increased or decreased
FEP†	Increased	Increased	Normal or increased
Marrow iron stores	Increased (in the reticuloendo-thelial cells of the bone marrow)	Absent	Absent or present, depend-ing on stores prior to recent blood loss

*TIBC = Total iron-binding capacity
†FEP = Free erythrocyte porphyrin

12

MONTHLY BLOOD LOSS

The most frequent cause of iron depletion in women in their reproductive years is the loss of blood in the menstrual flow. Approximately 1 mg of iron is lost from the body with each ml of blood. The appearance of clots, the necessity for "double padding," and the prolongation of flow beyond the usual five-day duration are associated with an excessive blood loss.

Several excellent studies on the quantitation of the menstrual flow exist. Fig. 12–2 shows patterns of menstrual blood loss in a population of 476 Swedish women. Their ages ranged from 15 to 50. Blood loss was carefully measured as alkaline hematin. For the series as a whole, the median menstrual blood loss was 30 ml. When patients with abnormal menses were excluded, the median rose to 33.2 ml, with the ninety-fifth percentile established at a bit over 76 ml per month. Changes in the iron-binding capacity were examined as an indication of impending iron depletion. It appeared that patients losing more than 60 to 80 ml of blood monthly regularly developed an increase in iron-binding capacity as an early sign of iron deficiency. Eleven per cent of the group examined exceeded this figure.

Similar results were obtained in a British study of 348 women. Nine per cent of those examined exceeded 80 ml of blood loss per month. The age range of women examined in this study was 17 to 45. The median value obtained was 27.6 ml, which rose to 37.9 ml when patients employing oral contraceptives or intrauterine devices were excluded from the study panel.

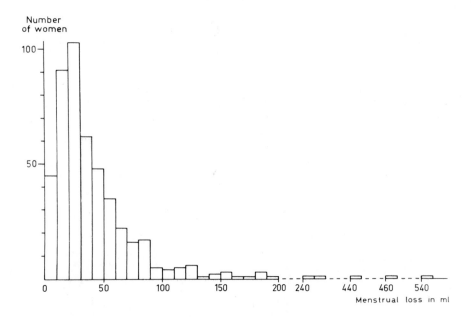

FIG. 12-2

Patterns of menstrual blood loss in 476 Swedish women. (From Rybo, G.: Clin. Haematol., 2:269, 1973.)

Factors predisposing to excessive menses were hereditary influences, parity (multiparous women had a higher degree of blood loss than nulliparous or primiparous women), age, and the presence of intra-uterine pathology, such as fibroids. The duration of the menstrual flow also influenced the degree of blood loss. Individuals with a duration of flow of more than six or seven days had a higher frequency of menorrhagia. The effect of antiplatelet agents such as aspirin on menstrual blood loss was not examined in these studies. One might anticipate a somewhat higher blood loss in those women who routinely employed aspirin or other compounds with antiplatelet activity during or immediately prior to the menses.

Reference: Rybo, G.: Clin. Haematol., *2*:269, 1973. Figure 12–2 reproduced with permission of publisher.

ABSORBED IRON REQUIREMENT

The chart below (Fig. 12–3) shows iron requirements in males and females of various ages.

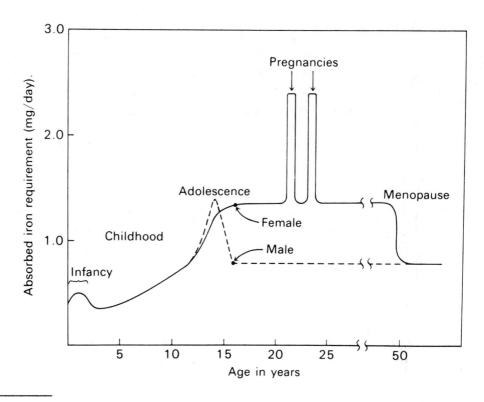

Reference: Wintrobe, M. M., et al. (Eds.): Clin. Hematol., 7th Edition. Philadelphia, Lea & Febiger, 1974, p. 647. Reprinted by permission.

PITFALLS IN THE THERAPY OF IRON DEFICIENCY ANEMIA

Therapy of iron deficiency anemia is relatively simple. In addition to mistakes in diagnosis, a number of common errors are made in the treatment of this disorder. Almost a third of patients treated for iron deficiency anemia "relapse." The common causes of relapse are provided in the following table. Twenty-nine relapses were observed in 100 patients treated for iron deficiency anemia. These patients were observed for three years or longer, and several patients had more than one identifiable cause for relapse.

Clearly the most common causes for the continued failure of iron therapy are lack of patient compliance and inadequate or an improperly administered iron dosage. Before you embark on an extended medical evaluation for the causes of "refractory" iron deficiency, the patient should be asked whether the iron is actually being taken. Ferrous iron is absorbed better than ferric iron, and its absorption is aided by the presence of succinic acid, absorbable iron chelates, and reducing substances such as ascorbic acid. Iron absorption is decreased in the presence of iron-binding substances, such as phytates and phosphates, which are found in food. Iron absorption is decreased by some 40 per cent in the presence of food. Thus, for maximal effect, iron should be given on an empty stomach. There appears to be no difference in the absorption or side effects of ferrous sulfate, gluconate, fumarate, or lactate when given in equivalent doses.

Iron is absorbed mainly in the proximal duodenum. Absorption decreases distally in the small intestine. When iron is released slowly, as from sustained-release capsules, the major site of iron absorption is bypassed. Thus, the gastrointestinal side effects of iron therapy are minimized by sustained-release capsules, but so are absorption and response to therapy.

Iron malabsorption *per se* is extremely rare in adults. It may occur when there is an extremely rapid gastrointestinal transit time or increased bulk, as may exist in established malabsorption syndromes. Similarly, iron malabsorption may accompany extensive gastric resection because of the changes in the relationships between the stomach and proximal duodenum. We have never observed iron malabsorption in an adult given the correct dose of iron, the appropriate preparation, and an appropriate dose schedule, unless there was an underlying malabsorption syndrome or a readily demonstrable anatomic defect. For doubters, a rise in serum iron two hours after the oral administration of the equivalent of 100 mg of elemental iron to the fasted subject should establish that the absorptive mechanism is functioning properly. Given a "refractory" patient, check whether the patient is taking the iron, whether you are giving enough iron in the proper manner, and whether the patient is continuing to bleed.

Patients with hemoglobin values of less than 8 grams/100 ml will show an increase of approximately 0.2 to 0.3 gram/day during the first 7 to 10 days of adequate iron therapy. As the hemoglobin rises, its rate of increase slows. A reticulocytosis is seen 48 to 72 hours after the beginning of therapy and reaches a peak 7 to 10 days afterward. A sustained reticulocytosis or a reticulocytosis in excess of 10 per cent usually does not occur.

Replacement therapy in the adult should be no less than one 325 mg tablet of ferrous sulfate three to four times daily, taken on an empty stomach. Therapy should be continued three to six months after attainment of a normal hemoglobin level in order to replenish iron stores. In the patient with continued excessive blood loss (i.e., menorrhagia), iron therapy should probably be continued indefinitely.

CAUSE	NUMBER	TOTAL
Inadequate iron supply		24
Therapy discontinued	21	
Dosage inadequate	2	
Intolerance to therapy	1	
Continuing blood loss		12
Menorrhagia	9	
Diverticulitis	2	
Undiagnosed alimentary bleeding	1	
Pregnancy	2	2
Malabsorption	4	4

12

Reference: Dagg, J. H., and Goldberg, A.: Clin. Haematol., 2:365, 1973.

ADMINISTRATION OF PARENTERAL IRON

Parenteral iron administration is usually not necessary. In certain states, however, where iron absorption is inadequate to replete iron stores, parenteral administration of iron may be indicated. Calculation of the amount of iron to be replaced may be done as follows:

$$(\text{Desired hemoglobin} - \text{patient's hemoglobin}) \times \frac{(\text{blood volume} \times \text{patient's weight})}{100}$$

$$\times \frac{\text{mg iron}}{\text{gram hemoglobin}}$$

where

hemoglobin is expressed as grams/dl

$$\text{blood volume} = \frac{70 \text{ ml}}{\text{Kg}}$$

patient's weight is expressed in Kg

3.38 mg of iron/gram hemoglobin

For example:

A 70 Kg patient has a hemoglobin of 7 grams/dl. To correct the hemoglobin to 14 grams/dl, administer:

$$\left(\frac{14 \text{ grams}}{\text{dl}} - \frac{7 \text{ grams}}{\text{dl}} \right) \times \frac{[70 \times 70]}{100} \times 3.38 = 1159 \text{ mg of Fe}$$

An additional 1000 mg should be administered to replenish tissue stores in males (600 mg in females).

Reference: Cline, M. J., and Territo, M. C.: Hematopoietic disorders. In Melmon, K. L., and Morrelli, H. F. (Eds.): Clin. Pharmacol., 2nd Edition. New York, Macmillan, Inc., 1978, p. 636.

VITAMIN B$_{12}$ AND FOLATE DEFICIENCY

	TOTAL BODY STORES	DAILY TURNOVER	TIME TO DEPLETION*
Vitamin B$_{12}$	5000 μg	1–5 μg	2.7–13.5 yrs
Folate	5000 μg	50 μg	100 days†

*Assuming normal stores at time deprivation begins.

†May be shortened by increased requirements (e.g., pregnancy, chronic hemolysis, malignancy) coexisting with deprivation.

TREATMENT OF DOCUMENTED VITAMIN B$_{12}$ AND FOLIC ACID DEFICIENCIES

Vitamin B$_{12}$ (cyanocobalamin or hydroxocobalamin)

1. 100 μg IM daily for 14 days, then
2. 100 μg IM twice weekly for 4 weeks, then
3. 100 μg IM monthly for life.

Folic Acid

1. Folic acid should not be used to treat megaloblastic anemia unless vitamin B$_{12}$ deficiency has been ruled out or vitamin B$_{12}$ is administered simultaneously. This will prevent exacerbation of the neurologic lesion of vitamin B$_{12}$ deficiency by inappropriate therapy with folic acid alone.

2. 1 mg orally a day.

3. An intravenous preparation of 15 mg of folic acid per ml is available for use in severely ill patients, patients with malabsorption or with intravenous hyperalimentation.

Reference: Williams, W. J., Beutler, E., Erslev, A. J., and Rundles, W. R.: Hematology. New York, McGraw-Hill Book Company, 1977, pp. 323, 344.

12

Pernicious — Meaning seriously harmful, it is derived from the Latin *perniciosus,* which consists of *per,* "through," and *nex, necis,* "death."

HALLMARKS OF HEMOLYSIS

The presence of hemolysis (i.e., a shortened red cell survival in the absence of bleeding) can often be detected by a number of laboratory determinations. Patients with hemolysis *need not be anemic,* as normal people can increase their red cell production six to eight times in the presence of premature destruction of red cells. (See table, pp. 389–391.)

Hallmark — Is a term derived from the official assay mark placed upon articles of gold and silver and used by the Goldsmith Company at Goldsmith's Hall in London. The Goldsmith's guild began in the eleventh century. The word hallmark appeared in the eighteenth.

TEST	COMMENT
1. Reticulocyte count	—The normal reticulocyte count is 0.5 to 1.5 per cent. —An absolute reticulocyte count $>75,000/mm^3$ suggests hemolysis. —The patient with hemolysis may have a normal or low reticulocyte count if the bone marrow is unable to respond appropriately to the shortened red cell survival.
2. Serum haptoglobin	—Haptoglobin binds to liberated hemoglobin *dimers* and the complex is cleared rapidly by the reticuloendothelial system. Thus, in hemolytic states, particularly those characterized by liberation of hemoglobin into the plasma, haptoglobin concentration is low. However, haptoglobin is an α-2-globulin, which rises in infection, inflammatory states, and malignant conditions. Thus, despite active hemolysis, the serum haptoglobin concentration may not be low, thereby limiting its usefulness as a diagnostic clue to hemolysis.
3. Hemoglobinemia	—When large quantities of hemoglobin are liberated into the plasma, hemoglobin *tetramers* are oxidized to methemoglobin and are measured as free plasma hemoglobin. In addition, the heme group then dissociates from the globin and binds to hemopexin. When the hemopexin is saturated, excess heme binds to albumin to form methemealbumin. The presence of methemealbumin implies a significant degree of intravascular hemolysis.

12

TEST	COMMENT
4. Hemoglobinuria/hemosiderinuria	—The hemoglobin dimers filtered at the glomerulus are reabsorbed by renal tubular cells and are converted to hemosiderin. When the tubular cells are desquamated into the urine, the urine sediment stained with Prussian blue will reveal the presence of hemosiderin.
	—When large quantities of hemoglobin dimers are filtered and the capacity of the tubules to reabsorb them is exceeded, the urine will be colored pink to red and will yield a positive test for occult blood. (Prussian blue stains only *nonheme* iron and cannot be used to stain the urine sediment for hemoglobin.)
5. Indirect bilirubin	—When hemolysis occurs, increased amounts of bilirubin are presented to the liver for conjugation and excretion. When the capacity of the liver to remove the increased amounts of bilirubin from the circulation is exceeded, the *indirect* bilirubin concentration rises.
	—In the absence of liver disease, the *total* serum bilirubin may rise to 3 to 5 mg/100 ml in hemolytic states (85 per cent indirect).
6. Serum lactic dehydrogenase (LDH)	—The serum LDH rises in cases of *intravascular hemolysis* (e.g., hemolytic transfusion reaction, heart valve hemolysis, G-6-PD deficiency, paroxysmal cold hemoglobinuria, march hemoglobinuria, malaria, hemolytic uremic syndrome, thrombotic thrombocytopenic purpura, burns, and *Clostridium welchii* infection), with *severe extravascular hemolysis* and with *megaloblastic anemias* caused by B_{12} or folate deficiency.

TEST	COMMENT
7. Carboxyhemoglobin	—For each mole of heme catabolized, a mole of carbon monoxide (CO) is liberated. Thus, in the absence of external exposure to CO, as in smoking or rush-hour expressway driving, an elevated carboxyhemoglobin (the CO liberated binds to hemoglobin-forming carboxyhemoglobin) represents increased heme degradation.
	—The carboxyhemoglobin (HbCO) determination is the most sensitive test of hemolysis if measured accurately. *Gas chromatography* represents the standard most exact method.
	—A normal HbCO level in *nonsmoking* adults is < 1 per cent.
8. Peripheral blood smear	—The presence of polychromasia and spherocytes suggests hemolysis.
	—Fragmented red cells, sickle cells, acanthocytes, "bite cells," and similar cells, when noted, should serve as clues to the cause of the hemolysis.

12

WHY DO ALL THOSE DIFFERENT HEMOGLOBINS MOVE IN THE SAME PLACES ON ELECTROPHORESIS? (or Everything that Moves like Sickle Hemoglobin May Not Be)

Hemoglobin variants of different structures may have identical or close to identical, electrophoretic mobility. The vast majority of variants of the adult hemoglobin molecule are single point mutations in the 141 or 146 amino acids that constitute the alpha and beta chains, respectively. The adult hemoglobin molecule is made up of two alpha and two beta chains. When an amino acid that is uncharged at the pH of electrophoresis is substituted for another neutral amino acid in either the two alpha or the two beta chains, no net change in electrophoretic mobility of the variant hemoglobin is observed. However, a neutral amino acid may be substituted for an acidic amino acid (aspartic or glutamic), with the loss of one charge "unit" per chain and the production of a hemoglobin with diminished anodal mobility.

Similar changes in charge occur when a basic amino acid (arginine, lysine, or histidine) replaces a neutral amino acid. When a basic amino acid replaces an acidic residue, two charge units are lost per abnormal chain. The loss in net negative charge that results decreases mobility toward the anode when current is applied. Thus, the electrophoretic mobilities of sickle hemoglobin (in which the neutral valine is substituted for the acidic glutamic acid in the sixth position of each of two beta chains) is virtually identical to the electrophoretic mobility observed for hemoglobin $G_{Philadelphia}$, in which a basic lysine has replaced the neutral asparagine. Conversely, hemoglobins having a more rapid anodal mobility than hemoglobin A will result from the conversion of basic amino acids to neutral or acidic amino acids.

Since the number of amino acids substituted are usually 2 in 574 (one each in the same site in both abnormal chains), and only substitutions involving relatively major changes in charge may be detected by casual clinical electrophoresis, the resulting electrophoretic patterns may prove highly repetitious despite the plethora of possible sites and apparent variety of substitution. The true differences between hemoglobins may be determined either by an observation of the special properties of the mutant hemoglobin (such as the sickling phenomena) or by close examination of the isoelectric point by more sophisticated techniques or peptide mapping. Since the delta chain of hemoglobin A_2 and the gamma chain of hemoglobin F differ from the normal beta chain in a number of sites, the electrophoretic mobility of hemoglobin A_2 and F are significantly different from that observed for hemoglobin A.

ADVERSE EFFECTS OF SICKLE CELL TRAIT

The morbidity from sickle cell trait is uncertain, as the literature abounds with case reports of sickle cell trait occurring in association with virtually every affliction. Some of the conditions likely to be associated with sickle cell trait are given below, along with those in which the association is thought to be due to chance. Many additional complications have been reported to have a statistical association with the trait (e.g., avascular necrosis of bone, delayed skeletal maturation, increased fertility), but further study is required to confirm these observations.

Conditions Unlikely to be Associated with Sickle Cell Trait
1. Shortened life expectancy.
2. Sudden death (with or without exertion).
3. Anemia.
4. Maternal or fetal complications of pregnancy (other than the higher incidence of urinary tract infection).
5. Complications from surgery or anesthesia if hypoxia is avoided (except for surgery conducted under tourniquet control).
6. Complications from flight in pressurized aircraft.
7. Cerebrovascular occlusions.
8. Leg ulcers.
9. Cardiopulmonary disease (including pulmonary infarction).
10. Hypertension.

Conditions Likely to be Associated with Sickle Cell Trait
1. Higher incidence of urinary tract infection in pregnancy.
2. Hyposthenuria.
3. Hematuria (but other causes should still be sought).
4. Renal papillary necrosis.
5. Splenic infarction at high altitudes (greater than 10,000 ft).
6. Decreased mortality from *Plasmodium falciparum* infection.

Reference: Sears, D. A.: Am. J. Med., *64*:1021, 1978.

12

THE HEINZ BODY

Heinz bodies are particles of denatured protein composed mainly of hemoglobin with some red cell stroma. They usually are seen as rounded red cell inclusions measuring between 0.3 and 2 microns in diameter. They are not demonstrable in Wright-stained smears but may be seen with May-Greenwald-Giemsa stain or phase contrast microscopy. Heinz bodies may also be demonstrated by vital staining with crystal violet, new methylene blue, or brilliant cresyl blue. After hemolysis of the red cell, Heinz bodies may be observed attached to the red cell membrane.

When present, Heinz bodies markedly limit red cell distensibility and thereby impose a selective survival disadvantage on the host cell in the microcirculation in general and in the spleen in particular. In addition, the presence of Heinz bodies appears to be associated with the presence of aggregates of cytoskeletal protein that also limit cell filterability. Membrane loss and membrane damage result from the extraction of Heinz bodies from red cells. Ultimately, the successive extraction of Heinz bodies and consequent membrane loss lead to the formation of spherocytes. Spherocytes, being rigid, nondistensible cells, are rapidly destroyed in the microcirculation. The inability of rigid Heinz bodies to traverse the intraepithelial slits of the spleen has been observed by electron microscopy. The inclusions are left behind in the perisinusoidal red pulp for ultimate phagocytosis by macrophages (Fig. 12–4).

The presence of Heinz bodies implies a failure of the red cell mechanisms to prevent oxidative denaturation of hemoglobin. One of the most important of these is the availability of reduced glutathione (a tripeptide consisting of cysteine, glutamic acid, and glycine). Oxidized glutathione is a double tripeptide, the halves of which are linked by conversion of the sulfhydryl groups of the two cysteines to a disulfide. Reduced glutathione is regenerated from the oxidized form by action of the hexose monophosphate shunt. Normally, about 10 per cent of the glucose metabolism of the red cell is directed to the hexose monophosphate shunt. Glucose is thus converted to glucose-6-phosphate, which is then dehydrogenated by glucose-6-phosphate dehydrogenase. The pathway is shown in Figure 12–5. The resultant conversion of NADP to NADPH (TPN to TPNH) is linked by glutathione reductase in a manner such that the NADPH supplies the hydrogen ion for the reduction of glutathione. The continued interconversion of reduced to oxidized glutathione supplies a regenerating, metabolically linked oxidative sink for the red cell.

In the absence of adequate amounts of glutathione to meet oxidative stress, mixed disulfides will form between glutathione and the cysteine in the ninety-third position on the beta chain of hemoglobin. The mixed disulfide is unstable and undergoes further reaction with sulfhydryl groups, which are usually buried in the interior of the hemoglobin molecule. The result of these interactions is the intracellular precipitation of an insoluble particle, the Heinz body. Ultimately, the Heinz body finds itself attached to the inner aspect of the red cell membrane.

In general, Heinz bodies may be found in those conditions in which hemoglobin is either unduly sensitive to oxidation (hemoglobin H and the unstable hemoglobinopathies) or in which glutathione is not adequately regenerated or synthesized (glucose-6-phosphate dehydrogenase deficiency or glutathione reductase deficiency). It may also be found where the red cell is subjected to continual oxidative stress (drug ingestion, liver or renal disease).

THE PERILS OF THE RED CELL IN THE MICROCIRCULATION

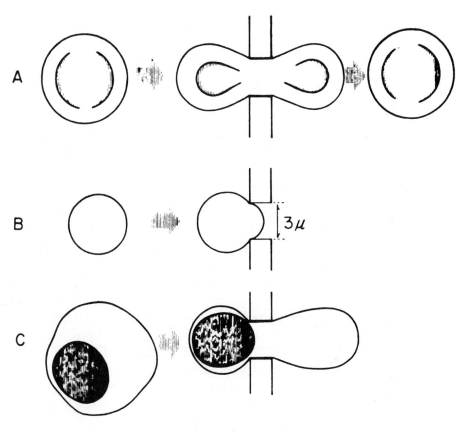

FIG. 12–4

12

A. *Salvation by distensibility.* Excess membrane allows the normal red cell to assume the shape of a distensible, malleable biconcave disk. Thus, a cell with a 7 to 8 micron diameter can slip through very small pores.

B. *Pity the poor rigid sphere!* Though small, it can't get anywhere.

C. *It's tough to be a Heinz body — or a red cell that owns one.* Following the "pitting" procedure shown, the membrane can reseal. A "bite" cell is formed (Fig. 12–6). Ultimately, continued membrane loss and resealing will produce a spherocyte.

HEXOSE MONOPHOSPHATE SHUNT

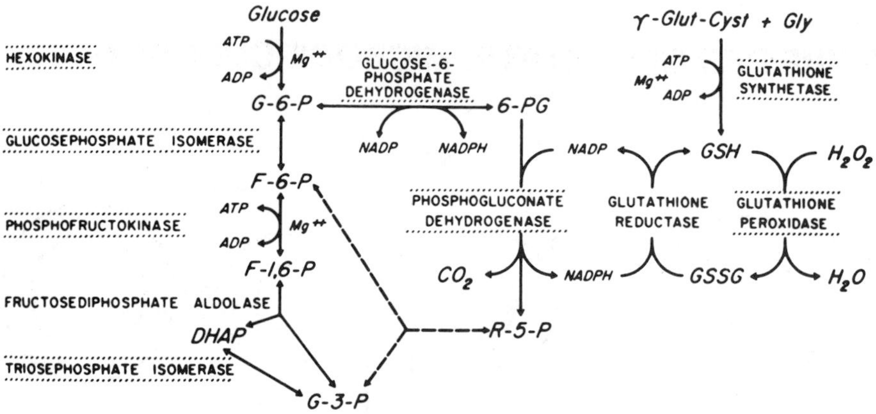

FIG. 12–5

The erythrocyte hexose monophosphate shunt.

The hexose monophosphate shunt and the early steps of the Embden-Meyerhof pathway of the erythrocyte are shown in Fig. 12–5. The shunt represents the only mechanism available to the erythrocyte for production of the NADPH (TPNH). For each mole of glucose metabolized, two moles of NADPH are generated by the action of glucose-6-phosphate dehydrogenase and phosphogluconate dehydrogenase. Reduced glutathione protects the red cell from oxidative injury and is regenerated from its oxidized form by the action of glutathione reductase in the presence of NADPH. Ribose phosphate may enter the Embden-Meyerhof pathway after conversion to fructose-6-phosphate (F-6-P) or glyceraldehyde-3-phosphate (G-3-P).

GLUCOSE-6-PHOSPHATE DEHYDROGENASE DEFICIENCY

A deficiency of erythrocyte glucose-6-phosphate dehydrogenase (G-6-PD) appears to be one of the most common inherited inborn errors of metabolism. In G-6-PD deficiency, diminished erythrocyte hexose monophosphate shunt activity results from a deficiency of the initiating and rate-limiting enzyme. A decrease in NADPH generation results and causes susceptibility to the formation of Heinz bodies.

"Normal" G-6-PD has been designated type B by electrophoresis. A large number of variants of the normal enzyme have now been described. Thus G-6-PD deficiency is a heterogenous disorder encompassing enzyme variants that may be unstable, synthesized in decreased quantity, or have altered affinity for substrates (G-6-P and NADP).

The most commonly encountered G-6-PD variant is the type A variant, which differs from normal G-6-PD by a single amino acid substitution. The type A variant is found in approximately 30 per cent of black American males but does *not* carry with it a significant decrease in enzyme activity. The A– type of G-6-PD is the most common clinically significant type of G-6-PD abnormality in the American black population. More than 10 per cent of black American males are affected. In the homozygote male, between 5 and 15 per cent of normal enzyme content of the red cell is present. Another commonly encountered G-6-PD mutation associated with enzyme deficiency is G-6-PD Mediterranean. The frequency of this gene among Northern Europeans is approximately 1 in 1000. On the other hand, almost 50 per cent of the males in a Kurdish Jewish population were found to be afflicted. Enzyme deficiency in this variant is even more severe, with homozygous erythrocytes having less than 1 per cent of the normal enzyme content.

The A– type of G-6-PD deficiency is associated with overt hemolysis only when the homozygote is stressed by oxidant metabolic products during an illness or by a variety of oxidant drugs. This enzyme variant is associated with decreased stability of the enzyme as the red cell ages. Thus, following exposure to an oxidant, the older, enzyme-insufficient cells are the first to hemolyze. Hemolysis of the more enzyme-replete, younger cell population soon follows. As these somewhat aged cells are replaced by enzyme sufficient reticulocytes, hemolysis is limited. This self-limiting feature of drug-induced hemolysis is not seen with the Mediterranean variant. In it the enzyme is far more unstable than in the A– variant, and the ability of the bone marrow and the reticulocyte to compensate is limited.

A screening test for G-6-PD deficiency may be falsely normal in the patient with the A– variant with a brisk reticulocytosis. If a patient with an active reticulocytosis and hemolysis is found *not* to have elevated levels of G-6-PD, G-6-PD deficiency should be suspected. It is probably easiest in this circumstance to study the patient when the

12

hemolytic episode has resolved.

While the mechanism for hemolysis involves the formation of a Heinz body, in the presence of high levels of oxidant stress or extremely low levels of enzyme, explosive intravascular hemolysis supervenes as excessive amounts of intracellular peroxide are formed. Hemoglobinuria is observed as a consequence. Remember G-6-PD deficiency is a sex-linked trait. In establishing the hereditary pattern in the family, male-to-male transmission does not occur. Some clinical differences between the A– and Mediterranean G-6-PD variants in male heterozygotes are outlined below.

	Gd^{A-}	$Gd^{MEDITERRANEAN}$
Steady state		
Activity of RBCs	5–15%	0–5 %
Activity of WBCs	100%	20%
Life span of RBCs	100 days	100 days
Hemolytic crisis		
Interval after exposure to hemolytic agent	24–36 hours	3–24 hours
Hemoglobinuria	Common	Constant
Jaundice	Common	Constant
Anemia	Moderate (rarely <6 grams Hgb)	Severe (often <6 grams Hgb)
Duration of hemolysis	Self-limited	Indefinite

Reference: McMillan, J., Nieburg, P., and Oski, F.: The Whole Pediatrician Catalog. Philadelphia, W. B. Saunders Company, 1977.

COMPOUNDS THAT HAVE INDUCED HEMOLYSIS IN G-6-PD-DEFICIENT ERYTHROCYTES

Analgesics:
    Acetanilid
    Acetylsalicylic acid*
    Phenacetin (acetophenetidin)*
Sulfonamides and sulfones:
    Sulfanilamide
    Sulfapyridine
    Sulfisoxazole (Gantrisin)*
    Thiazosulfone
    Salicylazosulfapyridine (Asulfidine)
    Sulfoxone*
    Sulfamethoxypyridazine (Kynex)
Antimalarials:
    Primaquin
    Pamaquin
Nonsulfonamide antibacterial agents:
    Furazolidone
    Nitrofurantoin (Furadantin)
    Chloramphenicol†
    Para-amino salicylic acid
Miscellaneous:
    Ascorbic acid††
    Vitamin K analogues
    Naphthalene
    Nalidixic acid
    Phenylhydrazine
    Probenecid
    Methylene blue*

---

*Slightly hemolytic in G-6-PD A– in large doses.
†Hemolytic in G-6-PD Mediterranean not in A–.
††Hemolytic in massive dose.

Reference: Beutler, E.: Glucose-6-phosphate dehydrogenase deficiency. In Williams, W. J. et al. (Eds.): Hematology. New York, McGraw-Hill Book Company, 1977, p. 471.

12

HEINZ BODIES, HEMOLYSIS, AND LIVER AND KIDNEY DISEASE

Hemolysis is often encountered in patients with active hepatic disease. A number of morphologic abnormalities of the red cell, including spur cells, acanthocytes, and stomatocytes, are found in these patients. The role of the spleen in remodeling these morphologically abnormal cells and inducing hemolysis has been noted. However, these morphologic abnormalities of the erythrocyte appear considerably less frequently than does clinical hemolysis. Acute hemolysis has also been observed in patients with active liver disease and G-6-PD deficiency. In 1958, Zieve described a hemolytic syndrome in patients with active alcoholic liver disease. Hemolysis tended to be rather long-lived, with a duration ranging from several weeks to several months. The pathogenesis of this disorder has never been clarified.

Recently, a markedly increased susceptibility of the erythrocytes to Heinz body formation has been demonstrated in patients with active liver disease. Despite the fact that the cells of patients with active hemolysis are generally younger, the average number of red cells with Heinz bodies after incubation with acetylphenylhydrazine was 47 per cent in patients with hepatic disease, as compared to 17 per cent in control groups. In each case, patients with overt hemolysis displayed markedly elevated Heinz body counts. In addition, the erythrocytes of patients with hepatic disease displayed significantly lower levels of reduced glutathione both before and after incubation with acetylphenylhydrazine. Erythrocyte G-6-PD glutathione peroxidase and transketolase were normal. When compared to normal erythrocytes, the glucose consumption of the patient's erythrocytes was increased. There was no difference in resting hexose monophosphate shunt activity or in the recycling of glucose through the hexose monophosphate shunt when erythrocytes from normal individuals were compared to those of patients. When the erythrocyte hexose monophosphate shunt was stimulated by methylene blue, a marked impairment in both total shunt activity and glucose reutilization by way of the shunt was observed in patients with hepatic disease (Fig. 12–5). Indeed, a continuum of shunt abnormalities ranging from a mild reduction of stimulated hexose monophosphate shunt activity to a combined decrease in both hexose monophosphate shunt and glucose recycling was observed. Patients with the lowest stimulated shunt metabolism and glucose recycling had the highest Heinz body counts, lowest reduced glutathione, and highest total glucose consumption.

With improvement in hepatic function, the abnormalities in Heinz body formation, erythrocyte reduced glutathione, and shunt metabolism returned to normal. In those patients with overt hemolysis, the improvement in the metabolic state of the erythrocyte correlated with the cessation of the premature red cell destruction. These studies strongly suggest that hemolysis in patients with liver disease may be mediated by the formation of intraerythrocytic Heinz bodies. The presumed cause of this disorder is the presence of a circulating oxidant during active hepatic disease. An apparently similar syndrome has been described in the erythrocytes of patients with renal failure, although its frequency seems to be lower than that observed in active hepatic disease.

While the biochemical mediator(s) of these syndromes are not yet clear, these studies provide a mechanism for heretofore unexplained premature red cell destruction observed in patients with active hepatic or renal disease. Due consideration should be given prior to the administration of potential oxidants to patients whose erythrocytes have a compromised ability to reduce oxidants and an increased tendency toward Heinz body–mediated hemolysis (see table, p. 398).

References: Smith, J. R., Kay, N. E., Gottlieb, A. J., and Oski, F. A.: Blood, *46*:955, 1975; Yawata, Y., Howe, R., and Jacob, H. S.: Ann. Intern. Med., *79*:362, 1973.

THE BITE CELL

Figure 12–6 shows examples of bite cells (arrows) from several patients with Heinz body hemolysis. The presence of red cells showing these morphologic changes should serve as a clue indicating ongoing formation of oxidatively denatured hemoglobin, i.e., Heinz bodies.

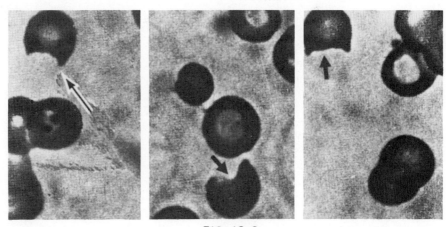

FIG. 12–6

The "bite" cell in G6PD deficiency. The red cell reseals after extraction of the Heinz body.

Reference: Greenberg, M. S.: Arch. Intern. Med., *16*:153, 1976. Figure reproduced with permission of author and publisher. Copyright 1976, American Medical Association.

DRUGS REPORTED TO CAUSE A POSITIVE DIRECT ANTIGLOBULIN TEST OR AN ANTIGLOBULIN POSITIVE HEMOLYTIC ANEMIA

Acetaminophen
α-Methyldopa (Aldomet)*
Aminopyrine (Pyramidon)
Antihistamines
Carbromal
Cephalosporins (Cephalothin, Cephaloridine, Cephalexin, Cefazolin)*
Chlorpromazine
Chlorpropamide
Dipyrone
Hydralazine
Insecticides
Insulin
Isoniazid
L-Dopa*
Mefenamic acid*
Melphalan (Alkeran)
Methadone
Para-Aminosalicylic acid
Penicillin
Phenacetin (acetophenetidin)
Quinidine
Rifampin
Stibophen
Streptomycin
Sulfonamides
Thiazides
Tolbutamide

---

*Most common.

THE NUCLEATED RED BLOOD CELL IN THE PERIPHERAL BLOOD

Nucleated red cells are normally found in the peripheral blood only in the fetus and the newborn. In the adult, the finding of a single nucleated red blood cell in the peripheral blood is cause for alarm, as it represents significant bone marrow stress. A recent prospective study reported a one-year mortality rate of 36 per cent for patients having nucleated red cells in the peripheral blood. The conditions most likely to cause nucleated red cells to appear in the peripheral blood are:

Hemorrhage
Hemolysis
Severe megaloblastic anemia
Myelophthisis
Severe hypoxemia
Miscellaneous: asplenia, electric shock

Reference: Editorial: J.A.M.A., *239*:91, 1978.

NAP OR LAP

The neutrophil alkaline phosphatase (NAP) (sometimes called the leukocyte alkaline phosphatase, LAP) is a useful test. It is usually evaluated histochemically by grading the staining of mature polymorphonuclear leukocytes (from 0 to 4) after incubation with a phosphate substrate. The value of the staining scores observed in the control and patient are reported for 100 cells counted. The NAP tends to be low in the acute nonlymphocytic leukemias. The greatest utility of the test is in distinguishing those conditions in which the NAP is clearly low or high.

Low NAP	*High NAP*
Typical chronic granulocytic leukemia	Leukemoid reaction
Paroxysmal nocturnal hemoglobinuria	Active inflammation (including
Infectious mononucleosis	active Hodgkin's disease)
Hypophosphatasia	Trisomy 21
	Polycythemia vera
	Primary myelofibrosis
	Post-splenectomy
	Estrogen therapy (and pregnancy)
	Adrenal corticosteroid therapy
	Rickets

12

THROMBOCYTOSIS

An elevated platelet count may be an extremely helpful laboratory finding. Consideration of the etiology of a platelet count above 400,000 per mm^3 will often help in determining the diagnosis.

1. Chronic inflammatory disease
    a. Collagen-vascular disease, particularly active rheumatoid arthritis
    b. Ulcerative colitis and regional enteritis
    c. Chronic granulomatous diseases
2. Blood loss or iron deficiency
3. Malignancy
    a. Carcinoma
    b. Hodgkin's disease
    c. Non-Hodgkin's lymphoma
4. Post-Operative
    a. Post-splenectomy
    b. After other surgical procedures
5. Response to drugs
    a. Vinca alkaloids
    b. Epinephrine
6. Response to exercise
7. "Rebound"
    a. Withdrawal of myelosuppressive drugs, including rebound from alcohol-induced thrombocytopenia
    b. Secondary to the therapy of B$_{12}$ or folic acid deficiency
8. The myeloproliferative disorders
    a. Polycythemia vera
    b. Chronic myelogenous leukemia
    c. Idiopathic myelofibrosis
    d. Essential thrombocythemia

Reference: Adapted from Williams, W. J.: Thrombocytosis. In Williams, W. J., et al.: Hematology. New York, McGraw-Hill Book Company, 1977, p. 1364.

PRIMARY THROMBOCYTOSIS/ESSENTIAL THROMBOCYTHEMIA

Primary thrombocytosis or essential thrombocythemia (ET) is considered one of the myeloproliferative disorders. However, ET has not been definitively shown to be a clonal stem cell disorder similar to its putative cousins polycythemia vera, chronic myelogenous leukemia (CML), and idiopathic myelofibrosis. Many patients thought to have ET may actually be cases of "bled-down" P. vera, CML in which the neutrophilic leukocytosis is not striking, or early myelofibrosis with minimal marrow and peripheral blood changes. Thus, many of the problems with the description of the disease and many of the claims for transition of ET to P. vera, CML, myelofibrosis, and acute myeloid leukemia may be examples of a faulty original diagnosis. Perhaps this annotation will help dispel some of the vagaries of nosology and natural history.

In an attempt to define the disorder, the P. Vera Study Group has first excluded all other known causes of thrombocytosis (see p. 404). Polycythemia vera is ruled out only after the patient's iron stores are repleted and the measured red blood cell mass remains normal. A bone marrow, a Ph^1 chromosome, and a leukocyte alkaline phosphatase (LAP) are obtained to rule out classical CML. Myelofibrosis is excluded by the absence of significant marrow fibrosis on bone marrow biopsy.

Patients who have at least two platelet counts above 1 million/μl and who are not excluded by the criteria above are thought to have ET. Although the average patient age is 62, the disorder may be seen in young patients. An apparently benign form of this disorder has been described in young females who do not have symptoms, develop no complications, and require no treatment. This small subgroup notwithstanding, the majority of patients are symptomatic and have a high incidence of both thrombotic and hemorrhagic (especially post-surgical) phenomena. Symptoms of pain, acrocyanosis, burning, numbness, and gangrene of the fingers and toes (possibly due to microthrombi in the digital vessels) are common. These signs and symptoms may respond to small daily doses of aspirin. Hepatomegaly is rare, and splenomegaly, which is present in about half of the patients, is usually only "scanomegaly."

Contrary to previous reports, only a slight leukocytosis is observed. As a rule, early WBC precursors and nucleated RBC are not seen; their presence should lead one to suspect one of the other myeloproliferative disorders. Leukocyte alkaline phosphatase tends to be normal in ET, and serum B_{12} tends to be elevated. In contrast in P. vera, the LAP is elevated in 70 per cent of cases and the B_{12} is elevated in only about 13 per cent. The bone marrow shows normal to moderately increased overall cellularity with markedly increased megakaryocytes and platelet clumps. Mature collagen is not seen on bone marrow biopsy, but slight to moderate increases in reticulin may be found.

Treatment depends upon many factors. Young asymptomatic patients may require no treatment. Older patients who are actively bleeding or clotting may require a rapid therapeutic reduction of platelet count, which may be achieved only by continuous plateletpheresis or injection of nitrogen mustard in full doses. Conventional wisdom appears to be that patients who are symptomatic with platelet counts over 1 million are candidates for myelosuppressive therapy. Alkeran and radiophosphorus appear to be equally effective when given in appropriate doses. Currently, control of the platelet count at 600,000/μl or below is the goal of therapy.

Alkeran: 10 mg/day for 5 days. 2 mg/day thereafter, with adjustment of dose according to blood count.

12

^{32}P: 2.9 millicuries/M^2 IV initially. May be repeated at 12-week intervals. A 25 per cent escalation of dose may be required at the twelfth week, or at subsequent doses, but the dose should never exceed 7 millicuries.

The ability of antiplatelet agents (aspirin and dipyridamole) to control the symptomatology and complications of ET is presently unknown, but it is the subject of ongoing study. Hydroxyurea, a myelo-suppressive agent that is thought to be neither as carcinogenic nor as mutagenic as the therapeutic agents currently employed is also under study.

It is important to note that many patients have abnormal platelet function both before and after therapeutic decrease in their platelet count. *In vitro* tests of platelet function serve as "markers" for this disease but do not correlate with clinical bleeding or thrombosis. Post-surgical bleeding may be a problem even for the successfully treated patient, and transfusion of fresh platelets may be needed in order to achieve hemostasis.

The long-term prognosis of these patients is unknown. Prompt objective and subjective improvement usually accompanies a decrease in platelet count. The improvement in transient ischemic attacks and claudication have, in particular, been impressive. Termination as acute leukemia has been described, as has "evolution" into P. vera, CML, and myelofibrosis. Whether these effects are due to the natural history of the disease or to therapy or indicate a faulty initial diagnosis is unknown. Many patients appear to require less myelosuppression after the first year of treatment. Thus, dose reduction should be a prominent thera-peutic goal to minimize the deleterious effects of prolonged myelo-suppression.

Thanks to Stephen Landaw, M. D., Ph.D., for this contribution.

POLYCYTHEMIA: VERA OR NOT VERA

The Polycythemia Vera and Myeloproliferative Disease Study Group is in the process of studying the natural history and therapy of 325 patients with P. vera. To some extent, the diagnosis of P. vera represents a diagnosis of exclusion. In this regard, an etiologic classi-fication of polycythemia is extremely useful.

I. Polycythemia vera

II. Secondary polycythemia (increased erythropoietin production)
  A. Physiologically appropriate (decreased blood oxygen saturation)
    1. High altitude

2. Chronic obstructive pulmonary disease
3. Postural hypoxemia
4. Cardiovascular shunt (right to left)
5. Pickwickian syndrome (massive obesity)
6. High-oxygen–affinity hemoglobinopathy and methemoglobinemia
7. Congenital decreased red cell DPG
8. "Smoker's" polycythemia

B. Physiologically inappropriate
   1. Tumor
      a. Renal cell carcinoma
      b. Cerebellar hemangioblastoma
      c. Hepatoma
      d. Uterine fibroid
      e. Adrenal cortical adenoma (and/or hyperplasia).
      f. Ovarian carcinoma
   2. Renal
      a. Cysts
      b. Hydronephrosis
      c. Bartter's syndrome
      d. Transplantation
   3. Cobalt
C. Recessive familial polycythemia

III. Relative polycythemia (also called stress, spurious polycythemia, pseudopolycythemia, Gaisböck's syndrome)

The diagnostic criteria employed in establishing a diagnosis of P. vera are given below. Patients must be polycythemic. The red cell volume requirement is quite conservative and excludes those patients with spurious or relative polycythemia. The diagnosis of polycythemia vera is made if categories A1, A2, and A3 are satisfied, or, alternatively, if A1 and A2 and two parameters from category B are present.

Category A

1. Total red cell volume
   Male $\geq$36 ml/kg
   Female $\geq$32 ml/kg
2. Art. O_2 Sat. $\geq$92%
3. Splenomegaly

Category B

1. Thrombocytosis
   Platelet count $>$400,000/mm^3
2. Leukocytosis $>$12,000/mm^3
   (No fever or infection)
3. Leukocyte alkaline phosphatase
   score (LAP) elevated.
   (No fever or infection)
4. Serum B_{12} ($>$900 pg/ml) or
   $UB_{12}BC^*$ ($>$2200pg/ml)

12

---

*Unsaturated B_{12} binding capacity.

A decision tree (Fig. 12–7) is quite helpful. The initial branch point of the tree involves the separation of true from relative polycythemia after determination of the red cell mass.

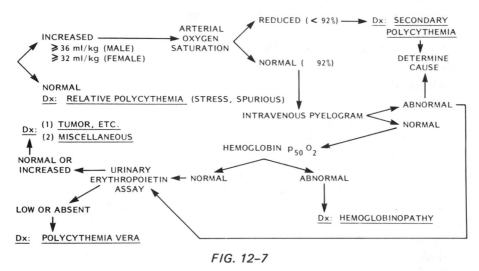

FIG. 12–7

Polycythemia decision tree. The decisions start with a determination of red cell mass.

The mean age of onset of the disease in this "pedigreed" group of patients is 60, with a range of 20 to 80 years. There are 20 per cent more males than females.

The major symptoms include headache, weakness, pruritus, and dizziness in 40 to 50 per cent of the patients. Excessive sweating, visual difficulties, weight loss, and paresthesias occur in approximately 30 per cent.

The principal findings on physical examination are plethora in 67 per cent, conjunctival plethora in 59 per cent, engorgement of the veins of the fundus in 46 per cent, a palpable liver in 40 per cent, and an enlarged spleen in 70 per cent. A systolic blood pressure of over 140 was found in 72 per cent and a diastolic pressure over 90 in 32 per cent.

The white blood count was increased above 12,000 in 43 per cent, and the platelet count above 400,000 in 64 per cent of the patients. The leukocyte alkaline phosphatase score was greater than 100 in 70 per cent. Examination of the bone marrow was extremely revealing in that fibrosis was present in more than one third of the cases, and stainable iron was absent in almost 100 per cent of the patients examined.

In general, it has not been difficult to arrive at a diagnosis of polycythemia vera when it is present. At times, the presence of associated disease such as a bleeding duodenal ulcer may mask the characteristic clinical and laboratory findings. More often than not, when difficulty is encountered in establishing a diagnosis, it is because the patient does not have polycythemia vera. Most often, occult arterial hypoxemia related either to nocturnal hypoventilation or smoking (see the following article) is the cause of the elevated red cell mass noted.

Reference: Berlin, N. I.: Diagnosis of polycythemia. Semin. Hematol., *12*:339, 1975. Fig. 12–7 reproduced with permission of author and Grune & Stratton, Inc.

"SMOKER'S" POLYCYTHEMIA

Excessive exposure to carbon monoxide is frequently encountered in contemporary life. In urban life levels of carboxyhemoglobin noted in drivers on the Los Angeles freeway or tunnel guards testify to the environmental hazards of the auto. In a rural environment, elevated ambient concentrations of carbon monoxide are encountered when burning charcoal in a confined space. Nonetheless, the levels of carbon monoxide in the atmosphere in general are usually small when compared to the levels found in the smoke of an inhaled cigar or cigarette.

The affinity of carbon monoxide for hemoglobin is extremely high, being some 350 times that of oxygen. Consequently, measurable levels of carboxyhemoglobin may be observed with only minimal ambient concentrations. The half-life of carbon monoxide in the body is some three to five hours. As a consequence of the displacement of oxygen by avid combination of carbon monoxide with hemoglobin, a functional anemia is produced in patients with elevated levels of blood carboxyhemoglobin. Since the portion of hemoglobin that is bound to carbon monoxide cannot combine with oxygen, the functioning hemoglobin is reduced by the percentage of measured carboxyhemoglobin. In addition, a shift in the oxygen-hemoglobin dissociation curve occurs, resulting in a hemoglobin with a higher affinity for oxygen. Consequently, for any given venous oxygen tension, less oxygen is delivered to the tissues.

The position of the oxygen-hemoglobin dissociation curve may be expressed as the mmHg of oxygen tension necessary to half-saturate

12

the hemoglobin molecule (P50). Normally, the P50 for hemoglobin at pH 7.2 to 7.4, 37°C, and pCO_2 of 40 mm is 27 to 29 mmHg. Hemoglobins with a high affinity for oxygen consequently have lower P50s, while those with low affinity have higher P50s. The presence of carbon monoxide produces a leftward shift in the oxygen-hemoglobin dissociation curve (high oxygen affinity). The relationship of blood carboxyhemoglobin and oxygen affinity is such that a decrease in the P50 of hemoglobin of 0.39 torr was observed for each 1 per cent increase in carboxyhemoglobin.

Elevated levels of blood carboxyhemoglobin are regularly observed in smokers who inhale. Those who are able to inhale cigar smoke appear to be the very worst offenders. Recently, the blood carboxyhemoglobin was found to be elevated in each of 22 smoking patients with polycythemia. Characteristically, a compensatory increase in red cell volume and a decrease in plasma volume was observed. Total blood volume tended to be normal. Thus, the majority of these patients were true polycythemics as a consequence of the hypoxemia secondary to their carbon monoxide exposure. These patients are distinguishable from patients with P. vera by the lack of splenomegaly, leukocytosis, elevated leukocyte alkaline phosphatase, and other stigmata usually encountered in the patient with polycythemia vera. In the past, these individuals have been recognized as being mesomorphic, hard-driving, aggressive smokers who were thought to have a relative, but not a true, polycythemia (due to a decrease in plasma volume). In those patients who could be cajoled to stop smoking the polycythemia disappeared.

Thus, before embarking on an extensive evaluation of a polycythemic patient, a thorough check of the patient's smoking history is mandatory. The patient should be questioned about inhaling, frequency, and type of smoking. Blood carboxyhemoglobin levels may be obtained from the laboratory. Beware! Most laboratory equipment is calibrated for "industrial" hazards. Carboxyhemoglobin levels are reported as abnormal only when they exceed 10 per cent. "Normal" blood carboxyhemoglobin should not exceed 1 per cent and represents the endogenous carbon monoxide produced in the normal attrition of aged red cells resulting from the oxidation of the alpha methene group of the porphyrin ring of hemoglobin. Blood carbon monoxide levels as low as 2 per cent are sufficient to produce a secondary polycythemia. Clinically, HbCO levels are lowest in the morning on arising and progressively increase during the course of a smoker's day. The smoking pattern of each individual, including his or her pattern of inhaling and the length of the cigarette or cigar smoked, individualizes the level of self-intoxication produced. Thus, variations in the level of poisoning may be observed in individuals whose smoking patterns appear similar.

Reference: Landaw, S. A., and Smith, J. R. New Engl. J. Med., *298*:6, 1978.

REPLACEMENT THERAPY IN FACTOR VIII AND FACTOR IX DEFICIENCY

Achieving adequate hemostasis in patients with hereditary deficiencies of Factor VIII or Factor IX requires awareness of certain points.

Dose: The dose of the coagulation factor is calculated in units. One unit is defined as the activity of the coagulation factor present in 1 ml of normal human male plasma.

Thus,

units to be administered = (desired factor concentration – initial factor concentration) $\times$ plasma volume $\times$ patient's weight (Kg)

Plasma volume = 41 ml/kg body weight
(if the hematocrit is nearly normal)

Thus, to correct a deficiency in a 70 kg person who has a level of 2 per cent of a coagulation factor by restoring 100 per cent of that factor: $(0.98) \times 41 \times 70 = 2812$ units to be administered. Note that the desired and initial factor concentrations are expressed as *decimals.*

Metabolic half-life: The factor must be given often enough to compensate for the decrease in plasma levels owing to its metabolism. *Each factor has a different metabolic half-life.*

Volume of distribution: Each factor has a different apparent volume of distribution, depending on the amount that diffuses into the extravascular space.

12

FACTOR	MINIMUM PLASMA CONCENTRATION TO ASSURE HEMOSTASIS	METABOLIC HALF-LIFE	EXTRAVASCULAR DISTRIBUTION	COMMENT
VIII	25–30%	12 hours	20–33%	Minimum levels of 25–30% usually assure hemostasis, but levels of 50–60% may be required for major surgery or severe trauma. One must *add* 20–33% to the calculated dose to account for extravascular leakage (e.g., calculate the dose to 125% when 100% is desired). Maintenance is *begun* approximately 6–8 hours after the initial dose. The maintenance doses are then given approximately every 6–12 hours. The exact dose, when to administer it, and total duration of therapy depend on the clinical circumstance.
IX	15–25%	24 hours	50%	One must add 50% to the calculated dose to account for extravascular leakage. The maintenance dose is administered every 24 hours. The exact dose and total duration of therapy depend on the clinical circumstance.

Reference: Williams, W. J., et al. (Eds.): Hematology. New York, McGraw-Hill Book Company, 1977, p. 1564.

PRODUCTS FOR THE THERAPY OF FACTOR VIII AND FACTOR IX DEFICIENCY

	APPROXIMATE UNITS (vial)	APPROXIMATE UNITS (ml)
Factor VIII		
1. Cryoprecipitate	60–140	3
2. Profilate (Abbott)	250	12
3. Hemofil (Hyland)	250, 750	25
4. Humafac (Parke Davis)	250	40
5. Factorate (Armour)	300	12
6. Koate (Cutter)	250	25
Factor IX		
1. Fresh frozen plasma		<1
2. Konyne (Cutter)	500	25
3. Proplex (Hyland)	500	17

EOSINOPHILIA

The presence of eosinophilia whether "relative" or absolute (>700 per μl) is important. Remembering the mnemonic NAACP (neoplasia, allergy, Addison's disease, collagen vascular disease, and parasites) will aid in the classification of the majority. A more complete list would be:

1. Neoplasm
    A. Hodgkin's disease
    B. Any tumor
    C. Myeloproliferative disorders
2. Allergy
    A. Asthma and hay fever
    B. Urticaria and hypersensitivity reactions
    C. Drug sensitivity
    D. Atopia
    E. Dermatitis — psoriasis, dermatitis herpetiformis, pemphigus
3. Adrenal insufficiency
4. Collagen vascular disease
    A. Periarteritis nodosa
    B. Polymyalgia rheumatica
    C. Other
5. Parasites
    A. Helminthic — trichinosis, ascariasis, hookworm, strongyloides, filariasis
    B. Toxocara (visceral larvae migrans)

12

6. Gastrointestinal disease
   A. Ulcerative colitis
   B. Regional enteritis
   C. Eosinophilic gastroenteritis
   D. Milk precipitin disease
   E. Protein-losing enteropathy
7. Sarcoidosis
8. Radiation therapy
9. Peritoneal dialysis
10. Hereditary familial eosinophilia
11. Idiopathic hypereosinophilic syndromes
    A. Loeffler's syndrome and pulmonary infiltration with eosinophilia (P.I.E.)

Thanks to Frank Oski for the mnemonic.

Reference: Finch, S. C.: Granulocytosis. In Williams, W. J., et al. (Eds.): Hematology. New York McGraw-Hill Book Company, 1977, p. 748.

A TIP ON EOSINOPHILIA

The entire clinical and laboratory picture should, of course, be taken into account in determining the etiology of eosinophilia. The morphology of the eosinophils on the peripheral smear may provide an important first diagnostic clue. In general, the causes of eosinophilia are either "myeloproliferative" or "reactive." Primary involvement of the eosinophils in the disease process, as exists in disorders of the granulocyte-erythroid-megakaryocytic cell line, often results in abnormalities in eosinophilic granulation (large granules, incomplete granulation) or in abnormalities in nuclear segmentation (pseudo–Pelger-Huet eosinophils). "Reactive" eosinophils are normal in morphology.

BONE MARROW NECROSIS

The clinical diagnosis of necrosis of the bone marrow is made infrequently. The aspirated specimen forms in clumps when smeared on slides. An eosinophilic proteinaceous haze, produced by the necrotic tissue, which partially obscures poorly stained cells in various stages of autolysis, is observed microscopically. Nutritional factors and toxins, as well as the compromise of the vasculature by expanding space-occupying intramedullary lesions, are involved in pathogenesis.

Laboratory findings are in part related to the underlying disease state. Patients are anemic and usually thrombocytopenic. Nucleated red cells are found in the peripheral smear. Schistocytes may be present.

The lactic dehydrogenase and alkaline phosphatase are almost invariably elevated. While the most frequent cause of marrow necrosis is intramedullary neoplasia, other etiologies must be considered.

Noninfectious

Hematologic malignancy of the bone marrow (acute leukemia, chronic myelogenous leukemia, "blastic crisis")
Sickle cell disease
Tumor necrosis
Caisson disease
Systemic lupus erythematosus
Antineoplastic drugs
Radiation
Shock and ischemia

Infectious

Bacterial sepsis (especially typhoid fever)
Fungal or acid fast infection of the marrow cavity

References: Caraveo, J., Trowbridge, A. A., Amaral, B. W., et al.: Am. J. Med., *60*:404, 1977, Keraly, J. F., and Wheby, M.: Am. J. Med., *60*:36, 1976.

FAVORABLE PROGNOSTIC FACTORS IN ACUTE LEUKEMIA

ALL*	ANLL**
Age (2–10 yrs)	Age ($<$ 40 yrs)
WBC count $<$ 50,000 μl	WBC count $<$ 50,000 μl
Absence of CNS leukemia	Absence of CNS leukemia
Absence of other major illnesses	Absence of other major illnesses
Good performance status	Good performance status
Presence of "null" type rather than "B" or "T" cell type	—
Absence of hepatosplenomegaly	Absence of Hepatosplenomegaly(?) Absence of previously treated malignancy (i.e., Hodgkin's, P. vera, ovarian cancer, chronic myelogenous leukemia, myeloma)

*Acute lymphocytic leukemia
**Acute nonlymphocytic leukemia

12

MORPHOLOGIC, HISTOCHEMICAL, AND IMMUNOLOGIC DIFFERENTIATION OF THE ACUTE LEUKEMIAS

The differentiation of acute lymphocytic leukemia (ALL) from the acute nonlymphocytic leukemias (ANLL) has important implications. Included in this latter group of disorders are acute granulocytic, myelo-monocytic, monocytic, promyelocytic leukemia and those cases of acute leukemia accompanied by marked dysplasia of the erythroid series (erythroleukemia or acute DiGuglielmo's syndrome). In evaluating acute leukemia, the data in the table on the opposite page may be helpful in differentiating ANLL from ALL. Of course, the demonstration of surface membrane immunoglobulin on, or rosette formation by, the blast cell will establish the lymphocyte as the cell of origin of the acute leukemia. Since the majority of cases of ALL involve lymphoblasts devoid of the usual surface markers (non-T, non-B, "null" lymphoblast), a negative test does not rule out ALL. Despite these aids, a few cases of acute leukemia still remain unclassifiable.

	ALL	ANLL
Morphology	—High nuclear-cytoplasmic ratio	—More cytoplasm
	—1 to 2 nucleoli	—2 or more nucleoli
	—Clumped chromatin	—Fine lace-like chromatin
	—Homogeneous cell population	—More heterogeneous cell population with microblasts
	—Round nuclei	—Auer bodies
		—Granules in primitive cells
		—Nuclear detail similar in blast and promyelocyte
		—Megaloblastosis and red cell dysplasia
		—Folded, indented nuclei (myelomonocytic)
Histochemistry	—Course granules or block positivity on PAS stains	—Positive erythroblasts (erythroleukemia) on PAS stains
		—Positive staining with Sudan black B
		—Esterase positive on alpha-naphthol acetate stains (myelomonocytic forms)
		—Positive staining for peroxidase activity
Immunology	—Surface membrane immunoglobulin present	—Experimental
	—Intracytoplasmic immunoglobulin present	
	—Immune or nonimmune rosette formation (monocyte Fc receptor must be excluded) present	

12

ELECTROLYTE ABNORMALITIES IN LEUKEMIA

Recent chemotherapeutic agents and improved support capabilities have allowed a majority of adult patients with leukemia to achieve remission. Concomitant with improved remission rates and longer survival is the awareness of electrolyte abnormalities associated with either the disease or the therapies employed. The table on the opposite page lists the most common abnormalities.

ELECTROLYTE ABNORMALITY	MOST COMMONLY SEEN WITH	POSTULATED MECHANISMS
Hypokalemia	Acute myelogenous leukemia	1. Renal potassium wasting secondary to elevated serum lysozyme
	Acute monocytic leukemia	2. Combination of gentamicin and cephalothin producing renal potassium wasting
		3. Carbenicillin produces renal potassium wasting because of the nonabsorbable anion effect
Hyperkalemia	Acute myelogenous leukemia	1. Rapid cell lysis associated with cytotoxic therapy
	Acute monocytic leukemia	2. Acute renal failure secondary to hyperuricemia
	Acute lymphocytic leukemia	3. Pseudohyperkalemia in patients with high leukocyte counts or high platelet counts; cell breakdown *in vitro* with release of potassium into the serum may falsely elevate the potassium level
	Chronic myelogenous leukemia	
Hypocalcemia	Acute lymphocytic leukemia	1. Chemotherapy-induced cytotoxicity with massive phosphate release
	Chronic lymphocytic leukemia	2. Hypoalbuminemia
	Acute myelogenous leukemia	3. Steroid therapy
		4. L-asparaginase therapy (pancreatitis)
		5. Uremia
Hypercalcemia	Acute lymphocytic leukemia	1. Production of PTH-like material by leukemic tissue
	Acute myelogenous leukemia	2. Production of osteoclast-activating factors
	Chronic myelogenous leukemia	3. Bone infiltration by leukemic tissue
	Chronic lymphocytic leukemia	
Hyperphosphatemia	Acute lymphocytic leukemia	1. Chemotherapy-induced cytotoxicity with massive release of phosphate; calcium may also fall.
Hyponatremia	Acute myelogenous leukemia	1. Syndrome of inappropriate ADH (SIADH)
		2. Drug-induced SIADH (e.g., for vincristine, cyclophosphamide)
		3. Diarrhea, emesis
		4. Sodium uptake by leukemic cells
Hypernatremia	Acute myelogenous leukemia	1. Diabetes insipidus due to leukemic infiltration of pituitary
	Acute lymphocytic leukemia	
	Chronic myelogenous leukemia	

Reference: O'Regan, S., Carson, S., Chesney, R. W., and Drummond, K. N.: Blood, 49:345, 1977.

12

ELECTRICITY, PARAPROTEINS, AND PROTEINS

There still appears to be a considerable mystique surrounding the origin of the homogeneous immunoglobulin peaks (paraproteins, or spikes) determined by serum protein electrophoresis. Contemporary structural biochemistry has taught us that antibody specificity is determined by alterations in the primary structure (amino acid sequence) in the variable, or N-terminal, end of both the light and the heavy chain of the immunoglobulin molecule. The C-terminal end of the immunoglobulin shows a greater degree of homology within each immunoglobulin subclass. From birth we are subjected to a variety of environmental insults, many of which prove to be antigenic. Thus, our immunoglobulins represent a slurry of molecules, each having a more or less unique amino acid sequence at the N-terminal, or antigen binding site, of the molecule.

Most routine electrophoretic assays performed in the clinical laboratory are done at a mildly basic pH. The mobility of molecules in an electrical field is determined by the sum total of acidic and basic charges. Since most amino acids are electrically neutral near a pH of 7, the electrophoretic mobility of the protein represents the net effect of the negative charges provided by the dicarboxylic amino acid content (glutamic and aspartic acids) and the positive charges contributed by the dibasic amino acids (lysine, arginine, and the imidizole group of histidine). Thus, the pattern obtained on densitometric tracings of immunoglobulin G, for example, represents the sum of a vast number of immunoglobulin G molecules, each directed against its own antigen and each having its own discrete electrophoretic mobility as a result of its amino acid composition.

The consequence of the proliferation of a single clone of actively secreting cells, be they B lymphocytes or plasma cells, is the elaboration of a markedly increased number of immunoglobulin molecules that are identical in every respect. The densitometric interpretation of this phenomenon is a single peak, which reflects the homogeneous nature of the electrophoretic mobility of identical molecules of protein.

BENCE-JONES PROTEINURIA

A spot testing of urine to determine "Bence-Jones protein" may not suffice when you are screening for urinary light chains. The Putnam heat test for urinary light chains (4 ml of centrifuged urine and 1 ml of 2 molar acetate buffer heated to 56°C in an incubation bath for 15 minutes produces a precipitate, which upon heating to 100°C disappears, then upon cooling reappears) has a sensitivity of 145 mg/dl.

The following chart shows the results obtained when urine specimens demonstrating monoclonal light chains by immunoelectrophoresis were checked against the findings obtained by the screening heat test.

True Positive Heat Test
(with a "spike" on urinary immunoelectrophoresis)

Per cent of all positive heat tests	Disease
68	Multiple myeloma
3.4	Amyloidosis
3.4	Adult Fanconi's syndrome
1.8	Hyperparathyroidism
3.4	Bence-Jones proteinuria only

False Positive Heat Test
(no "spike" on urinary immunoelectrophoresis)

Per cent of all positive heat tests	Disease
6.7	Connective tissue disease
5.0	Chronic renal failure
3.3	Lymphoma
1.5	Carcinoma
3.5	Miscellaneous diseases (FUO, iron deficiency anemia)

False negative heat tests (with a "spike" on urinary electrophoresis) also occur. The best way, therefore, to demonstrate the presence of light chain proteinuria is by immunoelectrophoresis of an aliquot of a concentrated 24-hour urine collection.

12

Reference: Perry, M. C., and Kyle, R. A.: Mayo Clin. Proc., *50*:234, 1975.

FORMULATION OF PARENTERAL ANTINEOPLASTIC AGENTS

There are always questions about the reconstitution, shelf stability, and administration of antineoplastic agents. The tabulation on pages 423–424 was prepared by Ms. Nancy Phillips, R. Ph., and has proved to be an extremely useful resource for us. The current version is an update as of November 1979.

DRUG (Brand name)	STORAGE BEFORE MIXING	HOW SUPPLIED	DILUENT	AMOUNT OF DILUENT	STABILITY AND STORAGE AFTER MIXING	ADMINISTRATION	SPECIAL PRECAUTIONS
m-AMSA* (acridinyl anisidine)	Refrigerate	75 mg	Diluent provided (lactic acid) Further dilute with D5W	13.5 ml 500 ml	8 hr	IV infusion over 30–60 min	†
L-asparaginase (Elspar)	Refrigerate	10,000 IU	Sterile water inj USP Sodium chloride inj USP	5 ml	8 hr–refrigerated	IV infusion in D5W or normal saline	Use only if clear; watch closely for anaphylaxis
5-Azacytidine*	Refrigerate	100 mg	Sterile water inj USP Further dilute with lactated Ringer's inj USP	19.9 ml	½ hr–concentrated 3 hours when further diluted	Continuous or intermittent IV	Fresh solutions must be prepared if infusing over 3 hours
Bleomycin (Blenoxane)	Room temperature	15 units	Sterile water inj USP Sodium chloride inj USP Dextrose inj 5% Bacteriostatic water inj	1–5 ml	7 days–refrigerated	IV push or IV infusion in D5W or normal saline	
Carminomycin*	Room temperature	10 mg	Sterile water inj USP	20 ml	10 days–refrigerated	IV push over 10–15 min	Protect from light †
Carmustine (BiCNU)	Refrigerate	100 mg	Absolute ethanol (provided) Sterile water inj USP	3 ml 27 ml	3 hr–room temperature 24 hr–refrigerated	IV infusion in normal saline or D5W over 1 hr	Protect from light †
Chlorozotocin*	Refrigerate	50 mg 200 mg	Sterile water inj USP Sodium chloride inj USP	5 ml 9.8 ml	3 hr–room temperature 24 hr–refrigerated	IV push over 10–15 min	
Cisplatin (Platinol)	Refrigerate	10 mg	Sterile water inj USP	10 ml	20 hr–room temperature	IV infusion in D5 ½ NS or normal saline	
Cyclophosphamide (Cytoxan)	Room temperature	100 mg 200 mg 500 mg	Bacteriostatic water inj (Paraben preserved only) or sterile water inj USP	5 ml 10 ml 25 ml	24 hr–room temperature 6 days–refrigerated	IV push	Shake well to dissolve
Cytarabine (Cytosar-U)	Room temperature	100 mg 500 mg	Diluent provided (bacteriostatic water) For intrathecal use, dilute 100 mg vial with 5 ml lactated Ringer's (preservative free)	5 ml 10 ml	48 hr–room temperature Infusion solutions may be stored at room temperature for 7 days	Continuous IV infusion in D5W or normal saline subcutaneous (maintenance) intrathecal	Discard solution in which a slight haze develops
Dacarbazine (DTIC)	Refrigerate	100 mg 200 mg	Sterile water inj USP	9.9 ml 19.7 ml	8 hr–room temperature 72 hr–refrigerated	IV push over 10–15 min or IV infusion in D5W	Protect from light †
Dactinomycin (Cosmegen)	Room temperature	0.5 mg	Sterile water inj USP (without preservative)	1.1 ml	Discard	IV push	Protect from light †
Daunorubicin* (Daunomycin)	Room temperature	20 mg	Sodium chloride inj USP	4 ml	8 hr	IV push over 10–15 min IV infusion in D5W or normal saline	†

12

DRUG (Brand name)	STORAGE BEFORE MIXING	HOW SUPPLIED	DILUENT	AMOUNT OF DILUENT	STABILITY AND STORAGE AFTER MIXING	ADMINISTRATION	SPECIAL PRECAUTIONS
Doxorubicin HCl (Adriamycin)	Room temperature	10 mg / 50 mg	Sodium chloride inj USP	5 ml / 25 ml	24 hr—room temperature / 48 hr—refrigerated	IV push over 10–15 min / IV infusion in D5W or normal saline	Protect from sunlight; shake well to dissolve †
5-Fluorouracil (Fluorouracil)	Room temperature	500 mg/10 ml	No dilution required	—	—	IV push	Check for precipitate (can be redissolved by warming)
Mechlorethamine HCl (Mustargen)	Room temperature	10 mg	Sodium chloride inj USP / Sterile water inj USP	10 ml	Use immediately after mixing	Inject into the tubing of a running IV infusion	Avoid skin contact †
Melphalan* (L-PAM)	Room temperature	100 mg	Diluents provided. Dissolve well in acid-alcohol solvent. Further dilute with phosphate buffer	1 ml / 9 ml	8 hr	IV push over 10–15 min	Protect from light
Methotrexate	Room temperature	5 mg/2 ml / 50 mg/2 ml	No dilution required when administered IV; for intrathecal use, dilute with preservative free lactated Ringer's solution to a concentration of 1 mg/ml			IV push intrathecal	
Methotrexate* (High dose)	Room temperature	1 gm (preservative-free)	Sterile water inj USP / Sodium chloride inj USP / Dextrose inj 5%	19.4 ml	1 week—room temperature	IV infusion in D5W, D5NS, or NS	
Mitomycin (Mutamycin)	Room temperature	5 mg / 20 mg	Sterile water inj USP	10 ml / 40 ml	7 days—room temperature / 14 days—refrigerated	IV push over 10–15 min	Protect from light †
Neocarzinostatin* (NCS, Zinostatin)	Refrigerate	2,000U/2 ml	No dilution required	—	—	IV push	Protect from light. Give Benadryl 50 mg IV before NCS IV push †
Rubidizone* (Benzoylhydrazone daunorubicine)	Room temperature	50 mg	Diluent provided (glycine buffer). Further dilute with D5W	4 ml / 500 ml	1 hr (reconstitute immediately before use)	IV infusion over 1 hr	Premedicate with Benadryl 50 mg IV †
Streptozotocin*	Refrigerate	1 gm	Sterile water inj USP / Sodium chloride inj USP	9.5 ml	8 hr	IV push	†
Vinblastine (Velban)	Refrigerate	10 mg	Bacteriostatic sodium chloride inj	10 ml	30 days—refrigerated	IV push	†
Vincristine (Oncovin)	Refrigerate	1 mg	Diluent provided (bacteriostatic NaCl)	10 ml	14 days—refrigerated	IV push	†
VM-26* (Teniposide)	Room temperature	50 mg/5 ml	Dilute in 10–20 volumes of normal saline or D5W (volume to volume dilution)	250–500 ml	4 hr when further diluted	IV infusion over 30 min–1 hr	Discard solutions with a precipitate
VP 16-213* (Etoposide)	Room temperature	100 mg/5 ml	Dilute in 20–50 volumes of normal saline (volume to volume dilution)	250–500 ml	1:20 dilution—30 min / 1:50 dilution—3 hr	IV infusion over 30 min	Discard solutions with a precipitate

*Experimental drugs (5/1/79).
†Potent vesicants—avoid extravasation.

IN SEARCH OF THE UNKNOWN PRIMARY CANCER

Among the most difficult diagnostic problems encountered by the physician is the evaluation of a patient with metastatic malignant disease from an unknown primary site. The two most common presentations of metastases from an unknown primary cancer are the involvement of a cervical node with squamous cell carcinoma and the involvement of any area of the body with either metastatic adenocarcinoma or metastatic undifferentiated carcinoma.

A systematic approach to the evaluation and treatment of patients with metastatic squamous cell carcinoma in a cervical lymph node has been generally accepted. This presentation, therefore, is the simpler of the two problems. If the initial examination fails to determine the primary site, direct inspection and palpation of the mucosal surfaces of the upper respiratory and alimentary tract under general anesthesia are performed. Random biopsies are taken of the nasopharynx, base of the tongue, tonsillar area, and pyriform sinuses as well as biopsies of any suspicious areas. If no primary site is located, therapy consisting of radical neck dissection and/or radiotherapy is recommended. When a primary site becomes manifest after initial therapy, the sites most often involved are the hypopharynx and oropharynx. Therefore, particular attention should be paid to these areas during examination under anesthesia. With aggressive treatment the three-year disease-free survival rate of these patients has ranged from 13 per cent to 48 per cent in various series. This wide range among series is due to differences in the criteria for inclusion of patients and in the exact therapy employed.

The patient with metastatic adenocarcinoma or undifferentiated carcinoma from an unknown primary site presents a more complex problem. A thorough initial evaluation must be completed before the diagnosis of carcinoma from an unknown primary site is accepted. This evaluation must include a careful review of the patient's history, physical examination, and baseline laboratory data as outlined below.

Initial Evaluation of Metastatic Adenocarcinoma or Undifferentiated Carcinoma

History
   Previous diseases and therapies
   Personal habits
   Industrial exposures to potential carcinogens
   Family history

Physical examination
   Always include careful examination of areas often overlooked or superficially examined: skin, thyroid, breasts, pelvis, prostate. (Include pap smear.)

12

Laboratory data

Complete blood count

Glucose, electrolytes, blood urea nitrogen, creatinine, calcium, phosphate, liver function tests, acid phosphatase

Stool examinations for blood (six times on red meat–free, high-residue diet)

Urinalysis—note particularly the presence of hematuria

The initial evaluation may elicit complaints arising from specific organ systems, permit the discovery of subtle abnormalities, or facilitate the identification of risk factors for particular types of cancer. Among the most common risk factors are contact with known carcinogens (smoking) and a positive family history of cancer. Women with a family history of breast cancer, for example, exhibit an incidence of breast cancer three to five times higher than that of the general female population. In addition, the initial evaluation provides an opportunity for the recognition of any paraneoplastic syndrome that may point to a particular cancer. For example, hypertrophic osteoarthropathy is most often seen in conjunction with lung cancer; hemolytic anemia is, at times, associated with gastric, breast, prostatic, and pancreatic cancers.

Initial Roentgenographic Studies, Chest X-Ray, and Mammography

A chest roentgenogram should be included as part of the initial evaluation. In addition, women who exhibit cancer from an unknown primary site should undergo mammography. In one breast cancer screening project ("HIP study"), it was found that a third of the breast cancers were detected on mammography alone and had not been found on physical examination. Since most of the cancers detected on mammography alone occurred in women over 50, this procedure is of particular importance in this group. It should be noted that in the same study 48 per cent of the breast cancers were detected on physical examination alone and were not visible on mammography. Thus, mammography and physical examination are complementary diagnostic tools.

A negative initial evaluation qualifies the metastatic cancer as a cancer from an unknown primary site. The following factors should be taken into account when attempts are made to locate the primary site:

1. **Relative frequencies of cancers arising from different primary sites.**

According to American Cancer Society estimates, cancers of the lung, prostate, and colon and rectum constitute more than 50 per cent of all cancers in men, while cancers of the breast, colon and rectum, and uterus are the most frequent in women.

However, these frequencies do not necessarily reflect the incidence of metastatic cancer arising from these sites. The incidence of metastatic cancer is more closely paralleled by the cancer mortality rates for each primary site, since most metastatic cancers are not curable at the present time. For example, although uterine cancer represents 14 per cent of all cancers in women, it accounts for only 7 per cent of cancer deaths in women each year because its potential for dissemination is less than that of certain other cancers.

2. **Relative frequencies with which cancers from particular primary sites metastasize.**

Cancers of the lung, colon and rectum, and other digestive organs account for 60 per cent of all male cancer deaths. Cancers of the breast, colon and rectum, other digestive organs, and lung account for 60 per cent of female cancer deaths.

3. **Relationship of patient age to the relative frequencies of different primary cancers.**

Lung cancer accounts for the largest number of cancer fatalities in men of all ages. In women younger than 75, breast cancer is the leading cause of cancer deaths, while in women over 75, colon and rectal cancer account for more cancer deaths.

4. **Relationship of the metastatic site or sites to the relative frequencies of different primary cancers.**

Primary cancers vary considerably in their propensity to metastasize to given sites.

Metastatic site	Primary cancer sites most frequently responsible
Brain	Lung, breast
Bone	Breast, lung, kidney, bladder, prostate
Lung	Breast, lung, colon, kidney, bladder
Liver	Breast, lung, colon, other digestive organs
Skin	Breast, lung
Peritoneal implants	Stomach, ovary, colon
Lymph nodes — supra-clavicular, axillary	Breast, lung, pancreas, stomach

These four factors are a guide to the usual relationships between a primary cancer and patient age, patient sex, metastatic potential, and common metastatic sites. However, within the subset of patients with an unknown primary cancer, both the frequencies and the metastatic patterns of many cancers probably differ from the expected. For example, in one study (Nystrom et al., 1977) of 264 patients with a referral diagnosis of metastatic carcinoma from an unknown primary site, the pancreas and lungs represented the most common cryptogenic primary sites. In this study, the primary site was ultimately established in 129 of the 264 cases. The diagnosis was established antemortem in 30 cases and following post-mortem examination in 99 cases. The distribution of primary cancer sites was: pancreas — 20 per cent, lung — 18 per cent, liver — 11 per cent, colon and rectum — 10 per cent, stomach — 8 per cent, kidney — 6 per cent, ovary — 4 per cent, prostate — 3 per cent, breast — 2 per cent, other sites — 1 per cent or less for each site. A similar study (Moertel et al., 1972) of 162 patients confirms the predominance of pancreatic primary sites among patients referred with the diagnosis of metastatic carcinoma from an unknown primary site. For 42 of the 162 patients, identification of their primary lesions had been made by the time of post-mortem examination. Pancreatic cancer was the primary lesion in 16 of the 42 cases (38 per cent). Thus, the frequency of carcinomas of the breast, colon, and rectum is less than expected in this subset of patients, while the frequency of pancreatic cancer is much greater than expected.

Similarly, deviations from the expected metastatic patterns of various cancers have been observed when these cancers initially presented as unknown primary cancers. In one study (Nystrom et al., 1977), it was found that the frequency of bone metastases was much greater than expected for primary pancreas and liver cancers and much less than expected for primary breast and prostate cancers in this subset of patients. The frequency of lung metastases was greater than expected for primary lung, ovary, and prostate cancers. The frequency of both liver and brain metastases was greater than expected for a primary prostate cancer.

Because of these deviations in the expected frequencies and metastatic patterns of particular cancers, attempts to find an unknown primary cancer often involve a large number of diagnostic tests. These tests should always be performed in order, with the least invasive and stressful tests preceding more stressful tests (see flow diagram).

Complete Evaluation for Unknown Primary Cancer

Thyroid scan

Chest x-ray → full lung tomograms → sputum cytologies → full lung bronchoscopy with selective cytologies

Mammograms → biopsy of any clinically suspicious area or any areas suspicious on mammography

Stools for blood → sigmoidoscopy → barium enema → colonoscopy → cytologic examination → UGI and small bowel x-rays → gastroscopy → cytologic examination

Abdominal sonogram or computerized axial tomography → cannulation of ampulla of Vater → cytologic examination

Liver scan → arteriography

Intravenous pyelogram → urine cytology → cystoscopy → arteriogram

Blind prostate biopsies

Pelvic sonogram or computerized axial tomography → laparoscopy

The following are pertinent to the complete evaluation.

1. A thyroid scan is most easily done prior to the use of iodinated compounds for other studies.

2. Chest x-rays can miss small lesions in the lung, particularly those hidden by osseous or soft tissue shadows. Stereoscopic AP views, full lung tomography, and computerized tomography can be helpful in delineating these lesions. Sputum cytologic examinations may be positive from an endobronchial lesion, with no mass present on chest film or tomography. Correctly performed sputum cytologic examinations are positive in almost 80 per cent of endobronchial carcinomas. If sputum cytologic examinations are positive, or if there is compelling evidence suggesting a lung primary site in the history or on physical examination, full lung bronchoscopy with selective washings and a post-bronchoscopy sputum examination is warranted.

3. A breast biopsy should be done if a suspicious lesion is either felt on physical examination or seen on mammography, since a significant percentage of breast cancer is diagnosed by one modality but not the other.

4. Examination of stools for blood is an excellent screen for cancers of the upper and lower gastrointestinal tracts if the correct procedures are used. Six stool specimens should be obtained from three consecutive evacuations in a patient on a high-residue, red meat–free diet. If six stool specimens obtained in this manner are negative, the probability of finding a bowel primary is much reduced.

Since two thirds of colon and rectal cancers can be identified with sigmoidoscopy, it should be the next procedure. An upper gastrointestinal x-ray examination or a barium enema should not be performed unless the patient's stools are positive for blood. The routine use of diagnostic contrast roentgenography in patients with unknown primary cancers has been shown to be of little value (Nystrom et al., 1979). While approximately 60 per cent of patients subsequently found to have cancers of the upper and lower gastrointestinal tract had positive contrast roentgenograms, the false positive and false negative rates were high (approximately 40 per cent each).

5. A pancreatic tumor may be delineated by a sonogram of the abdomen or computerized axial tomography of the abdomen. Cannulation of the ampulla of Vater is a technically difficult procedure that is performed only in select medical centers.

6. A hepatoma can be diagnosed with a fair degree of certainty on the basis of its arteriographic appearance. Arteriography should be considered if the liver scan is suggestive of hepatoma. A high level of α-fetoprotein provides additional evidence suggesting a hepatoma.

7. Urinary cytologic examinations are more likely to be positive with lower urinary tract cancers than with renal cell cancer. If an intravenous pyelogram suggests a renal mass, arteriography may be in order. The arteriographic appearance of a renal cell carcinoma is characteristic and can provide a probable diagnosis.

12

8. A blind prostate biopsy should be done if there is an elevated level of acid phosphatase or other factors suggesting a primary prostate cancer. Prostate cancer most frequently occurs in the area of the prostate that is least easy to palpate.

9. While a sonogram or a computerized axial tomogram of the pelvis may help to identify masses in the pelvic region, a laparoscopy or laparotomy may be necessary to confirm a suspected diagnosis.

Finally, can one justify such rigorous evaluations to find an unknown primary cancer? Two considerations favor such an approach. First, many cancers have specific therapies to which a significant percentage of patients will respond. Patients who respond will both feel better and have a greater chance of prolonged survival than untreated patients or patients who receive therapy that is ineffective for their particular disease. Thus, discovery of a primary cancer may allow potentially effective therapy for the patient. Second, if a patient is identified as having a particular cancer for which there is no effective therapy, the patient can be offered experimental therapies as part of programs aimed at the discovery of new and effective cancer treatment.

Our thanks to Sandra Ginsberg, M.D., who provided this contribution.

References: Jesse, R., Perez, C., and Fletcher, A.: Cancer, *31*:854, 1973; Nystrom, J. S., Weiner, J. M., Heffelfinger-Juttner, J., et al.: Semin. Oncol., *4*:53, 1977; Moertel, C. G., Reitemeier, R. H., Schutt, A. J., and Hahn, R. G.: Cancer, *30*:1469, 1972; Nystrom, J. S., Weiner, J. M., Wolf, R. M., et al: J.A.M.A., *241*:381, 1979, Moertel, C. G.: Editorial. Ann. Intern. Med., *91*:646, 1979.

CLINICAL AND PATHOLOGIC STAGING OF CANCERS

Staging systems attempt to organize clinical and pathologic information about tumor dissemination into prognostically and therapeutically significant categories. Cancer staging assumes increased importance as more effective therapy for disseminated cancer is developed and as the utility of adjuvant therapy is demonstrated for specific disease stages. The optimal therapy of many cancers is dependent upon the stage of the cancer at the time of diagnosis. Correct staging may require the aggressive use of invasive procedures, as, for example, laparotomy in the staging of Hodgkin's disease.

Shown below are the staging systems currently in use for several common tumors: breast cancer, lung cancer, and ovarian cancer. Invasive, aggressive staging employed in these disorders defines both the prognosis and the nature of therapy.

Breast Cancer

Survival in breast cancer is related to the stage of the cancer at the time of diagnosis. Patients with stage I and II disease have longer rates of disease-free survival than do patients with stage III or IV disease. However, 80 to 85 per cent of women with stage II breast cancer ultimately die from their cancer despite standard surgical therapy with or without post-operative irradiation. Recently, improvement in disease-free survival rates has been obtained with adjuvant chemotherapy in premenopausal women with stage II disease. The optimal therapeutic approach to stage III breast cancer is under investigation at the present time.

The following TNM classification for breast cancer has been recently established by the American Joint Committee for Cancer Staging.

TNM Classification

Primary Tumor (T)
  Clinical-diagnostic classification

TX		Tumor cannot be assessed
T0		No evidence of primary tumor
TIS		Paget's disease of the nipple with no demonstrable tumor *(Note: Paget's disease with a demonstrable tumor is classified according to size of the tumor)*
T1*		Tumor 2 cm or less in greatest dimension
	T1a	No fixation to underlying pectoral fascia and/or muscle
	T1b	Fixation to underlying pectoral fascia and/or muscle
T2*		Tumor more than 2 cm but less than 5 cm in its greatest dimension
	T2a	No fixation to underlying pectoral fascia and/or muscle
	T2b	Fixation to underlying pectoral fascia and/or muscle
T3*		Tumor more than 5 cm in its greatest dimension
	T3a	No fixation to underlying pectoral fascia and/or muscle
	T3b	Fixation to underlying pectoral fascia and/or muscle
T4		Tumor of any size with direct extension to chest wall or skin *(Note: Chest wall includes ribs, intercostal muscles, and serratus anterior muscle but not pectoral muscle)*
	T4a	Fixation to chest wall
	T4b	Edema (including peau d'orange), ulceration of the skin of the breast, or satellite skin nodules confined to the same breast
	T4c	Both of above
	T4d	Inflammatory carcinoma

*Dimpling of the skin, nipple retraction, or any other skin changes, except those in T4b, may occur in T1, T2, or T3 without changing the classification.

Post-surgical treatment–pathologic classification

TX		Tumor cannot be assessed
T0		No evidence of primary tumor
TIS		Preinvasive carcinoma (carcinoma *in situ*), non-infiltrating intraductal carcinoma, or Paget's disease of nipple
T1		Same as clinical-diagnostic classification
		i. Tumor ≤ 0.5 cm
	T1a	ii. Tumor > 0.5 cm and ≤ 1.0 cm
	T1b	iii. Tumor > 1.0 and ≤ 2.0 cm
T2		
	T2a	Same as clinical-diagnostic classification
	T2b	
T3		
	T3a	Same as clinical-diagnostic classification
	T3b	
T4		
	T4a	
	T4b	Same as clinical-diagnostic classification
	T4c	
	T4d	

Nodal Involvement (N)

Clinical-diagnostic classification

NX		Regional lymph nodes cannot be assessed clinically
N0		No palpable homolateral axillary nodes
N1		Movable homolateral axillary nodes
	N1a	Nodes not considered to contain growth
	N1b	Nodes considered to contain growth
N2		Homolateral axillary nodes considered to contain growth and fixed to one another or to other structures
N3		Homolateral supraclavicular or infraclavicular nodes considered to contain growth or edema of the arm*

Post-surgical treatment–pathologic classification

NX		Regional lymph nodes cannot be assessed clinically
N0		No metastatic homolateral axillary nodes
N1		Movable homolateral axillary metastatic nodes not fixed to one another or other structures
	N1a	Lymph nodes with only histologic metastatic growth

*Edema of the arm may be caused by lymphatic obstruction, and lymph nodes may then be unpalpable. Homolateral internal mammary nodes considered to contain growth are included in N3 for surgical-evaluative classification and post-surgical treatment–pathologic classification.

N1b   Gross metastatic carcinoma in lymph nodes
- i. Micrometastasis 0.2 cm or less in diameter
- ii. Metastasis (more than 0.2 cm in diameter) in one to three lymph nodes
- iii. Metastases to four or more lymph nodes
- iv. Extension of metastasis beyond the lymph node capsule
- v. Any positive node more than 2 cm in diameter

N2   Homolateral axillary nodes containing metastatic tumor and fixed to one another or to other structures

N3   Homolateral supraclavicular or infraclavicular nodes containing tumor or edema of the arm*

Distant Metastasis (M)

MX	Not assessed
M0	No (known) distant metastasis
M1	Distant metastasis present

Stage Grouping

In Situ Cancer (*in situ* lobular, pure intraductal, and Paget's disease of the nipple without palpable mass)

TIS

Invasive Cancer

Stage I	T1a or T1b	N0 or N1a	M0
Stage II	T0	N1b	M0
	T1a or T1b	N1b	M0
	T2a or T2b	N0 or N1a or N1b	M0
Stage III	T1a or T1b	N2	M0
	T2a or T2b	N2	M0
	T3a or T3b	N0 or N1 or N2	M0
Stage IV	Any T4	Any N	Any M
	Any T	N3	Any M
	Any T	Any N	MI

Lung Cancer

With squamous cell carcinoma, adenocarcinoma, and large cell anaplastic carcinoma of the lung, there is a relationship between the stage of lung cancer, as defined below, and survival. Stage I cancers and some stage II cancers can be surgically resected in an apparently complete manner. However, the five-year survival rate, even in stage I

---

*Edema of the arm may be caused by lymphatic obstruction, and lymph nodes may then be unpalpable. Homolateral internal mammary nodes considered to contain growth are included in N3 for surgical-evaluative classification and post-surgical treatment—pathologic classification.

disease, is less than 50 per cent. Survival is shorter with stage II and III disease than with stage I disease. The survival rate in small cell anaplastic ("oat cell") carcinoma is not related to stage. Less than 10 per cent of patients treated with surgery or radiation therapy survive two years with stage I, II and III small cell anaplastic carcinoma. This poor survival rate reflects the propensity of this cell type of lung cancer to spread hematogenously, creating micrometastases throughout the body. Improved survival rates in small cell anaplastic carcinoma have resulted from the use of chemotherapy.

The following TNM classification for lung cancer has been established by the American Joint Committee for Cancer Staging.

TNM Classification

Primary Tumor (T)

TX	Tumor proven by the presence of malignant cells in bronchopulmonary secretions but not visualized roentgenographically or bronchoscopically; also, any tumor that cannot be assessed
T0	No evidence of primary tumor
TIS	Carcinoma *in situ*
T1	Tumor 3.0 cm or less in greatest diameter, surrounded by lung or visceral pleura, and without evidence of invasion proximal to a lobar bronchus at bronchoscopy
T2	Tumor more than 3.0 cm in greatest diameter, or a tumor of any size that either invades the visceral pleura or has associated atelectasis or obstructive pneumonitis extending to the hilar region. On bronchoscopy, the proximal extent of demonstrable tumor must be within a lobar bronchus or at least 2.0 cm distal to the carina. Any associated atelectasis or obstructive pneumonitis must involve less than an entire lung, and there must be no pleural effusion
T3	Tumor of any size with direct extension into an adjacent structure, such as the parietal pleura, the chest wall, the diaphragm, or the mediastinum and its contents; also, any tumor demonstrated bronchoscopically to involve a main bronchus less than 2.0 cm distal to the carina, or any tumor associated with atelectasis or obstructive pneumonitis of an entire lung or pleural effusion

Nodal Involvement (N)

N0	No demonstrable metastasis to regional lymph nodes
N1	Metastasis to lymph nodes in the peribronchial or the ipsilateral hilar regions or both, including direct extension
N2	Metastasis to lymph nodes in the mediastinum

Distant Metastasis (M)

MX   Not assessed
M0   No (known) distant metastasis
M1   Distant metastasis present

Stage Grouping

Occult stage

TX N0 M0   Occult carcinoma with bronchopulmonary secretions containing malignant cells but without other evidence of the primary tumor or evidence of metastasis to the regional lymph nodes or distant metastasis

Stage I

TIS N0 M0   Carcinoma *in situ*
T1 N0 M0   Tumor that can be classified T_1 without any metastasis or with metastasis
T1 N1 M0   only to the lymph nodes in the peri-
T2 N0 M0   bronchial and/or ipsilateral hilar region; also, a tumor that can be classified T2 without any metastasis to nodes or distant metastasis (*Note:* TX N1 M0 and T0 N1 M0 are also theoretically possible, but such a clinical diagnosis would be difficult, if not impossible, to make. If such a diagnosis is made, it should be included under stage I.)

Stage II

T2 N1 M0   Tumor classified as T2 with metastasis only to the lymph nodes in the peribronchial and/or ipsilateral hilar region

Stage III

T3 with any N or M   Any tumor more extensive than T2,
N2 with any T or M   any tumor with metastasis to the
M1 with any T or N   lymph nodes in the mediastinum, or any tumor with distant metastasis

12

Ovarian Cancer

The five-year survival rate of patients with ovarian cancer is related to the stage of the disease at the time of diagnosis. Following treatment with surgery alone, the five-year rate in stage I disease is 67 per cent; in stage II, 24 per cent; and, in stage III, 1 per cent. Based on relapse patterns, it is thought that patients with stage II and III disease have a high incidence of post-surgical microscopic residual disease. Also, patients with advanced, measurable ovarian carcinoma have an excellent response to chemotherapy. Consequently, it is recommended that patients with stage II and III ovarian cancer receive adjuvant chemotherapy.

The International Federation of Gynecology and Obstetrics (FIGO) has established the following staging system for ovarian cancer.

Stage I	Growth limited to the ovaries	
A	Growth limited to one ovary; no ascites	
	1. No tumor on the external surface; capsule intact	
	2. Tumor present on the external surface, or capsule ruptured	
B	Growth limited to both ovaries; no ascites	
	1. No tumor on the external surface; capsule intact	
	2. Tumor present on the external surface, or capsule(s) ruptured	
C	Tumor either stage IA or IB, but with ascites or positive peritoneal washings	
Stage II	Growth involving one or both ovaries, with pelvic extension	
A	Extension or metastases to the uterus or fallopian tubes	
B	Extension to other pelvic tissues	
C	Tumor either stage IIA or IIB, with ascites or positive peritoneal washings	
Stage III	Growth involving one or both ovaries, with intraperitoneal metastases outside the pelvis or positive retroperitoneal lymph nodes; tumor limited to the true pelvis, with histologically proven malignant extension to small bowel or omentum	
Stage IV	Growth involving one or both ovaries, with distant metastases; if pleural effusion is present, there must be positive cytology to allot a case to stage IV; parenchymal liver metastases indicate stage IV	
Special category	Unexplored cases that are thought to be ovarian carcinoma	

Ascites is peritoneal effusion that, in the opinion of the surgeon, is pathologic or clearly exceeds normal amounts.

This article was prepared in collaboration with Sandra Ginsberg, M.D.

Reference: Henderson, I. C. and Canellos, G. P.: N. Eng. J. Med., *302*:17, 1980. Carr, D. T. and Mountain, C. I.: Semin. Oncology, *1*:229, 1974. Day, T. and Smith, J. P.: Semin. Oncology, *2*:217, 1975. Tobias, J. S. and Griffiths, C. T.: N. Eng. J. Med., *294*:818, 1976.

Results can always be improved by omitting controls.

13
INFECTIOUS DISEASE

FEVER OF UNKNOWN ORIGIN (FUO)

Uncovering the diagnosis in patients with fever of unknown origin has been a fascinating chapter for the medical sleuth. "Pedigreed" cases fulfill the criteria given below. In these cases fever is the presenting sign and symptom. Associated symptoms are limited to malaise, fatigue, chills, and weight loss.

1. an illness of greater than three weeks duration.
2. several febrile episodes of greater than 101°F.
3. diagnosis uncertain after a week of study or after the completion of a "routine" diagnostic evaluation.

Common things occur commonly.
The race may not always be to the swift nor the battle to the strong, but it's a good idea to bet that way.
When you hear hoofbeats, think of horses, not zebras.
Place your bets on uncommon manifestations of common conditions rather than common manifestations of uncommon conditions.

Bacteria — From the Greek *bakterion,* meaning "little staff."

The Series

The differential diagnosis of FUO presented in the table on the following pages is adapted from Jacoby and Swartz, who in turn adapted it from findings in the classic monograph by Petersdorf and Beeson. Where possible, the diagnoses established in five contemporary studies of patients with FUO are provided. Included are two series from university hospitals (A,B), a series from a community hospital (C), a series from a referral hospital in Cairo, Egypt (D), and a surgical series (E):

A. Petersdorf, R. G., and Beeson, P.: Medicine, *40*:1, 1961.

B. Jacoby, G. A., and Swartz, M. N.: New Engl. J. Med., *289*:1407, 1973.

C. Gleckman, R., Crowley, M., and Esposito, A.: Am. J. Med. Sci., *274*:21, 1977.

D. Hassan, A., and Farid, Z.: New Engl. J. Med., *290*:807, 1974.

E. Geraci, J. E., Weed, L. A., and Nichols, D. R.: J.A.M.A., *169*:169, 1959.

13

DIFFERENTIAL DIAGNOSIS OF FUO	SERIES A[1] (100 patients)	SERIES B[2] (128)	SERIES C[3] (34)	SERIES D[4] (139)	SERIES E[5] (70)	NEWER DIAGNOSTIC APPROACHES
I. *Infection*	36%	40%	18%	60%	33%	Improved culture techniques, counter immunoelectrophoresis
A. Systemic						
1. Tuberculosis (especially extrapulmonic)	11	—	6	16	7	Fluorescent stain for mycobacteria
2. Subacute bacterial endocarditis	5	—	—	—	—	Echocardiography, serology
3. Miscellaneous infections	2	—	—	—	—	—
a. Cytomegalovirus	—	—	—	—	—	Serology
b. Toxoplasmosis, histoplasmosis	—	—	—	—	—	Serology
c. Brucellosis	1	—	—	3	3	—
d. Psittacosis	2	—	—	—	—	Serology
e. Disseminated mycosis	—	—	—	—	—	Serology
f. Parasitic (e.g., malaria, kala-azar)	1	—	—	3	—	—
g. Enteric pathogens (e.g., salmonella)	—	—	—	22	—	—
B. Localized						
1. Hepatic	—	—	—	—	—	Sonography, computerized axial tomography, radionuclide (TC or gallium) scan
a. Liver abscess (bacterial, fungal, amebic)	2	—	—	2	3	Serology (amebic abscess)
b. Cholangitis	5	—	—	—	1	ERCP, "skinny" needle cholangiogram
2. Other visceral infections	—	—	—	—	—	Sonography, computerized axial tomography, gallium scan and Selenomethionine scan
a. Pancreatic abscess	—	—	—	—	—	—
b. Tubo-ovarian abscess	—	—	—	—	—	—
c. Empyema of gallbladder	—	—	—	—	—	—
d. Pericholecystic abscesses	—	—	—	—	—	
3. Intraperitoneal infections	4	—	—	—	—	Sonography, computerized axial tomography, gallium scan
a. Subhepatic abscesses	—	—	3	—	—	Combined liver and lung scan
b. Subphrenic abscesses	—	—	—	—	—	—
c. Paracolic abscesses	—	—	—	—	—	—
d. Appendiceal abscesses	—	—	3	—	—	—
e. Other abscesses	—	—	—	—	—	—

DIFFERENTIAL DIAGNOSIS OF FUO	SERIES A[1] (100 patients)	SERIES B[2] (128)	SERIES C[3] (34)	SERIES D[4] (139)	SERIES E[5] (70)	NEWER DIAGNOSTIC APPROACHES
4. Urinary tract	–	–	–	–	1	Sonography, computerized axial tomography, gallium scan, renal scan
a. Pyelonephritis	3	–	–	9	–	–
b. Renal carbuncle	–	–	–	–	–	–
c. Perinephric abscess	–	–	–	–	–	–
d. Prostatic abscess	–	–	–	–	–	–
5. Osteomyelitis	–	–	6	–	–	Bone scan
II. *Neoplasia*	19%	20%	9%	14%	30%	Bone marrow biopsy, sonography, computerized axial tomography, gallium scan
A. "Hematologic"	8	–	–	9	14	Serology (paraprotein), identification of monoclonal lymphocytic populations
B. "Nonhematologic"	7	–	–	–	16	Serology (e.g., alpha feto-protein, CEA), ERCP, radioimmunoassay for hormone identification in paraneoplastic syndromes
III. *Collagen-vascular disease**	15%	15%	9%	10%	7%	Serology, angiography, tissue immunofluorescence (i.e., skin, kidney)
IV. *Other causes*	23%	17%	29%	4%	16%	
A. Other granulomatous diseases (atypical acid fast, leprosy, sarcoid)	2	–	–	2	11	angiotensin converting enzyme
B. Inflammatory bowel disease	–	–	–	–	–	Endoscopy, air contrast enema with high viscosity, high density barium, double contrast small intestinal enema
C. Pulmonary embolization	3	–	9	–	–	–
D. Drug fever/hypersensitivity	4	–	–	–	–	
E. Factitious fever	3	–	3	–	–	Electronic thermometers, urine temperature
F. Active hepatocellular disease	–	–	15	2	4	Serology
G. Miscellaneous rare diseases	6	–	–	–	–	–
1. Familial Mediterranean fever	5	–	–	–	–	Rectal biopsy (amyloid)
2. Whipple's disease	–	–	–	–	–	Gastrointestinal biopsy
3. Atrial myxoma	–	–	–	–	–	Echocardiography
V. *Undiagnosed*	7%	8%	35%	12%	14%	

*Temporal arteritis included.
[1] From a referral hospital in New Haven Conn., 1961.
[2] From a referral hospital in Boston. Mass. 1973.
[3] From a community hospital in Boston, Mass. 1977.
[4] From a referral hospital in Cairo, Egypt, 1974.
[5] From a referral hospital (surgical) in Rochester, Minn., 1959.

13

Notes on Diagnosis

1. The per cent of cases falling into the major diagnostic categories is rather consistent. Infection, neoplasia and collagen-vascular disease ultimately account for some 80 per cent of diagnoses made. A similar situation prevailed in studies published in the years preceding the report of Petersdorf and Beeson. In general, common diseases are represented in less common presentations.

2. A definitive diagnosis could not be reached in about 10 per cent of the cases. This figure was highest in the community hospital series and resulted from the disappearance of fever during the course of the diagnostic evaluation. Presumably these cases would never reach the university hospital. Their inclusion in the diagnostic head count probably dilutes the incidence of malignancy and infection in the community hospital series.

3. The influence of referral patterns, prior screening, and diagnostic time at risk is reflected in the higher incidence of malignancy observed in the surgical series.

4. The influence of geographic and other demographic factors is clearly evident in the high incidence of enteric infections observed in Cairo, Egypt. A multitude of factors, including socio-economic and racial factors, the endemic incidence of pathogens (i.e., histoplasmosis, coccidioido- and blastomycosis, malaria, and leishmania), the age of the patient population at risk, and referral patterns, will influence the frequency with which a specific diagnosis is made.

5. The best diagnostic approach in some patients is "watchful waiting" after a period of initial evaluation. Just how much evaluation and how much waiting must remain individualized. The appropriate decision depends on the urgency in making the diagnosis and an assessment of the risk and the cost/benefit ratio of any new evaluation. The option of "watchful waiting" appears most likely to be exercised in those patients who retrospectively are shown to have a noninfectious cause for the FUO.

6. Similar considerations govern the use of therapeutic trials. The possibility that the contemplated trial will inadequately treat the patient or obscure the diagnosis is an important consideration that must be entertained prior to the initiation of any such trial.

7. In the majority of cases, a definitive culture or biopsy is necessary. We, like others, have in the past advocated the use of biopsy and culture in aggressively pursuing a diagnosis. In large measure, the "blind" biopsy and culture were previously directed by clinical intuition. Where appropriate, these procedures may now be directed by objective findings provided by the newer diagnostic modalities.

8. These newer diagnostic tools are listed in the last column as they apply to the individual diagnoses. One must be impressed by their aggregate efficacy and utility.

Our diagnostic acumen has also been sharpened by a more complete understanding of many of the disease processes (e.g., granulomatous hepatitis) and our greater facility with well-established diagnostic techniques (e.g., liver biopsy).

9. With these considerations in mind, the checklist should prove helpful. Remember, tuberculosis still lives!

Additional suggested reading: Geraci, J. E., Weed, L. A., and Nichols, D. R.: J.A.M.A., *169*: 1306, 1959; Molavi, A., and Weinstein, L.: Med. Clin. North Am., *54*:379, 1970; Deller, J. J., and Russell, P. K.: Ann. Intern. Med., *66*:1129, 1967; Simon, H. B., and Wolff, S. M.: Medicine, *52*:1, 1973.

SUTTON'S LAW

While on ward rounds, William Dock, M. D., discovered that every study except the appropriate one had been performed on the patient being discussed. He therefore suggested that Sutton's Law be followed. By way of definition, he noted that Willy Sutton, the bank robber, was asked why he always robbed banks, rather than hotel clerks, filling stations, or other easy marks. "That's where the money is," Sutton replied. Sutton's Law had actually become fairly common medical parlance prior to its formalization in the article by Drs. Beeson and Petersdorf (see preceding article). Lest Mr. Sutton become too romantic a figure, it should be remembered that at least one unsolved murder is connected with the story—that of the young man who provided the information leading to Sutton's final capture and imprisonment.

FEVER OF UNKNOWN ORIGIN OF GREATER THAN ONE YEAR'S DURATION (100 Cases)

Infection	11 per cent
Urinary	6
Tuberculosis	2
Malaria	1
Trypanosomiasis	1
Subdiaphragmatic abscess	1
Neoplastic	2 per cent
"Reticulum cell sarcoma"	1
Carcinoma of the colon	1
Collagen-vascular diseases	6 per cent
Juvenile rheumatoid arthritis	6 per cent
Miscellaneous	64 per cent
No fever (circadian)	15
Factitious	10*
Unknown	17
Sarcoid	5
Hepatitis	3

13

---

*Many were health professionals.

Granulomatous hepatitis	7
Vasculitis	7
Erythema multiforme	3
Familial Mediterranean fever	5
Type II hyperlipidemia	1
Weber-Christian disease	1
Whipple's disease	1
Regional enteritis	5
Enterocolitis	1
Cyclic neutropenia	1
Hypothalamic disorders	2
Bromism	1

Reference: Wolff, S.: Personal communication (with thanks).

TUBERCULIN SKIN TESTING

The purpose of tuberculin skin testing is to identify those persons who may have been exposed to the tubercle bacillus and thus have become sensitized to extracts of the organism. The two methods currently used are the Tine test and the Mantoux test. Certain points to note regarding each are provided.

Tine Test

— Multiple-puncture technique.
— The tuberculin extract is not standardized.
— Requires less skill to administer.
— *Interpretation:* Presence of *papules* requires a Mantoux test to verify the test as a true positive. Presence of *vesicles* is considered a true positive.

Mantoux Test

— Is the method of choice.
— Uses a standardized mixture of proteins derived from the tubercle bacillus called PPD-S.
— PPD-S contains *Tween 80* to reduce adsorption to glass and plastic containers.
— PPD-S is supplied in 3 strengths:
   a. *First strength* contains 1 *Tuberculin Unit (TU).*
   b. *Intermediate strength* contains *5 TU.*
   c. *Second strength* contains *250 TU.*
— In general, the stronger the clinical impression that the patient has *active* tuberculosis, the lower the dose of PPD-S applied.
— *Method:* 0.1 ml of 5 TU of PPD-S (this is the strength usually applied) is administered intradermally with a 26- or 27-gauge needle. A 6 to 10 mm wheal should be produced.
— *Interpretation:* the test is read *48 hours* after administration.

- A positive response requires *induration*.
- Most positive responses will have both erythema and induration.
- Erythema without induration is not considered a positive response.

Results
- Induration of 10 mm or more is a positive response representing past or present infection.
- In general, the larger the reaction, the more likely that active tuberculosis is present.
- Induration of 5 to 9 mm usually reflects exposure to an atypical mycobacterium.
- Induration of 4 mm or less is a *negative reaction*. No repeat test is indicated unless the patient has had recent exposure to tuberculosis.

false positives
- Atypical mycobacterium 5 to 9 mm (doubtful reactions should be skin-tested with PPD-B to distinguish those patients sensitized to the atypical mycobacterium. In this circumstance the patients will react more strongly to PPD-B than PPD-S).
- Previous administration of *BCG vaccine*.
- *Frequent* prior tuberculin skin testing.

false negatives
- Poor technique or materials.
- *Miliary tuberculosis: presence of a pleural effusion caused by active tuberculosis. Generalized anergy* (can be tested with a panel of skin tests that include mumps, *Candida albicans,* and streptokinase-streptodornase).
- Recent vaccination with live virus.
- Acute viral illnesses.

Thanks to Paul Cohen, M.D., for assisting in the preparation of this material.

THERAPY OF TUBERCULOSIS

*Antituberculous Programs**

Program A — Isoniazid and ethambutol for 18 months.†
Program B — Isoniazid and ethambutol for 18 months, with streptomycin for the first two to three months.
Program C — Isoniazid and rifampin for 12 to 18 months.
Program D — Isoniazid and rifampin for 18 months, with streptomycin for first two to three months, or with ethambutol for at least three months.
Program E — Isoniazid and rifampin for six to nine months.††

13

---

*Take drugs orally before breakfast for optimal absorption.
†Safest regimen during pregnancy.
††Experimental in this country.

Indications for Various Antituberculous Drug Programs

Pattern of disease	Drug program
Minimal-moderate pulmonary	A
Pleural disease	A
Cavitary pulmonary	B, C, or D
Severe miliary disease	B, C, or D
Meningitis	D or B
Pericarditis	B, C, or D
Peritonitis	
Genito-urinary	
Musculoskeletal	
Lymphadenopathy	A, B, or C
Enteritis	
Hepatitis	
Laryngitis	

The adverse effects associated with each of the commonly used antituberculous drugs are noted in the table on the following page.

TEXT CONTINUED ON PAGE 448

Antituberculous Drugs

DRUG	DOSAGE FOR ADULTS	ADVERSE EFFECTS	DETECTION OF ADVERSE EFFECTS
Isoniazid	5 mg/kg (up to 300 mg) daily as a single dose, oral or intramuscular; add pyridoxine (B6) 50–100 mg daily orally	Hepatitis: may be fatal if drug continued after its onset Hypersensitivity Peripheral neuritis and seizures (if pyridoxine deficient)	Educate patient about symptoms of hepatitis; test for SGOT/SGPT, bilirubin, and alkaline phosphatase — if greater than three times normal, stop isoniazid
Ethambutol	15 mg/kg daily in a single oral dose; if severe infection is present, administer 25 mg/kg for first one to three months	Optic neuritis: diminished visual acuity and green color perception (rarely, when dose is 25 mg/kg daily or less); reversible if drug is stopped	Check for baseline visual acuity and color discrimination
Streptomycin	15 mg/kg daily (up to 1 gram) intramuscularly for 30 to 60 days, followed by twice weekly doses for one to two months	Ototoxicity Vestibular toxicity Nephrotoxicity (increased danger in elderly and patients with renal disease) Allergic reaction	Check baseline audiogram; educate patient about eighth nerve dysfunction; bimonthly tests of BUN and creatinine
Rifampin	10 mg/kg daily in one single oral dosage (up to 600 mg per day)	Hepatitis (increased probability if combined with isoniazid) Thrombocytopenia Flu-like syndrome Increased metabolism of anticoagulants and oral contraceptives Orange urine (and other body fluids) If patient is receiving isoniazid and rifampin and develops clinical hepatitis, both drugs should be discontinued.	Educate patient about symptoms of hepatitis; test for SGOT/SGPT, bilirubin, and alkaline phosphatase — if greater than three times normal, stop rifampin

13

Indications for the Addition of Corticosteroids to Antituberculous Chemotherapy in the Treatment of Tuberculosis*

1. Meningitis with subarachnoid block.
2. Pericarditis.
3. Fulminant miliary disease.
4. Hypersensitivity to antituberculous drugs.

---

*Prednisone dosage: 0.5 mg per kg daily for at least two to three weeks.

Notes on the Management of Patients with Tuberculosis

1. Notify the local department of public health about all new cases of tuberculosis.

2. All close contacts of the tuberculous patient must have skin tests. Household contacts younger than 5 years old should be considered for isoniazid therapy.

3. Sputum stains and cultures should be monitored every two to four weeks until they become negative.

4. Patients should be seen monthly throughout their period of therapy.

5. Patients should be carefully and repeatedly warned about the dosages and toxicity of the drugs they are taking.

6. The patient should be instructed to discontinue isoniazid and/or rifampin and call the physician if 48 to 72 hours of anorexia, nausea, vomiting, or malaise are encountered.

7. The recommended treatment period should be completed even if a patient appears to be "cured" at an earlier time.

8. Drug susceptibility tests should be done on all organisms obtained from patients who do not respond to treatment. The addition of only one drug to a failing program is a serious error when drug resistance exists. A tuberculosis specialist should be consulted.

9. Drug susceptibility testing should be undergone by all patients who may have contracted tuberculosis in Asia. There is a higher incidence of isoniazid resistance in the Orient!

10. A patient may be discharged from the hospital after two weeks of anti-tuberculous chemotherapy if:

   a. The patient is clinically stable, and appropriate diagnostic studies requiring hospitalization have been completed.

b. The patient is considered reliable to take medications, keep follow-up appointments, and comply with the other instructions provided.

c. The patient is not highly infectious (i.e., far-advanced pulmonary disease).

d. Ziehl-Neilsen stains of sputa reveal either a small number of organisms or a definite reduction in the number of organisms.

References: Johnston, R., and Wildrick, K.: Am. Rev. Resp. Dis., *109*:636, 1974; Comstack, G. W., and Edwards, P.: Am. Rev. Resp. Dis., *111*:573, 1975; Byrd, R. B., Horn, B. R., Solomon, D. A., et al.: Ann. Intern. Med., *86*:799, 1977.

Our thanks to Dr. Paul Cohen for this contribution.

CHEMOPROPHYLAXIS OF TUBERCULOSIS INFECTION

Populations at Risk

The probability of active tuberculosis developing in patients at high risk can be significantly decreased by prophylactic therapy with isoniazid. Prophylactic isoniazid is thought to act by decreasing the bacterial population in clinically asymptomatic patients with undetectable disease. In patients with a positive tuberculin skin test, isoniazid is given as presymptomatic treatment for an established infection prior to its progression to active disease. Isoniazid administration can be associated with severe and, at times, irreversible hepatic dysfunction. Priorities, therefore, must be set for preventive therapy. The following factors should be taken into consideration before embarking on a chemoprophylaxis program:

1. The risk of developing tuberculosis compared with the risk of isoniazid toxicity (see table on following page).

2. The ease of identifying and supervising the care of persons for whom chemoprophylaxis is indicated.

3. The likelihood of that person infecting others.

13

Risk of Developing Tuberculosis Versus Risk of Isoniazid Hepatitis

POPULATION	RISK
Risk of developing active tuberculosis	
Close contacts: *skin test negative	2.5% for the first year*
skin test positive	5.0% for the first year*
Positive skin test and abnormal x-ray	1.0–4.5% per year (risk of reactivation)
Recent skin test converters	5.9% for the first year
Risk of "severe" isoniazid liver injury	
Younger than 20	Rare
Ages 20–34	0.3%
Ages 35–40	1.2%
Older than 50	2.3%

*Of documented active cases.

Indications for Isoniazid Chemoprophylaxis

The following recommendations of the American Thoracic Society on isoniazid use are based on a comparison of the risk of isoniazid hepatitis (the most serious complication of isoniazid therapy) to the potential benefit of preventive therapy. Chemoprophylaxis is indicated for:

1. Household members and other close contacts of persons with recently diagnosed tuberculosis.
   Comment: Contacts who have Mantoux tuberculin skin test readings of 5 mm or more should receive preventive therapy.
   Contacts with *negative tuberculin skin test:* Children who are in contact with bacteriologically active patients are at highest risk. They should receive preventive therapy for three months and then be retested. If the skin test remains negative and the exposure has ended, therapy can be discontinued. If the skin test becomes positive, a 12-month course of therapy should be completed. For adult contacts with negative skin tests, the state of infectiousness of the source case versus the risk of drug side effects should be considered. If therapy is not initiated, the contact should be retested in three months.

2. Established positive skin test reactors who have an abnormal chest roentgenogram and who have not had adequate past treatment.

3. Newly infected persons.
   Comment: A newly infected person is defined as one who has had a tuberculin skin test conversion within the previous two years.

4. *Special clinical situations.* The following situations variably increase the risk of developing active disease and *may* require chemoprophylaxis in the patient with a positive skin test:
    a. Therapy with steroids.
    b. Immunosuppressive therapy.
    c. Some hematologic malignancies such as leukemia and Hodgkin's disease.
    d. Diabetes mellitus
    e. Silicosis.
    f. Post-gastrectomy.

5. Other positive skin reactors:
    a. Persons younger than 35 years who are positive on skin tests. Chemoprophylaxis should be instituted even in the absence of one of the aforementioned risk factors.
    b. Chemoprophylaxis is *mandatory* for children through age 6 who have a positive skin test.
    c. In persons older than 35 who have a positive skin test but none of the aforementioned risk factors, the risk of hepatitis precludes the use of *routine* chemoprophylaxis. Preventive therapy should be considered if there is a high probability of serious consequences for contacts who may become infected.

Therapeutic Program

The chemoprophylaxis program consists of:

Adults: 300 mg isoniazid administered as a single dose daily for 12 months.

Children: 10 mg/kg per day, not to exceed 300 mg/day for 12 months.
    Contraindications to isoniazid therapy are:
    a. Previous isoniazid-associated liver damage.
    b. Severe adverse reactions to the drug, such as fever, chills, and arthritis.
    c. Acute liver disease of any etiology.

Relative contraindications include chronic liver disease. Alcohol used daily and pregnancy increase the risk of isoniazid hepatitis.

Though isoniazid has no documented harmful effects on the fetus, new mothers are at increased risk for tuberculosis during the post-partum period. Therefore, preventive therapy can be delayed until after delivery.

Pyridoxine is given to all patients receiving isoniazid.

Monitoring Patients

The following guidelines are recommended for adequate monitoring of patients:

13

1. Advise patients of the symptoms associated with isoniazid toxicity. (See Therapy of Tuberculosis, p. 445.)

2. Advise patients to discontinue use of the drug immediately and report to you if toxic symptoms occur.

3. Routine monthly evaluations should include close questioning for any symptoms of isoniazid toxicity.

4. Routine monthly SGOT determinations are mandatory.

It is worth noting that approximately 30 per cent of patients on chemoprophylaxis will have transient elevations of the SGOT, which usually occur within the first six months of therapy. In the majority of cases, the SGOT will return to normal despite continued use of isoniazid.

Current recommendations include: (a) discontinuing the isoniazid in any symptomatic individual, regardless of the level of SGOT elevation, and (b) stopping the isoniazid in any *asymptomatic* individual with an SGOT elevation exceeding three times the normal value. Recent studies have indicated that progressive liver damage will result if isoniazid is continued in patients with marked elevations of the SGOT.

References: American Thoracic Society: Am. Rev. Resp. Dis., *110*:371, 1974; Mitchell, J. R., et al: Ann Intern. Med., *84*:181, 1976; Byrd, R. B., Horn, B. R., et al: J.A.M.A., *241*: 1239, 1979.

IMMUNIZATION IN ADULTS

Immunization programs to prevent and treat disease are usually thought of as being for children. The internist or family physician may not be aware of the current recommended immunization procedures for adults. The chart on pages 453–457 outlines the available and recommended immunization policies for adults. (Superscript numbers correspond to entries listed on the chart under the "Comments" heading.)

TEXT CONTINUES ON PAGE 458

DISEASE	PRE-EXPOSURE	POST-EXPOSURE	COMMENTS
Tetanus	*History of Tetanus Immunization* — Clean Minor Wounds | Doses	Td[1]	TIG[2]
Unknown	Td	No
0–1	Td	No
2	Td	No
≥3	Td[3]	No | *History of Tetanus Immunization* — Wounds Other than Clean Minor Wounds | Doses	Td	TIG
Unknown	Td	Yes
0–1	Td	Yes
2	Td	Yes
≥3	Td[5]	No[4] | Primary immunization should be carried out as follows for all individuals who are uncertain whether they have ever been immunized. TD–3 doses IM with 4–6 weeks between first and second dose and 6–12 months between second and third dose.	For clinical tetanus, supportive care is the key to therapy. TIG is administered IV, and 3000–10,000 U are given. Td given as in primary immunization.	1. Administer adsorbed adult tetanus-diphtheria (Td) toxoid IM *without* pertussis vaccine, because of the high incidence of untoward CNS reactions with pertussis vaccine in adults, except as indicated on page 463. 2. TIG–*Human* tetanus immune globulin; the dose is *250 Units* intramuscularly. 3. Unless it has been 10 years or less since last toxoid dose. 4. Unless wound is more than 24 hours old. 5. Unless it has been 5 years or less since last toxoid dose.

TABLE CONTINUES ON FOLLOWING PAGES

13

DISEASE	PRE-EXPOSURE	POST-EXPOSURE	COMMENTS

Rabies	Persons at high risks of exposure to wild animals should receive duck embryo vaccine (DEV):
	
	a. Two 1 ml injections one month apart and booster 6 months after second dose
		Clean wound with soap and water. Then scrub with aqueous benzalkonium chloride.
		
		Active immunization with DEV:
		a. 23 doses subcutaneously in abdomen or lateral thigh
		b. 1 dose BID for 7 days and 1 dose daily for 7 days
		    or
		    1 dose daily for 21 days.
		c. Last 2 doses are given 10 and 20 days after completion of 14- or 21-day series.
		
		Passive immunization recommended for all bites in which rabies cannot be excluded and for nonbite exposures to animals suspected of having rabies:
		a. *Human:* antirabies globulin — 20 IU/kg.
		b. Infiltrate 50% locally into wound.
			6. Rabies contracted by humans if virus penetrates skin or gains access to mucous membranes.
			
			7. Wild skunks, foxes, raccoons, bats are considered rabid administer vaccine if patient is bitten. Rats, mice, chipmunks, rabbits are not considered rabid; vaccine not indicated.
			
			8. Domestic animal: if healthy and vaccinated, confine for 10 days. If it is ill during confinement, kill and have brain examined.
			
			9. If domestic animal bites and escapes, try to capture it and learn circumstances surrounding bite. If animal can't be found, start treatment after 12 hours if circumstances are suspicious. Can wait 48 hours if victim provoked the attack.
			
			10. Local reactions to DEV are common and are *not* indications for stopping immunization.
			
			11. Greater than 1% incidence of anaphylaxis with DEV; therefore, obtain history for allergy to avian products.
			
			12. If patient is bitten, tetanus prophylaxis as indicated.

Disease			Notes
Diphtheria	(See Tetanus)	For clinical diphtheria, diphtheria antitoxin is given in doses of 20,000–80,000 units IM or IV depending on severity of infection[13,14]	13. Diphtheria antitoxin is horse globulin, and sensitivity tests to horse serum must be done. 14. Additional dose given if patient doesn't improve within 24 hours after start of therapy.
Rubella	—	Rubella vaccine[15] given as a single subcutaneous injection to adolescent girls[16] and young women[16]	15. Live attenuated virus. 16. Recommended *only* if the women: a. Are shown to be susceptible by hemagglutination inhibition testing *and* b. If the women agree not to become pregnant for *3 months* after immunization.
Influenza	—	Vaccine recommended for high-risk groups[17]	17. High-risk groups are those persons with chronic debilitating conditions, such as congenital and RHD, ASHD, COPD, cystic fibrosis, diabetes mellitus, chronic renal disease, and persons over 65 years old.
Hepatitis	—	Human immune serum globulin *hepatitis A.* 0.02 ml/kg to total of 2 ml[18,19,20] *Hepatitis B* – 0.04 ml/kg to a total 4 ml; indications same as for Hepatitis A[21]	18. Made from pooled plasma. 19. Given to persons exposed to hepatitis A: household contacts, school contacts, institutional contacts, and persons with common needle exposure; also given in food-borne, water-borne outbreaks.

TABLE CONTINUES ON FOLLOWING PAGES

13

DISEASE	PRE-EXPOSURE	POST-EXPOSURE	COMMENTS
Hepatitis (continued)			20. Should be given within 1–2 weeks of exposure.
			21. May be useful in preventing some non-A, non-B, post-transfusion hepatitis.
			22. Hepatitis B immune globulin is commercially available. It is recommended *only* for one-time exposure to *blood-containing hepatitis B virus* either by accidental needle stick or by contact with mucous membranes. It is administered twice — as soon as possible after exposure, but within 7 days of exposure, and again 25–30 days after the first injection. The dose is 0.05–0.07 ml/kg. A single dose may cost as much as $150.
Botulism	—	Botulism antitoxin[23]	23. Several types of antitoxin are available. Antitoxin is horse globulin, and testing for sensitivity to horse serum is necessary. a. Toxin type unknown—administer trivalent antitoxin (types A,B,E). b. Toxin known—give bivalent anti-toxin (A,B) or monovalent (E). c. One vial given IV, one vial IM.

Measles	—	Measles immune globulin, 0.05–0.1 ml/kg, or standard immune globulin, 0.25 ml/kg[24]	24. Measles vaccine not indicated in adults. Immune globulin given to immuno-suppressed patients exposed to a person with measles within 6 days of exposure.
Polio	(See comment 25)	Nonvaccinated adults exposed to a case of polio should receive immune serum globulin, 0.35 ml/kg; should be given within a few days of exposure	25. Vaccine not routinely recommended for adults in the United States. Persons with high-risk jobs (sanitation men, medical personnel) who are suscepti-ble should be immunized with 3 doses of trivalent oral polio vaccine.

13

Certain active immunization procedures are *not indicated* in adults. They are those for measles, pertussis, smallpox, and polio.

Contraindications to immunization:

1. Live viral or bacterial vaccines (e.g., rubella, mumps, polio, yellow fever, vaccinia, and BCG) are contraindicated in immunosuppressed patients.
2. Pregnancy is a contraindication to rubella vaccine and to any other live vaccine. Pregnancy not a contraindication to treatment with immune globulin, toxoid vaccines, or inactivated vaccines.

References: Rimland, D., McGowan, J. E., and Shulman, J.: Ann. Intern. Med. *85*:622, 1976; Corey, L., Hattwick, M. A. W., and Rubin, R. J.: Postgrad. Med., *59*:887, 1976.

ANTIMICROBIAL PROHYLAXIS: RHEUMATIC FEVER VERSUS INFECTIVE ENDOCARDITIS

There is some confusion as to why prophylactic antimicrobial agents are administered to patients who have had an episode of rheumatic fever or currently have rheumatic heart disease. Patients with a well-documented history of rheumatic fever or Sydenham's chorea or those who show evidence of rheumatic heart disease should receive *continuous* antimicrobial prophylaxis directed against the group A beta-hemolytic Streptococcus. The aim of this therapy is to prevent a recurrent episode of rheumatic fever with its potential risk of additional cardiac damage.

Prevention of Recurrent Rheumatic Fever

I. Benzathine penicillin G: 1,200,000 units intramuscularly every 4 weeks.[1]

II. Penicillin G: 200,000 or 250,000 units orally twice a day.[2]

III. Sulfadiazine: 1000 mg once daily for patients weighing more than 60 pounds; 500 mg daily for patients weighing less than 60 pounds.[3]

IV. Erythromycin: 250 mg orally twice daily.[4]

Comments:
1. Risk of recurrence lower after parenteral prophylaxis than after oral.
2. Taken 30 minutes prior to eating or 60 minutes after.
3. Sulfadiazine contraindicated in late pregnancy.
4. For patients allergic to both penicillin and sulfonamides.
5. Duration of prophylaxis in patients with clinical rheumatic valvular disease is for life. Patients with rheumatic heart disease with prosthetic valves should continue to take prophylaxis for life. Patients without valvular heart disease should receive prophylaxis until age 20 or for 5 to 10 years after their last episode of rheumatic fever.

Antibiotic therapy aimed at preventing infective endocarditis is recommended for patients with cardiac lesions—which predispose to endocarditis, when these patients undergo procedures associated with bacteremia. Thus, patients being treated with continuous antimicrobial prophylaxis to prevent rheumatic fever recurrences should also receive prophylaxis against bacterial endocarditis. Remember, penicillin-resistant organisms are produced by penicillin prophylaxis of rheumatic fever. Therefore, penicillin is *not* an effective drug for prevention of endocarditis in these patients. Antimicrobial therapy aimed at preventing infective endocarditis should be given to patients with the following cardiac abnormalities:

1. Rheumatic heart disease.
2. Congenital heart disease.
   a. Most lesions except for ostium secundum atrial septal defects, and large ventricular septal defects.
3. Acquired (degenerative) heart disease.
   a. Calcific aortic stenosis.
   b. Calcified mitral annulus.
   c. Damage to valves from a previous episode of endocarditis.
4. Syphilitic heart disease.
5. Idiopathic hypertrophic subaortic stenosis.
6. Marfan's syndrome.
7. Prosthetic intracardiac devices.
8. Mitral valve prolapse syndrome.
   a. At present the prevalence of this syndrome is too great and the attack rate of endocarditis too low to justify antibiotic prophylaxis for all patients. It is thus uncertain which of these patients should receive prophylaxis.
9. Patients with arteriovenous fistulas (e.g., hemodialysis patients).

The chart shown on the following pages outlines the recommended antibiotic therapy for preventing infective endocarditis relative to certain procedures. Superscript numbers correspond to the "Comments" listed on the far right of the chart.

TEXT CONTINUES ON PAGE 462

13

Prevention of Infective Endocarditis

PROCEDURE	ORAL	PARENTERAL	COMMENT
Dental extraction Periodontal surgery Any dental procedure that may induce gingival bleeding (including professional cleaning)	1. Phenoxymethyl penicillin, 2.0 grams orally, 30 minutes before the procedure followed by 500 mg orally every 6 hours for 48 hours[2]	1. Aqueous penicillin G, 2,000,000 units IM, and procaine penicillin G, 600,000 units IM, and streptomycin, 1.0 gram IM, 30 min. prior to the procedure	1. Prior to procedures in oropharynx and upper airway, prophylaxis is aimed at preventing bacteremia with *Streptococcus viridans.*
Nasotracheal intubation Nasotracheal suctioning Rigid tube bronchoscopy[1]	2. Erythromycin, 500 mg orally, 1½–2 hours prior to the procedure, then 250 mg orally every 6 hours for 11 additional doses[3]	2. Vancomycin, 500 mg IV over 30 minutes, starting 1 hour prior to procedure[3] and oral erythromycin	2. The parenteral methods are preferred for patients with prosthetic valves or those taking daily oral penicillin for rheumatic fever prophylaxis.
		3. Cefazolin, 1.0 gram IM and streptomycin, 500 mg IM, 30 minutes before the procedure and every 8 hours for two additional doses[3]	3. In patients allergic to penicillin.
Genitourinary or lower abdominal[4,5]	1. Ampicillin, 3.5 grams orally, and Probenecid, 1 gram orally 1–2 hours prior to procedure; then ampicillin (1 gram) orally every 6 hours for 4 doses and gentamicin (80 mg) IM 1 hour prior to procedure; repeat gentamicin once 12 hours later	1. Ampicillin, 1 gram IV or IM 30 minutes prior to procedure and 8 and 16 hours later, and gentamicin, 80 mg IM 30 minutes before the procedure and 8 and 16 hours later	4. Prophylaxis in these circumstances is aimed at preventing bacteremia with enterococcus.

5. There are conflicting data on whether to use prophylaxis in susceptible patients undergoing sigmoidoscopy, barium enema, and colonoscopy. Susceptible patients undergoing urologic instrumentation or obstetrical or gynecologic procedures should receive antimicrobial prophylaxis.

6. In patients allergic to penicillin.

7. Prophylaxis is aimed at preventing bacteremia with *Staphylococcus aureus.*

8. Parenteral antimicrobials are advisable when there is a high probability of staphylococcal bacteremia.

2. Cefazolin, 1 gram IM 30 minutes prior to the procedure and 8 and 16 hours after the procedure, and gentamicin as described in point 1[6]

3. Vancomycin, 1 gram IV over 30 minutes, starting 1 hour prior to the procedure and gentamicin, 80 mg IM, 30 minutes prior to procedure; repeat both once 12 hours later[6]

1. Cefazolin, 1 gram IM 1 hour prior to procedure, then every 8 hours for 72 hours[8]

Surgical manipulation of infected cutaneous tissue[7]

1. Dicloxacillin, 500 mg orally, 1 hour prior to procedure, then 500 mg every 6 hours for 72 hours

References: Committee on Prevention of Rheumatic Fever and Bacterial Endocarditis of American Heart Association: Circulation, *55*:1, 1977; Sipes, J. N., et al.: Annu. Rev. Med. 28:371, 1977; Everett, D. E., and Hirschmann, J. V.: Medicine, *56*:61, 1977; Committee on Prevention of Rheumatic Fever and Bacterial Endocarditis of American Heart Association: Circulation, *56*:139a, 1977.

13

MENINGOCOCCAL PROPHYLAXIS

Chemoprophylaxis for persons in contact with cases of meninogococcal disease is required to avoid a high rate of secondary cases. The design of a chemoprophylaxis program must consider the population at risk and the antibiotics necessary for adequate prophylaxis. The current Center for Disease Control guidelines for such a program in a nonepidemic setting are enumerated below.

1. All *close contacts* of a case of meningococcal disease should *receive prophylaxis*. A close contact is defined as an individual "who *slept and ate* in the *same dwelling* as the *index case*." Therefore, all household members are considered close contacts, as are all day care nursery contacts.

School contacts, contacts on public transportation, casual contacts and hospital contacts are *not* considered close contacts. An important exception is anyone who has administered mouth-to-mouth resuscitation to a patient with meningococcal disease.

2. Close contacts should receive chemoprophylaxis as soon as possible. All members of a household should receive prophylaxis simultaneously.

3. If the pathogenic strain of meningococcus is sensitive to sulfa, adequate prophylaxis consists of 1 gram of sulfadiazine twice daily for two days.

4. If the sensitivities of the infecting strain are unknown, or if the stain is sulfa-resistant, administer 600 mg of rifampin every 12 hours for four doses. Minocycline therapy is also considered adequate chemoprophylaxis. However, because of the high incidence of adverse vestibular reactions, minocycline is not the drug of choice.

For any contact who develops objective signs of meningococcal disease, appropriate therapy consists of prompt hospitalization and initiation of intravenous penicillin G (or chloramphenicol) while blood and cerebrospinal fluid cultures are being analyzed.

Reference: McCormick, J. B., and Bennett, J. V.: Ann. Intern. Med., *83*:883, 1975.

ACUTE EPIGLOTTITIS

Adults are sometimes only large children when it comes to upper airway infections. Acute infectious epiglottitis can rapidly progress to complete upper airway obstruction in the adult, although it is much more common in children. The diagnosis is easy to make if one thinks of it; but who thinks of acute epiglottitis when one sees a dyspneic adult? When dyspnea is associated with symptoms and signs pointing to the upper airway, such as sore throat, hoarseness, stridor, and inspiratory retractions, acute epiglottitis should be considered.

A lateral soft tissue x-ray of the neck that reveals the enlarged epiglottis will confirm the diagnosis. Failure to make the diagnosis carries a high probability that the patient will die. Attempts at direct visualization of the area should be avoided, since such manipulation may produce acute, complete airway obstruction.

The initial treatment of acute epiglottitis should be intubation to insure airway patency. Blood cultures are obtained. Antibiotic therapy directed against *Hemophilus influenzae* should be started. Standard respiratory care should be undertaken in an intensive care unit. The intubation should be performed by a skilled intubationist in an operating room with the personnel and equipment for emergent tracheostomy at hand, since intubation of such patients is often very difficult. The decision to extubate the patient should be based on resolution of the epiglottic swelling confirmed by a lateral soft tissue x-ray of the neck or by direct visualization.

Reference: Ward, C. R., Benumof, J. C., and Shapiro, H. M.: Chest, *71*:93, 1977.

PROLONGED BRONCHITIS IN AN ADULT— CONSIDER "WHOOPING COUGH"

In 1977 there were 1,915 cases of pertussis reported in the United States. The widespread use of pertussis vaccine since the 1940's has led to the erroneous conclusion that adults do not contract the disease. Recent research has suggested that 11 to 38 per cent of the cases of whooping cough occurring in epidemic situations involved adults. In one study, the attack rate was 95 per cent in individuals who had been vaccinated 12 or more years prior to exposure to pertussis. Thus, there appears to be a loss of vaccine-induced immunity with time, which in turn, may lead to an increased incidence of the disease in previously vaccinated adults.

Pertussis in the adult produces a spectrum of clinical manifestations ranging from mild respiratory infection with prolonged symptoms of bronchitis to severe paroxysmal coughing associated with an inspiratory whoop. Hence, mild disease may go unrecognized, and the patient may spread the disease via infected droplets of respiratory tract secretions. In addition, previously immunized individuals may not demonstrate the lymphocytosis that is characteristic of the disease.

Adults then should be considered susceptible to infection with *Bordetella pertussis*, although the symptoms may not be that of classic "whooping cough." Indeed *B. pertussis* or *B. parapertussis* infection should be considered in an adult with prolonged symptoms of bronchitis. A nasopharyngeal swab plated on Bordet-Gengou agar is required for isolation of *Bordetella pertussis*. Antibiotics do not affect the clinical course of pertussis but they can eradicate *B. pertussis* from the respira-

13

tory tract and are, therefore, useful in preventing further spread of the disease from infected patients. Erythromycin (1 to 1½ grams by mouth daily for 14 days) is recommended for patients and for susceptible close contacts. In epidemic situations, medical personnel should receive booster doses of 0.2 ml of available pertussis vaccine to prevent both the clinical disease in the personnel and its spread from personnel to hospital patients.

Reference: Linnemann, C. C., and Nasenbeny, J.: Ann. Rev. Med., *28*:179, 1977.

EXTRACARDIAC MANIFESTATIONS OF BACTERIAL ENDOCARDITIS

The patient with bacterial endocarditis presents both a diagnostic and a therapeutic challenge. The myriad manifestations of the disease result from the hemodynamic, embolic, and immunologic sequelae of the endovascular infection.

The following review of the more common extracardiac manifestations may serve as an aid in diagnosis and management of this disease.

MANIFESTATION	COMMENT
I. Renal	
1. Microscopic hematuria and proteinuria	1. Biopsy
2. Occasionally azotemia	a. Focal glomerulonephritis *or*
3. Abnormalities usually resolve with effective antimicrobial therapy	b. Diffuse proliferative glomerulonephritis
II. Neurologic	
1. Major neurologic complications are:	1. Neurologic complications occur in 25–40% of patients with bacterial endocarditis
a. *Cerebral infarction* in region of middle cerebral arteries secondary to emboli (most common neurologic complication)	2. The mortality of patients with neurologic complications is > 50%
b. Meningeal signs and symptoms	3. Embolic phenomenon are usually seen in endocarditis due to *S. aureus, Pneumococcus, Enterobacteriaceae,* and *anaerobic streptococci*
c. Seizures	4. *Mitral valve* endocarditis produces *major cerebral emboli more frequently* than *aortic valve* endocarditis
d. Intracranial hemorrhage	
e. Large macroscopic brain abcesses are uncommon	5. Mycotic aneurysms occur more frequently in the *early* course of *acute* endocarditis than *late* in the course of *subacute* endocarditis
f. *Microscopic* brain abcesses are *common* and reflect multiple microemboli	6. Cerebrospinal (CSF) fluid exam tends to reflect the nature of the infecting organism; i.e., virulent organisms are more likely to produce meningitis with a purulent CSF than are less virulent organisms, which are likely to produce a sterile "aseptic" CSF
III. Musculoskeletal	
1. Arthralgia — usually in shoulder, knee, hip	1. Musculoskeletal findings are seen in approximately 44% of patients with bacterial endocarditis
2. True synovitis	
a. Ankle, knee, wrist most frequent	
b. Usually sterile	
c. Biopsy shows acute inflammatory changes	

13

MANIFESTATION   COMMENT

III. Musculoskeletal (*continued*)
  3. Low back pain
     a. Often severe
     b. Often demonstrates spinal
        tenderness and decreased
        range of motion
     c. X-rays usually normal
     d. Usually not secondary to
        disc space infection
  4. Myalgias — often localized to
     thighs and calves
  5. Miscellaneous
     a. Clubbing of the digits
     b. Hypertrophic osteo-
        arthropathy
     c. Avascular necrosis of hip

IV. Skin
  1. Petechiae
  2. Osler's nodes
  3. Janeway lesions
  4. Periungual erythema
  5. Subungual "splinter" hemorrhages

V. Hematologic
  1. Anemia
  2. Thrombocytopenia (in the
     absence of disseminated
     intravascular coagulation)
  3. Monocytosis
  4. Splenomegaly
  5. Plasmacytosis of the bone
     marrow
  6. Disseminated intravascular
     coagulation

VI. Serologic
1. Elevated erythrocyte sedimentation rate
2. Elevated serum gamma globulins
3. Positive rheumatoid factor
4. Positive antinuclear antibody
5. Circulating immune complexes
6. Presence in serum of cryo-globulins
7. Low serum complement

1. Titers of circulating immune complexes highest in patients with:
   a. Right-sided endocarditis
   b. Extravascular manifestations
   c. Signs of infection for more than four weeks

References: Pruitt, A. A., Rubin, R. H., Karchmer, A. W., and Duncan, G. W.: Medicine, *57*:329, 1978; Churchill, M. A., Geraci, J. E., and Hunder, G. G.: Ann. Intern. Med., *87*:754, 1977; Bajer, A. S., Theofilopoulos, A. N., Eisenberg, R., et al.: N. Engl. J. Med., *295*:1500, 1976.

SPONTANEOUS BACTERIAL PERITONITIS (SBP)

Patients with cirrhosis and ascites are prone to develop bacterial infection of the ascitic fluid. As this syndrome of "spontaneous bacterial peritonitis" has become more frequently recognized, certain features have emerged that may aid in treatment of these patients. The table on the following pages identifies some of those features.

13

Features of SBP

FEATURES	COMMENTS
Clinical	
Fever (63–68%)	Fever *absent* in a third of cases.
Abdominal pain or rebound tenderness (42–70%)	Abdominal signs *absent* in 20–50% of cases.
Increasing ascites (75%)	
Mortality (57–96%)	
Poor prognostic signs	
a. Increasing hepatic encephalopathy.	
b. More than 85% polymorphonuclear leukocytes in the peripheral blood or ascitic fluid.	
c. Serum bilirubin greater than 8 mg/dl.	
d. Serum albumin less than 2.5 g/dl.	
Invasive procedures (endoscopy, paracentesis, intra-arterial Pitressin) account for the source of infection in only a *minority* of patients with SBP.	

Laboratory

Cloudy ascitic fluid (86–92%)

Positive gram stain (22–24%)

Peripheral blood leucocytosis (72%)

Ascitic fluid leucocytosis (>300 cells/mm^3)

Gram stain usually negative.

Found in 90–96%. An ascitic fluid leucocytosis of more than 300 cells/mm^3 does not necessarily imply infection, however. A count of more than 1000 cells/mm^3 with more than 80% polymorphonuclear leukocytes usually does mean infection. For counts between 300 and 1000 cells/mm^3 the clinician must weigh the benefits and risks of presumptive antibiotic therapy until culture reports are known.

Bacteriology

Enteric organisms (75%)
(i.e., *E. coli,* Klebsiella species, *Streptococcus faecalis, B. fragilis, γ*-Streptococcus, *Clostridium perfringens*)

Nonenteric organisms (25%)
(Pneumococcus, group B Streptococcus, *Staphylococcus aureus*)

E. coli is the most frequently recovered organism (33–57%); Klebsiella species, Pneumococcus, and *Strep. faecalis* are each recovered with almost an equal frequency (10–20%).

Staphylococcus aureus, B. fragilis, group A Streptococcus, *Clostridium perfringens, Pasteurella multocida,* and other gram negative rods are recovered less frequently (3–7%).

References: Weinstein, M. P., Iannini, P. B., Stratton, C. W., and Eickhoff, T. C.: Am. J. Med., *69*:592, 1978; Correia, J. P., and Conn, H. O.: Med. Clin. North Am., *59*:963, 1975; Conn, H. O.: Gastroenterology *70*:455, 1976.

13

PERINEPHRIC ABSCESS

Rupture of an abscess from within the renal parenchyma into the perinephric space is almost always the inciting event in the development of a perinephric abscess. Approximately two thirds of intraparenchymal renal abscesses arise by direct extension from a focus of pyelonephritis; the other third develops by hematogenous spread, often from sites of skin infection.

The mortality rate of perinephric abscess is 40 to 50 per cent. The mortality rate for patients admitted to medical services is *twice* that of patients admitted to surgical services, reflecting a delay in the making of the correct diagnosis on nonsurgical services. The most frequent admitting diagnoses for patients who are admitted to a medical service and ultimately are shown to have a perinephric abscess are *fever of unknown origin, sepsis,* and *acute pyelonephritis.*

Awareness of this syndrome and its clinical features should facilitate earlier diagnosis and appropriate therapy and hence improve survival rates.

A. *Incidence*
1. 1.3 cases/year/100,000 admissions (Parkland Memorial Hospital, 1970 to 1974).

B. *Sex distribution*
1. The frequency is *slightly greater* in *males* than in *females.*

C. *Age*
1. Perinephric abscess is seen in all age groups.

D. *Associated disorders*
1. The most common associated disorders are:
   a. Genito-urinary stones.
   b. Diabetes mellitus.
   c. Antecedent soft tissue or skin infection.

E. *Organisms*
1. The organisms usually isolated from either the abscess cavity or the blood are:
   a. Gram negative aerobic bacilli (especially *E. coli* and Proteus species) in 60 per cent of cases.
   b. *Staphylococcus aureus* in 15 per cent.
   c. Miscellaneous organisms or no organisms in 15 to 25 per cent.

F. *Clinical features*
1. *Fever* is present in 85 to 95 per cent of patients on admission.
2. A *flank mass* or *flank tenderness* is present in 65 to 75 per cent of patients on admission.

3. *Dysuria* is present in 33 to 40 per cent of patients at the time of admission.
4. *Gross hematuria* occurs in only 5 per cent of patients.
5. Most patients complain of *being sick* for *more than five days* before seeking medical attention.

G. *Laboratory findings*
   1. The BUN is usually normal.
   2. The *urinalysis* is usually *abnormal*.
      a. Pyuria (66 to 85 per cent of cases).
      b. Proteinuria (33 to 42 per cent).
      c. Microscopic hematuria (10 to 32 per cent).
   3. *Positive cultures*
      a. Abscess cavity (96 per cent).
      b. Blood (20 to 40 per cent).
      c. Urine (66 to 80 per cent).
   4. The *sedimentation rate* is *elevated* in only *a third* of the cases.
   5. The white blood count is greater than 10,000/mm^3 in 75 per cent of patients.

H. *Radiographic findings*
   1. The most important radiographic finding is *loss of renal mobility*. The normal kidney moves approximately 2 to 6 cm during the change from expiration to inspiration, or from a supine to an upright position.
   2. The disease is usually *unilateral.*
   3. The most frequent abnormalities seen on an intravenous pyelogram are:
      a. Diminished or no visualization of the involved kidney.
      b. Dilatation of the calyces.
      c. Genito-urinary stones.
   4. The use of ultrasound and computerized axial tomography are now the noninvasive studies most likely to yield a finding of a fluid-filled perinephric lesion.

I. *Distinguishing a perinephric abscess from acute pyelonephritis*

13

	Perinephric abscess	*Acute pyelonephritis*
Flank or abdominal mass	May be present	Absent
Duration of symptoms prior to admission	5 days or more	Less than 5 days
Duration of fever while receiving antibiotics	5 days or more	Less than 4 days

J. *Treatment*
   1. The treatment of perinephric abscess is *prompt surgical drainage* and administration of appropriate parenteral antibiotics.

Reference: Thorley, J. D., Jones, S. R., and Sanford, J. P.: Medicine, *53*:441, 1974.

CSF LDH ACTIVITY AND MENINGITIS

Bacterial meningitis demands prompt institution of the correct therapy. Current antibiotic therapy has markedly reduced the morbidity and mortality rates from meningitis. Nevertheless, the distinction between viral and bacterial meningitis remains one of the more difficult medical problems we face. Until the proper cultures have had a chance to grow, physicians must still rely on analysis of a few precious drops of spinal fluid for the diagnosis. Yet, the CSF white count and differential and total protein and glucose concentrations may not correctly categorize all cases of bacterial meningitis. Indeed, early in the course of viral meningitis, a polymorphonuclear pleocytosis may occur in the CSF. The likelihood of correctly classifying and managing cases of meningitis can be increased by determining the level of CSF LDH activity.

If the CSF LDH activity is greater than 70 units/ml, the meningitis is presumed to be bacterial in origin; if it is less than 30 units/ml, the meningitis is presumed to be viral, chemical, or of other origin. The gray zone between 30 to 70 units/ml may reflect partially treated bacterial infection. However, other conditions, such as cerebrovascular accident, meningeal leukemia, and metastatic tumor to the CNS, can produce a high LDH.

CSF LDH isoenzymes from patients with bacterial meningitis are predominantly isoenzymes 4 and 5. Those patients with aseptic meningitis have isoenzymes 1 and 2.

Reference: Feldman, W. E.: Am. J. Dis. Child, *129*:77, 1975.

FEVER, INFECTION, GRANULOCYTOPENIA, AND CANCER CHEMOTHERAPY

Contemporary, aggressive, multiagent chemotherapy of malignant disease is often ablative to normal bone marrow function. Prolonged periods of marrow aplasia or hypoplasia and consequent granulocytopenia and thrombocytopenia commonly arise in the course of therapy for adult acute leukemia. As therapy for other hematologic and solid malignancies becomes more intensive, these problems will undoubtedly be encountered with increasing frequency. While the availability and use of platelet transfusion have markedly improved the therapy and prophylaxis of thrombocytopenic bleeding, infection in the granulo-cytopenic host remains a major problem.

Approximately 75 per cent of treatment deaths in patients treated for acute leukemia are infective. The fatal infection proves to be bacterial in 75 per cent of the cases. The prime factor predisposing to infection is absolute granulocytopenia, and the number of infective febrile episodes endured by the patient can be directly related to the patient's degree of granulocytopenia. Patients with less than 500 granulocytes/mm^3 are at markedly increased risk. A favorable outcome to therapy, moreover, can be related to the imminence of marrow recovery.

In the granulocytopenic host, the clinical signs and symptoms characteristic of infection other than fever may not be present, at least initially. Thus, all too frequently, the physician is faced with a febrile, granulocytopenic patient who does not exhibit a specific site or organism as the source or cause of the infection. Nonetheless, more than two thirds of these febrile episodes can be shown to be infective. Disseminated infection and pneumonia account for about 60% of infections in patients with acute leukemia. In a third of the febrile episodes, the etiology of the fever cannot be identified, but the febrile episode can only occasionally be shown to be noninfectious. The high frequency with which bacteremia is coupled with fever and the relationship of bacteremia to the total granulocyte count are shown in the data drawn from a study by Sickles et al. It should be underscored that the etiology of the febrile episodes were usually established by rigorous and aggressive use of surveillance cultures, serologic techniques, diagnostic procedures, and necropsy. In most institutions, the etiology of the febrile episode cannot be documented with such frequency.

Bacteremic Episodes in Granulocytopenic Patients Undergoing Cancer Therapy as a Function of the Absolute Granulocyte Count and Site of Infection

SITE OF INFECTION	ABSOLUTE GRANULOCYTE COUNT					
	0–100 mm^3		*101–1000 mm^3*		*> 1000 mm^3*	
Pharynx	5/15	(33%)	1/10	(10%)	0/6	(0%)
Skin	4/19	(19%)	1/8	(13%)	2/24	(8%)
Anorectal region	6/13	(46%)	1/5	(20%)	0/3	(0%)
Urinary tract	5/9	(56%)	2/7	(29%)	5/38	(13%)
Lung	23/42	(55%)	7/34	(21%)	10/58	(17%)
Total	43/100	(43%)	12/64	(19%)	17/129	(13%)

Data from Sickles et al. (1975). See Selected References at end of article.

13

The most common offending organisms are gram negative bacilli and include *Klebsiella pneumoniae, E. coli, Pseudomonas aeruginosa,* and the Enterobacter group. These pathogens appear to account for up to 80 per cent of all proven infections and approximately half of those with fatal outcome. The relative attack rate for each particular organism varies among treatment centers.

There is a rising incidence of infections due to resistant organisms such as *Serratia marcescens* and previously unusual gram positive bacilli such as *B. cereus.* Infections with Candida, Aspergillus, and the Phycomycetes group and with *Pneumocystis carinii* and Toxoplasma are increasingly common. The diagnosis and specific therapy for intercurrent infection in patients with acute leukemia are further complicated by the increased susceptibility of these patients to viral infection.

A mortality rate of 20 to 40 per cent from untreated bacterial sepsis may be anticipated in the first 48 hours of infection in the compromised granulocytopenic host. Close observation of temperatures is thus mandatory in the group at risk.

Thus, fever in the granulocytopenic host is associated with a high frequency of bacterial sepsis, a paucity of associated signs of infection, and a rapid and frequent mortality. Consequently, sustained (two or more consecutive) temperatures of greater than 101°F that are not otherwise explicable are an urgent indication for antimicrobial therapy — even in the site-negative, organism-negative patient who is granulocytopenic. After appropriate cultures and clinical evaluation, no less than broad-spectrum coverage for gram negative and gram positive organisms is mandatory. The most commonly employed antibiotic combinations are a cephalosporin and an aminoglycoside, carbenicillin (or ticarcillin) and an aminoglycoside or cephalosporin, or carbenicillin and aminoglycoside. As a specific organism or site of infection emerges, therapy should be tailored to more specific indications.

In patients in whom a specific infective site or organism is identified, the duration of therapy presents less of a dilemma than in the febrile patient who continues to be site-negative, organism-negative for the source of the pyrexia. More than three quarters of this latter group will prove to be apparently antibiotic responsive. Since recrudescence of an underlying infection following premature termination of antibiotics leaves the granulocytopenic patient with a poor prognosis, antibiotics are generally continued for a minimum of 7 to 10 days. The nonresponsive patient who continues to be febrile without an apparent source or identifiable organism represents a difficult therapeutic dilemma. Both the timing of the reassessment of the patient by culture after discontinuing antibiotics and the level of diagnostic intervention must remain individualized. Clearly, it is just such a patient in whom a diagnosis of generalized fungal infection should be considered.

The use of white blood cell transfusions has recently been shown to be efficacious in supporting patients during periods of granulocytopenia and infection and will play an increasing role in supportive care in the ensuing decade. Stringent patient isolation in "life islands" and prophylactic antibiotics directed against enteric pathogens have their advocates but have not seen widespread use.

The measures that may be *routinely* employed in the prevention of infection deserve particular attention. Given the magnitude and seriousness of the problem, these procedures, which are within the scope of each treatment facility, should be rigorously followed (see below).

Selected references: Bodey, G. P., and Rodriguez, V.: Semin. Hematol., *15*:221, 1978; Bodey, G. P., Whitecar, J. P., and Middleman, E.: J.A.M.A., *218*:62, 1971; Gurwith, M. J., Brunton, J. L., Lank, B. A., et al.: Am. J. Med., *64*:121, 1978; Ketchell, S. J., and Rodriguez, V.. Semin. Oncol., *5*:167, 1978; Levine, A. S., Schimpff, S. C., Graw, R. G., and Young, R. C.: Semin. Hematol., *11*:141, 1974; Sickels, E. A., Greene, W. H., and Wiernik, P. H.: Arch. Intern. Med., *135*:715, 1975.

Luria's Law:
Three antibiotics equal one fungal infection.

GENERAL PRINCIPLES OF THE PREVENTION OF INFECTION IN THE GRANULOCYTOPENIC HOST

Reduce acquisition of organisms from the hospital environment.
   Avoid hospitalization when ambulatory care will suffice.
   Avoid crowding in treatment facilities.
   Enforce strict hygiene among physicians, nurses, aides, and other contacts. Handwashing!
   Decrease contacts with nonessential personnel.
   Remove the patient from the general hospital environment at periods of greatest risk (mask and gown isolation, laminar air-flow rooms).

Avoid invasive procedures where possible.
   In-dwelling intravenous or arterial lines or in-dwelling catheters should not be employed except when absolutely necessary.
   Change "butterfly" needles, tubing, and intravenous bottles daily.
   Take scrupulous care of intravenous sites.
   Use oral temperatures whenever possible; avoid rectal administration of medications.
   Use blood and blood products screened for hepatitis-associated antigens.

Reduce numbers of colonizing organisms and sites of colonization.
   Remove or reduce the number of catheters and episodes of venipuncture.

13

Bolster the host defense mechanisms.

Support good personal hygiene and employ preventive medicine in the intervals between therapy (good dental hygiene, remove carious teeth).

Promptly treat intercurrent infections.

Use active antibacterial immunization (pneumococcal vaccine).

Employ passive immunization where appropriate.

Encourage adequate nutrition and exercise.

Improve respiratory toilet.

Treat comorbid disease (e.g., heart failure).

Decrease the patient's time at risk.

Appropriately and aggressively treat the primary disease in such a manner as to avoid the untoward effects of multiple courses of suboptimal therapy.

Adapted from Levine et al. (1974).

RATIONAL USE OF GENTAMICIN

The aminoglycosides are highly effective against a wide range of gram negative bacillary infections. However, they have the lowest ratio of therapeutic to toxic serum concentrations of the most commonly used antibiotics. Therefore, their use must be closely monitored. Since these drugs are excreted almost solely by renal mechanisms, patients with changing or diminished renal function are at an increased risk for toxicity. The following will aid in establishing reasonable dosage schedules for patients with *stable* renal function.

1. *The loading dose* is based on lean body mass and is independent of the patient's renal function.

2. *The estimated maintenance dose* is based on an approximation of the creatinine clearance (which can be estimated from the patient's serum creatinine and the creatinine clearance nomogram) and on the dosage interval chart.

3. The dose calculated from step 2 is used until a more accurate assessment of the patient's creatinine clearance is made from a 24-hour

urine collection. An *adjusted maintenance dose* is then established, based on the measured creatinine clearance and the dosage interval chart.

4. The development of possible renal toxicity should be monitored by measuring the serum creatinine every two or three days while the patient is on therapy.

LOADING DOSE	EXPECTED PEAK SERUM LEVEL BASED UPON ONE-HALF HOUR IV INFUSION
2.0 mg/kg	6 - 8 μg/ml
1.75 mg/kg*	5 - 7 μg/mι
1.5 mg/kg	4 - 6 μg/ml
1.25 mg/kg	3 - 5 μg/ml
1.0 mg/kg	2 - 4 μg/ml

*(Recommended for most moderate to severe systemic infections.)

FIG. 13–1

Gentamicin dosing charts.

PERCENTAGE OF LOADING DOSE REQUIRED FOR DOSAGE INTERVAL SELECTED :			
Cr. Clear.	8 hrs.	12 hrs.	24 hrs.
90	90%	-	-
80	88	-	-
70	84	-	-
60	79	91%	-
50	74	87	-
40	66	80	-
30	57	72	92%
25	51	66	88
20	45	59	83
15	37	50	75
10	29	40	64
7	24	33	55
5	20	28	48
2	14	20	35
0	9	13	25

(Shaded areas indicate suggested dosage intervals)

13

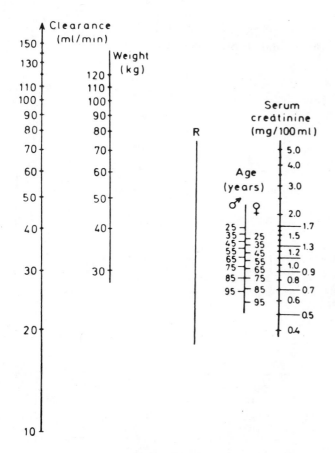

FIG. 13-2

Nomogram for rapid evaluation of endogenous creatinine clearance. With a ruler, join weight to age. Keep ruler at crossing point of line marked "R." Then move the right-hand side of the ruler to the appropriate serum creatinine value and read the patient's clearance from the left side of the nomogram.

Guidelines to the Use of Serum Levels

1. The pharmacokinetics of these aminoglycosides are *extremely unpredictable* in the individual patient and may be further altered by fever, hepatic dysfunction, and the other intercurrent diseases. *Therefore, serum levels should be monitored to assure efficacy and avoid toxicity.*

2. The potential for drug accumulation and toxicity is greatest in patients with changing renal function or severe renal insufficiency (especially creatinine clearances of less than 10 ml/min). Serum levels must be employed in the management of such patients.

References: Hull, H. J., and Sarubbi, F. A.: Ann. Intern. Med., *85*:183, 1976. Fig. 13–1 reproduced with permission of author from Hull, H. J., and Sarubbi, F. A.: Ann. Intern. Med., *85*:188, 1976; Fig. 13–2 reproduced with permission of author and Lancet from Siersbaek-Nielson et al.: Lancet, *1*:1133, 1971.

Tuchman's Rule:

"In assessing the frequency of events from their recorded accounts, Tuchman's rule applies: 'The fact of being reported multiplies the apparent extent of any deplorable development by five to tenfold'."

Barbara Tuchman

DANGER: FALSE POSITIVE GRAM STAIN

The Gram stain is a valuable tool. To avoid errors in its interpretation, a preliminary evaluation of the stained specimen should include:

1. *Assess adequacy of specimen.*
   a. Check for the presence of polymorphonuclear leucocytes, the hallmark of acute bacterial infection.
   b. Check for significant numbers of epithelial or other cell types that may indicate an inadequate specimen.
   c. Check for presence of alveolar macrophages, which may indicate an adequate specimen (sputum).

2. *Assess technical adequacy.*
   a. If the smear is too thick, artifacts, including excessive decolorization, may be present.
   b. Check to see whether the smear is adequately decolorized. Consider the smear properly decolorized if gram positive bacteria are found next to properly decolorized leucocytes (nucleus of the leucocyte must have the color of the *red counter stain;* i.e., the leucocytes are gram negative). If only gram negative organisms are present and there is a concern about excessive decolorization, check the thicker part of the smear, where decolorization may be marginal. Purplish cells will be present. If red-stained bacteria are nearby, this will confirm that these organisms are gram negative and not present because of excessive decolorization.

To insure proper interpretation, the following points are worth emphasizing.

Caveats in Interpretation

1. In acute infections, diagnostic microscopic fields usually contain only one or two types of bacteria near inflammatory cells.
   a. Avoid interpreting minor morphologic variations of a single organism as multiple types of organisms.
   b. Exceptions to this rule include infections that are secondary to contamination from heavily colonized areas (e.g., peritonitis from a ruptured diverticulum).

2. Ignore contaminating flora.
   a. Areas near epithelial cells may abound with varied types of contaminating organisms. These organisms usually constitute the normal flora of the contaminating area (e.g., mouth flora in a sputum specimen).

13

3. Beware of artifacts.
    a. Precipitated crystal violet stain may appear as gram positive organisms.
    b. Old or antibiotic-treated bacteria that are normally gram positive may show variable staining or even appear to be gram negative.
4. Examine the background to avoid missing small organisms.
    a. Hemophilus and Bacteroides are both small, pleomorphic gram negative organisms that may blend into the background.
    b. Nocardia and Actinomyces are weakly gram positive and delicately filamentous. They may be overlooked if you're not careful.
5. Examine several areas of the smear.
    a. Be certain the organism that predominates in one field does so for the entire smear.
6. Identify more than two organisms before making any decisions.
    a. A low concentration of organisms can occur in early or partially treated meningitis.
    b. The study of more than a single smear is usually more productive than an overzealous examination of one.

Despite all precautions, false positive Gram stains occur. That is, organisms will be present on smear, but cultures will be consistently negative. The following circumstances can lead to this type of false positive Gram stain:

1. Use of an unoccluded needle to perform lumbar puncture.
2. Sterile broth and commercial transport media contaminated with nonviable bacteria.
3. Storage of slides in an alcohol bath.
4. Contaminated Gram stain reagents.
5. Use of crystal violet reagent that has precipitated.

References: Ericsson, C. D., Carmichael, M., Pickering, L. K., et al.: South Med. J., *71*: 1524, 1978; Gardner, P., and Provine, H.: Hospital Practice, October 1974; Hoke, H. C., Batt, J. M., Mirrett, S., et al.: J.A.M.A., *241*:478, 1979.

THE BUG AND THE DRUG—A CHECKLIST TO PREVENT ANTIBIOTIC FAILURES

The outcome of the battle between microbial pathogen and host often appears favorable for the pathogen despite what the clinician feels is appropriate antibiotic therapy. By considering the factors listed below, an accurate assessment of why the therapy appears to be failing can be made. An assumption is made that appropriate cultures and sensitivities have been obtained.

The Human Factor

Wrong diagnosis (most common reason for antibiotic failure)
Poor patient compliance
Errors in prescribing and carrying out drug schedules
Contaminated intravenous lines

The Drug Factor

Inadequate dose
Interval between doses too long
Inappropriate route of administration
Incompatability of drugs mixed in intravenous fluids
Interference with gastrointestinal absorption by another drug
Administration of a bacteriostatic drug when a bactericidal drug would be more appropriate
Drug fever
Inadequate drug penetration into sites of infection (e.g., cephalosporins and clindamycin penetrate poorly into the central nervous system)

The Host Factor

Phlebitis at the intravenous site
Abscess in the intramuscular site
Drainage of purulent material required
Debridement of necrotic tissue required
Removal of a foreign body required
Relief of an obstructed passageway required
Coexisting serious disease
Normal variation in the clinical course
Compromised host

The Pathogen Factor

Drug resistance
Superinfection

13

Reference: Gardner, P.: Hospital Practice, *11*:41, 1976.

TREATMENT OF GONORRHEA AND SYPHILIS

Gonorrhea

TYPE	DRUG	DOSE	ALTERNATIVE
Anogenital and urethral	Procaine penicillin G *and* probenecid	4.8 million U IM (total dose) in several sites at one visit. 1 gram orally 15 minutes prior to injection	Spectinomycin (2 grams IM — 1 dose) Tetracycline (1500 mg orally — 1 dose, then 500 mg QID for 4 days) Amoxicillin (3 grams orally) *and* probenecid (1 gram orally) Ampicillin (3.5 grams orally) *and* probenecid (1 gram orally)
Pelvic inflammatory disease Outpatient	Procaine penicillin G *and* probenecid *followed* by ampicillin *or* ampicillin *plus* probenecid *followed* by ampicillin	Same as for anogenital 500 mg orally QID for 10 days 3.5 grams orally (1 dose) 1 gram orally 500 mg orally QID for 10 days	Tetracycline (1500 mg orally — 1 dose, then 500 mg QID for 10 days)
Hospitalized patients	Crystalline penicillin G *followed* by ampicillin	20 million U IV daily until clinical improvement 500 mg orally QID (at least 10 days)	Tetracycline (1500 mg orally — 1 dose, then 500 mg QID for 10 days)
Bacteremia and/or arthritis	Crystalline penicillin G *or* ampicillin *plus* probenecid *followed* by ampicillin	10 million U IV daily for at least 3 days 3.5 grams orally (1 dose) 1 gram orally 500 mg orally QID for at least 7 days	Tetracycline (1500 mg orally — 1 dose, then 500 mg QID for at least 7 days) Erythromycin (500 mg orally QID for 5 days)
Meningitis	Crystalline penicillin G	At least 10 million U IV daily for at least 10 days	
Endocarditis	Crystalline penicillin G	At least 10 million U IV daily for at least 3–4 weeks	
Pharyngitis	Procaine penicillin G *plus* probenecid	Same as for anogenital	

Notes:
1. Patients known to be infected with strains resistant to high levels of penicillin should be given spectinomycin.
2. Pregnant women are treated with the same regimen of penicillin G, amoxicillin, or ampicillin as other patients. For penicillin-allergic pregnant females, erythromycin (not Estolate) is the drug of choice for initial therapy. The failure rate with the use of erythromycin approaches 25 per cent. Follow-up cultures are highly recommended.
3. Alternative therapy for meningitis in penicillin-sensitive individuals involves chloramphenicol.
4. Alternative therapy for endocarditis in penicillin-sensitive individuals may involve either documentation of penicillin sensitivity or use of a cephalosporin.

Syphilis

STAGE	DRUG	DOSE	ALTERNATIVE
Early (primary, secondary, or latent less than a year)	Benzathine penicillin G *or* procaine penicillin G	2.4 million U IM (1 dose) 600,000 U IM daily for 8 days	Tetracycline (500 mg QID for 15 days)
Late (more than one year's duration, cardiovascular)	Benzathine penicillin G *or* procaine penicillin G	2.4 million U IM weekly for 3 doses 600,000 U IM daily for 15 days	Tetracycline (500 mg orally QID for 30 days) Erythromycin (500 mg orally QID for 30 days)
Neurosyphilis	Benzathine penicillin G *or* procaine penicillin G *or* crystalline penicillin G	2.4 million U IM weekly for 3 doses 600,000 U IM daily for 15 days 2 million to 4 million U IV every 4 hr for 10 days	Tetracycline (500 mg orally QID for 30 days) Erythromycin (500 mg orally QID for 30 days)

Reference: The Medical Letter, *19*:105, 1977.

13

GENITAL HERPES

The pattern of herpes simplex infection in humans is changing. In the past, genital herpes was caused by "type 2 virus" and oral herpes by the type 1 virus. Now 20 per cent of genital herpes is caused by type 1 virus. Furthermore, herpetic keratitis and pharyngitis from type 2 virus have begun to appear. Type 1 virus as a cause of neonatal herpes infection is being reported more frequently. Herpetic infection of the hands is now caused by both viral types with equal frequency. Wow!

Currently, there is only symptomatic treatment for active genital herpes. A thin coating of zinc oxide will help prevent irritation by sweat and urine. Steroid creams won't help the lesions but will reduce edema and pain. There is no cure for recurrent herpes (endogenous reinfection or reactivation). One can advise patients about how to prevent dissemination:

1. In the absence of active lesions, no precautions are necessary.
2. Lesions distant from oral or vaginal orifices should be covered with a Band-Aid during sexual relations.
3. For lesions near the vaginal orifice or on penis:
    - With a partner who has no past history of genital herpes, a condom should be used.
    - With a *casual* partner who has had genital herpes, contraceptive foam should be used, and the genitals cleaned with soap and water after sex. Foam is virucidal.
    - With a regular partner who has had genital herpes, no precautions are required (exogenous reinfection is rare).
4. Abstinence.

Reference: Chang, T.: J.A.M.A., *238*:155, 1977.

GENITAL ULCERS

Pity the patient with ulcerative disease of the genital region. Urine, salty sweat, friction, and secondary infection all lead to inflamed, edematous, raw, and tender tissues. Many home remedies may lead to tissue maceration and further inflammation.

A proper physical exam includes the following areas: eyes, mouth, skin, regional lymph nodes, anus and rectum, and possibly the joints and nervous system. The genitals should be cleaned of any ointments or salves prior to examination and culture. The prudent physician will don gloves before performing the genital examination.

Scrapings for Gram stain and swabs for culture should be obtained. In venereal infections it is not uncommon to have more than one disease process occurring simultaneously. The appropriate media (i.e., Thayer-Martin) should be used to culture for gonorrhea; a serologic test for syphilis should be obtained. Look for the elusive painless syphilitic chancre. A not-so-elusive chancre is shown in Figure 13–3.

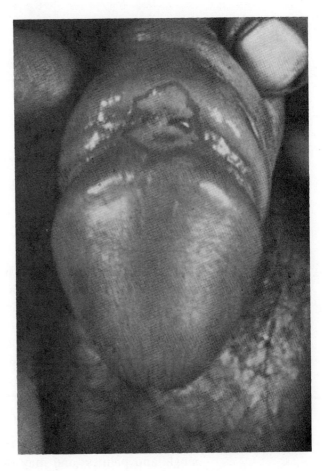

FIG. 13–3

A typical luetic chancre. Note the typical indurated rolled margin. The dark-field examination was positive.

The following are the differential considerations when seeing a patient with genital ulcers.

Reiter's Syndrome

Erosive and exudative plaques can be seen over the scrotum and penis, as well as the more common balanitis circinata of the glans. The triad of conjuctivitis, urethritis, and arthritis with negative cultures suggests this diagnosis.

Bowen's Disease and Queyrat's Erythroplasia

When located on the penis or vulva, they are practically identical, giving a bright red, sharply defined, velvety plaque that looks denuded (but really is not). Regional lymph nodes should be examined for metastases, and a history of arsenic contact should be explored.

13

Carcinoma of the Genitals

Remember, any ulcer or lesion could be a carcinoma, with or without infection. One's suspicions are increased with a lesion that does not heal.

Scabies

One often sees small excoriated papules on the penis or vulva and in the entire genital region. Pruritic lesions in the popliteal fossae, at the waistline, and other sites of pressure, and in the interdigital webs of hands and feet are strongly suggestive of this diagnosis.

Fixed Drug Eruption (Tetracycline)

Tetracycline (in particular) can cause red patches, plaques, and ulcers on the glans penis.

Granuloma Inguinale

The disease starts as a macule that develops into a papule. The surface erodes, presenting a velvety, red, painless granuloma. This exuberant, granulomatous tissue begins on the vulva or glans, later spreads to the shaft or vagina, and then moves to the perianal area. It frequently becomes secondarily infected, producing painful ulcers. The etiologic agents are gram negative, immobile, encapsulated Donovan's bodies.

Syphilis

The chancre is the earliest manifestation of syphilis. It tends to be single and painless and may occur anywhere. However, multiple lesions are not rare. Pain may occur with secondary infection. There is usually one satellite bubo, which is rubbery and painless. A dark-field examination that demonstrates the spirochete is diagnostic in the genital area (but not in the mouth).

Trauma

Ulcers and erosions anywhere in the genital area are frequently the result of trauma. The patient's story to explain the lesion is frequently bizarre, but often true (e.g., a tear from a zipper, dental braces causing abrasion, bites).

Genital Herpes

One sees clusters of eroded vesicles and ulcers on the glans; vesicles and ulcers on the shaft. In the female there may be vesicles on the mucosa of the labia and adjoining skin. These break, forming shallow painful erythematous ulcers. There may be regional lymphadenopathy. The diagnosis is strongly suspected when "giant cells" and inclusion bodies are seen microscopically. The Pap stain will show these details nicely.

Chancroid

This begins as a vesicle-pustule that breaks down rapidly, leaving a shallow, saucer-shaped ulcer with a red margin. It is painful and ragged and develops a grayish odious exudate. Painful bubos are present (usually unilaterally). The causative organism is *H. ducreyi,* a gram negative bacillus seen in "railroad track" double chains on Gram stain.

Behçet's Syndrome

This syndrome is characterized by vulvar, scrotal, and penile ulcers that are well-demarcated and deep. The ulcers heal with scarring. Ulcer recurrences are common. The disease is rare but should be considered when uveitis is combined with oral and genital ulcers. CNS involvement may also be present.

MEDICAL ADVICE FOR TRAVELERS TO FOREIGN COUNTRIES

Physicians may be asked by their patients for recommendations regarding precautions to be taken while traveling in foreign countries, as well as for specific information about immunizations. The physician should inquire about the patient's destination, as immunization requirements vary according to both the country being entered and the place from which the traveler departed.

Diphtheria and tetanus (TD) immunization should be brought up to date. If the person plans to travel to rural areas of developing countries, a booster dose of *trivalent oral polio vaccine* is recommended for those who have completed the primary series. If the traveler has not received the entire primary series, it should be completed according to the recommended schedule.

Smallpox vaccine is necessary only for travel to Somalia (as of 1977) and to countries still requiring an International Certificate of Vaccination as a condition for entry. Most countries requiring a certificate of vaccination will waive the requirement for children under a year old. If a physician believes that vaccination should not be performed for medical reasons, a signed and dated statement of the reasons written on the physician's letterhead will usually suffice to waive the requirement. Skin disorders (such as eczema or other forms of chronic dermatitis), pregnancy, altered immune states (as in leukemia, lymphoma, and dysgammaglobulinemias), immunosuppressive therapy, and radiation are *strong contraindications* to smallpox vaccination.

13

Cholera immunization is not recommended as prophylaxis for travelers heading for countries that do not require the vaccination for entry. Travelers to countries requiring evidence of cholera vaccination should receive *one* injection of the vaccine before leaving the United States.

Yellow fever vaccination is recommended for all travelers to endemic areas in South America and Africa. Several countries in Africa require evidence of vaccination from all entering travelers. A number of countries require certification of vaccination from travelers coming from infected areas. The vaccine must be approved by the World Health Organization and given at a designated yellow fever vaccination center.

Chemoprophylaxis for *malaria* consists of chloroquine phosphate in a dosage of 500 mg (300 mg base) orally once a week beginning a week before arrival in an endemic area. The drug is continued during the stay and for six weeks after departure. Malaria chemoprophylaxis is strongly recommended for travelers to areas where malaria is transmitted. Physicians should contact the Center for Disease Control for the most recent recommendations concerning travel to areas where the chloroquine-resistant *Plasmodium falciparum* is found.

Typhoid vaccination is not required for international travel, but it is recommended for persons who plan to travel or reside in areas of the world that are highly endemic for typhoid.

Serum immune globulin may be recommended for protection against hepatitis A, depending on where the traveler plans to go and how long he will be there. General measures regarding beverages, food, diarrhea, and insects are discussed in several excellent references, including those listed on the opposite page which also provide detailed immunization policies for all countries.

References: Health Information for International Travel — Supplement to MMWR Volume 28, July 1979; Warren, K. S., and Mahmond, A. A. F.: J. Infect. Dis., *133*:596, 1976.

IMMUNOLOGIC TESTS IN THE DIAGNOSIS OF INFECTIOUS ILLNESS

ORGANISM (or disease)	TEST	COMMENT
Streptococcus	Anti–streptolysin O titer	Antibodies to streptolysin O appear approximately 7 days after the onset of acute streptococcal *pharyngitis* in 70–80% of cases. Peak levels are attained 2–4 weeks later and may remain at high titers for weeks to months. A *rising* titer suggests recent infection. One may see a *false positive* reaction with liver disease.
	Streptozyme test	Measures antibodies against *five* streptococcal enzymes. More *sensitive* than the ASO titer, and therefore may be useful in the diagnosis of post-streptococcal glomerulonephritis and acute rheumatic fever.
Staphylococcus aureus	Anti–techoic acid antibody	Identifies patients with bacteremia due to *S. aureus*. May be useful in patients with negative blood cultures due to previous antibiotic therapy.
Pneumococcus	Quellung reaction	Type-specific antibody reacts with the capsule of the Pneumococcus, causing it to swell. Swelling is observed microscopically.
	Counterimmunoelectrophoresis (CIE)	Can be used to evaluate cerebrospinal fluid, blood, and urine. *Less sensitive than culture* for diagnosis of meningitis (85% vs. 55%). Allows one to make the diagnosis *rapidly*.
Neisseria species	Counterimmunoelectrophoresis	Used to diagnose *meningococcal meningitis*. Less sensitive than culture of CSF.
	Latex agglutination test / Microflocculation test / Indirect fluorescent antibody test	All three are used in the attempt to diagnose *N. gonorrhoeae* infection. All have high incidence of false positives and false negatives. Isolation of organism is the only sure way to establish the diagnosis.
Hemophilus influenzae, type B	Counterimmunoelectrophoresis	CSF and blood can be used. Comments are the same as for Pneumococcus and Meningococcus.
Mycoplasma pneumoniae	Cold agglutinins	Fifty per cent of patients with pneumonia secondary to *M. pneumoniae* develop significant titers during second to fourth week of illness. Titers disappear by sixth to eighth week. However, the test is not specific, and the sensitivity is only 50%.

13

TABLE CONTINUES ON FOLLOWING PAGES

ORGANISM (or disease)	TEST	COMMENT
	Complement fixation test	If *paired sera* are obtained during the *acute* and *convalescent phases* of the illness, a rise of fourfold or greater in titer is diagnostic of recent infection. A serum obtained during convalescence with a titer of 1:64 or greater is highly *suggestive of recent* infection.
Syphilis	VDRL RPR Wasserman reaction	All detect a *serum globulin complex, reagin,* induced by infection with the treponeme. May see biologic false positives in (a) febrile illnesses, (b) leprosy, (c) connective tissue diseases, (d) sarcoidosis, and (e) drug addiction. These tests *can be quantified* and used to assess response to therapy. Most patients treated adequately for *primary* syphilis become seronegative. Fewer patients treated adequately for secondary syphilis become seronegative. Many patients with late or latent syphilis remain seropositive despite adequate therapy. The VDRL and RPR are also employed as screening tests for syphilis and to diagnose neurosyphilis (i.e., VDRL or RPR performed on CSF).
	FTA–ABS TPI	Both are more sensitive than the above tests in detecting early, late, and latent syphilis. They are performed if the VDRL or RPR is positive. They remain positive despite adequate therapy.
Salmonella	Widal reaction	Agglutinins against O and H antigens appear at the end of the first week and peak during the third week of infection in Salmonella-induced enteric fever. A fourfold rise or more in the O agglutinin titer in *nonimmunized* individuals *suggests,* but doesn't prove, infection. Cross-reactivity between different Salmonella species is common; therefore, the test lacks specificity.
Legionella pneumophilia	Indirect fluorescent antibody test (IFA)	A fourfold change of titer or a single titer of 1:128 or greater of the IFA test implies recent infection. By six weeks, all persons with recent infection show fourfold increases in titer. Cross-reactivity in patients with tularemia, plague, psittacosis, leptospirosis, and possibly *Mycoplasma pneumoniae* infections may occur.

Organism/Disease	Test	Description
Rickettsia rickettsii (Rocky Mountain spotted fever)	Weil-Felix test	Antibody in serum of patients with Rocky Mountain spotted fever agglutinates a suspension of Proteus OX-19. The antibodies develop *late* in the course of the illness; therefore, the test is used to *confirm* a *suspected diagnosis*, but presumptive diagnosis and institution of therapy are decisions made on clinical grounds.
	Complement fixation test	Early antibiotic therapy may suppress the complement fixation response.
	Indirect hemagglutination test / Indirect fluorescent antibody test	Both may be superior to the complement fixation test.
Histoplasmosis	Complement fixation test	Two types of antigens are used in the tests: (a) the *histoplasmin mycelial antigen* and (b) the *whole yeast antigen*. In *primary pulmonary histoplasmosis*, whole yeast antibody appears 10–21 days after exposure; Histoplasmin *mycelial antibodies* are important in *chronic* disease when yeast antibody titers may be absent. *Mycelial* antibody titers of 1:8 or greater reflect active infection. However, some patients with active disease may have lower *mycelial* titers. Persistent *yeast* antibody titers of 1:32 or greater are a bad prognostic sign. Complement-fixing antibodies are nonspecific and may be observed in patients with blastomycosis or coccidioidomycosis. Skin testing with *mycelial antigen* will cause the complement fixation test to become positive in 10–20% of patients with a positive skin test. The antibody titer induced by skin testing is usually 1:32 or less. Antibodies appear within 15 days of skin testing and may persist for up to 6 months.
	Immunodiffusion	The M and H bands refer to precipitin reactions to *mycelial antigen only*. The *M band* appears *early* in the course of illness and may persist after clinical illness subsides. The M band may become *positive* after *skin testing*. The *H band* is specific for active disease, since it is *not inducible* by *skin testing*.
	Latex agglutination	Latex agglutination is rapid but insensitive. If the latex agglutination test is positive, a complement fixation test should be performed to confirm the diagnosis.
	Skin test	The histoplasmin skin test is *not useful* in helping to make the diagnosis of *active* disease in adults.

TABLE CONTINUES ON FOLLOWING PAGES

13

ORGANISM (or disease)	TEST	COMMENT
Blastomycosis	Complement fixation	The reactions are transient and inconsistent. The sensitivity is poor.
	Agar gel double diffusion	Highly specific.
Aspergillosis	Agar gel diffusion	Precipitins found in almost *100%* of patients with *aspergillomas* and in *65–70%* of patients with *allergic* pulmonary aspergillosis. *Forty per cent* of patients with active pulmonary tuberculosis have a positive precipitin titer. There are no useful serologic tests to help in making the diagnosis of invasive aspergillosis.
Cryptococcosis	India ink of CSF	Too insensitive to exclude the diagnosis if negative. Easy to do and diagnostic if positive.
	Latex agglutination to detect cryptococcal antigen	The test on CSF is rapid and sensitive (*5–15% false negative rate* in patients with cryptococcal meningitis). A *false positive* reaction may occur in patients with *rheumatoid arthritis* or *chronic lymphocytic leukemia*. Hence a rheumatoid factor test should be done on the serum of all patients with a positive latex agglutination test for cryptococcal antigen in their CSF. The latex agglutination test for antigen may be performed on the serum of patients with cryptococcal meningitis.
Coccidioidomycosis		The antigen used for the tests is a culture filtrate of the *mycelial phase* of *Coccidioides immitis.*
	Tube precipitin test	Tube precipitins are highly specific and are useful in acute illness and acute exacerbations of chronic infection. Tube precipitins are positive in almost 80% of patients within two weeks of the onset of symptoms. Tube precipitins decline to zero after 6 months.
	Latex agglutination	Latex agglutination is useful in acute illness and acute exacerbations. It is a rapid and sensitive test but lacks specificity. If positive, an additional test must be done to confirm it.
	Immunodiffusion	The immunodiffusion test is *sensitive* but nonspecific. It becomes positive

	Complement fixation test	This test becomes positive 4–6 weeks after the onset of symptoms. The antibody response peaks at 2–3 months. A complement fixation titer of 1:2 or greater may indicate active disease. In coccidioidal *meningitis*, about 25% of patients have *negative* complement fixation in the CSF and positive tests in the serum.
Candidiasis	Precipitin reaction	The Candida precipitin reaction is very *specific* but is *not sensitive* enough (it is falsely negative in 25-40% of patients with disseminated candidiasis).
	Agglutinating antibody test	Agglutinating antibodies may be found in patients with systemic candidiasis; however, they are also found in patients with superficial candidal infection and in healthy individuals, thereby limiting their diagnostic utility.
Epstein-Barr (E-B) virus	Monospot test	A 4% saline suspension of *formalinized horse red cells serves* as the *antigen.* One drop of the horse cell suspension is added to the patient's serum. Coarse granulation indicates a positive reaction. This test is both *sensitive* and *specific.* The mono spot becomes positive during the first week of illness. Eighty per cent are positive by the third week of illness.
	Heterophile antibody test	Heterophile antibodies are antibodies that agglutinate sheep red cells. Heterophile antibodies may be found in (a) infectious mononucleosis, (b) serum sickness, (c) normal individuals, and (d) other viral illnesses. However, the heterophile antibodies in infectious mononucleosis are *not completely removed* by absorption with *guinea pig kidney;* they are *completely removed* by absorption with *beef red cells.* The heterophile antibodies both in persons with serum sickness and in healthy persons are *completely removed* by absorption with *both guinea pig kidney* and beef red cells. These facts form the basis for the differential heterophile antibody test.
	Epstein-Barr virus titers	The need for E-B virus titers is limited to heterophile and monospot-negative patients. At present, no practical E-B virus test is available to aid in making a prospective diagnosis of Epstein-Barr virus disease.

TABLE CONTINUES ON FOLLOWING PAGES

13

ORGANISM (or disease)	TEST	COMMENT
Rubella	Hemagglutination inhibition test (HI)	The test is employed (a) in the evaluation of *pregnant women* who have been *exposed to rubella*, (b) in the detection of *susceptible women* for the purposes of *vaccination*, and (c) in the *assessment* of the *response to vaccine*. A HI titer of 1:8 or less within 10 days of exposure to rubella indicates susceptibility. A HI titer of more than 1:8 implies *probable* immunity to infection (see below).
		An increase of fourfold or greater in titer indicates a recent infection. *Reinfection* has occurred when there has been at least a fourfold increase in the pre-existing titer. Reinfection is less frequent in those with natural immunity than in those who have been vaccinated; reinfection probably does not occur in those with HI antibody titers of greater than 1:64.
Entamoeba histolytica (amebiasis)	Indirect hemagglutination test	The indirect hemagglutination test is the *most sensitive* of all the tests used in the serologic diagnosis of amebiasis. The test is *positive* in *95%* of patients with *hepatic abscesses* and *85%* with *intestinal amebiasis.* The test is usually *negative* in *asymptomatic cyst passers.*

Toxoplasma gondii	Cellulose acetate diffusion test	This test is used for rapid diagnosis in life-threatening situations.
	Sabin-Feldman dye test	The organism is stained by methylene blue dye *except* when it has been previously exposed to antitoxoplasmosis antibodies. The test is specific but expensive and potentially dangerous to laboratory personnel, as the test requires the use of live organisms. Dye test antibodies persist for many years. An elevated dye test titer (1:256 or greater) and a negative complement fixation test suggest either recently acquired infection or the residua of a previous infection (see below).
	Complement fixation antibody test	Complement fixation antibodies are slower to develop than dye antibodies and disappear more rapidly.
	Indirect hemagglutination test (IH)	The IH test is specific but time-consuming. The IH titers often parallel the dye test.
	Indirect fluorescent antibody test (IFA)	The IFA test is both specific and sensitive. IgM fluorescent antibodies appear in the first week of infection and reach a peak within 3–4 weeks. A titer of greater than 1:80 or a twofold increase in the IgM antibody titer implies active or recent infection.

References: Weinstein, A. J., and Farkas, S.: Med. Clin. North Am., *62:*1099, 1978; Sanford, J. P.: N. Engl. J. Med., *300:*654, 1979.

13

LESS USUAL MANIFESTATIONS OF INFECTIOUS MONONUCLEOSIS

Although the typical signs and symptoms of infectious mono-nucleosis are familiar to the clinician, there are a number of unusual clinical features of the disease that are not as well appreciated. You should be on the alert for the complications listed below when treating a patient with infectious mononucleosis.

Respiratory Complications

Airway obstruction (dramatic relief with steroids)
Interstitial pneumonitis
Pleural effusion

Cardiac Complications

ECG abnormalities (prolonged PR interval and repolarization abnormalities)
Pericarditis
Myocarditis

Hepatic Dysfunction

Abnormal liver function tests (common)
Hepatic necrosis (very rare)

Glomerulonephritis

(Immunologic, not related to associated streptococcal pharyngitis)

Splenic Rupture

Hematologic Complications

Hemolytic anemia (anti-i antigen)
Thrombocytopenia (may be severe)
Neutropenia

Neurologic Complications

Aseptic meningitis (approximately 25 per cent of patients will have spinal fluid abnormalities without clinical meningitis)
Encephalitis
Meningoencephalitis
Acute cerebellar syndrome
Cranial neuropathies

Transverse myelitis
Peripheral neuropathies
Guillain-Barre syndrome (may be descending)
Psychiatric disturbances

Although many of these complications are potentially serious and very disturbing to both the patient and the clinician, it is important to realize that in almost all cases they resolve without lasting damage. Most of these complications respond dramatically to therapy with corticosteroids.

THE BAND-AID BOX

Wide-eyed and frightened, they appear with white knuckles clutching the metal Band-Aid box. Their gaze is intense and expectant.
You suspect what is in the box without having them tell.
"Is it alive?" you ask phlegmatically.
Frequently residents of the Band-Aid box include the following:

Crab Lice (Phthirus pubis)

This small (1 mm), round, reddish-brown louse causes itching. Transmission is by close personal contact. On close examination, the crab louse is found in the pubic area with its head buried in a hair follicle or clutching two adjacent hairs. The dark nits are frequently difficult to find. Crabs may infest the chest and axillary hair *as well as the eyelashes. Treatment:* 25 per cent benzyl benzoate or gamma benzene hexachloride on two successive days. Infested eyelashes are treated with daily applications of yellow oxide of mercury.

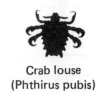

Crab louse
(Phthirus pubis)

Scalp Lice (Pediculus humanus var. capitis)

This long (up to 4 mm), slender, white louse causes pruritus and excoriations with frequent secondary infection. The densest involvement is posteriorly, behind the ears. There may be tender occipital nodes as well as excoriated bites on the neck and shoulders. You may not find the adult louse, but the small white nits glued to hair shafts are obvious. Nits fluoresce under Wood's light. *Treatment:* Gamma benzene hexachloride shampoo for two days, repeated in a week. Comb out nits with a fine-toothed comb.

13

Head or body louse
(Pediculus humanus
var. capitis or corporis

Body Lice (Pediculus humanus var. corporis)

The adult louse is 1 to 4 mm long and lives, loves, and lays eggs (nits) in the seams of clothing. This louse feeds on the body, leaving an urticarial wheal with a hemorrhagic central punctum.

Examination of the skin reveals parallel linear excoriations that are often secondarily infected. *Treatment:* Thorough laundering of clothes and bedding. Iron all seams. Bedding and clothing may be dusted with 10 per cent DDT powder.

Pinworms (Enterobius vermicularis)

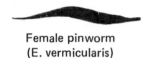

Female pinworm
(E. vermicularis)

The patient may find small white worms at the anal orifice in the early morning hours. Infestation produces intense perianal pruritus, which leads to excoriations, lichenification and infection. Bruxism and nightmares are common. The diagnosis is usually made by identifying ova on transparent tape that has been pressed to perianal skin at bedtime. *Treatment:* Pyrvinium pamoate (Povan, Vanquin), 50 mg or 5 mg/kg as a single dose, or piperazine citrate 65 mg/kg for 8 days. The Medical Letter has recently recommended pyrantel pamoate (Banminth) (11 mg/kg) as a single oral dose therapy.

Maggots (Fly Larvae)

Maggot

Rarely, maggots will be picked from an open sore, the nose, or ear canal or from the stool.

Fish Tapeworm (Diphyllobothrium latum)

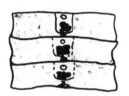

Fish tapeworm
(D. latum)

This is a very large cestode that produces enormous numbers of yellowish eggs. It has been an occupational disease of Jewish housewives who taste raw ground fish to check seasoning when making gefilte fish. Thus, its incidence may be decreasing (at least in this population). Immobile white flat segments may be found in the stool. Treatment is with niclosamide, 2 grams orally in a single dose. The tablets should be chewed thoroughly.

Beef Tapeworm (Taenia saginata)

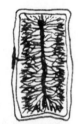

Beef tapeworm
(T. saginata)

Gravid, white, mobile segments of this worm may be passed in the stool. *Treatment:* Quinacrine, 200 mg every 5 to 10 minutes for four dosages, on an empty stomach. This is followed by a magnesium sulfate purge two to four hours later. Niclosamide, 2 grams p.o., may also be employed.

Roundworm (Ascaris lumbricoides)

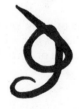

Roundworm
(A. lumbricoides)

Ascaris lumbricoides is characterized by an elongated, cylindrical, nonsegmented, translucent, flesh-colored body 15 to 35 cm long. A cosmopolitan worm, ascaris infects 25 per cent of the world's population. One or more worms may be passed in the stool or, less frequently, vomited. Worms have been known to crawl out of the nose, ear, and umbilical fissures! *Treatment:* Piperazine citrate syrup 3 to 4 grams,

(30 to 40 ml) one time only. Pyrantel pamoate may also be employed as single-dose therapy (11 mg/kg with a 1 gram maximum dose).

Debris

Vegetable particles, such as seeds (corn), stems, and celery, and other debris, like dirt, gravel, stringy fuzz, and cellophane, can be swollen and decolored by passage through the alimentary canal. Even a normal person would be alarmed, and the person with parasitophobia will be in panic! *Treatment:* Show the patient the characteristics of the debris by hand lens or dissecting microscope.

Miscellaneous

Products of conception, menstrual blood clots thought to be products of conception, "grape-like bodies" of hydatidiform mole, fragments of tampons, and clotted mucus and blood from cystitis have all made it to the Band-Aid box.

LEGION AND LYME

Contemporary epidemiology usually gets little "ink" in either the medical literature or the lay press. In the past few years, however, description of two new disease entities — Legionnaire's disease and Lyme arthritis — has generated new respect for physicians practicing the subspecialty of medical detective.

Legionnaire's Disease

During July 1976, 147 patients were hospitalized in Pennsylvania hospitals with an acute respiratory syndrome. Twenty-nine of these patients died (20 per cent). All the patients had attended an American Legion convention held in a Philadelphia hotel between July 21 and 24, 1976. Hence the name Legionnaire's disease.

Since that time, a gram negative bacillus has been isolated and serologically identified as the cause of the epidemic. It has been named *Legionella pneumophilia.* This organism has been shown to be the cause of outbreaks of pneumonia in Washington, D.C. (1965), Nottingham, England (1977), and Spain (1977). Cases from all over the United States have now been reported. As more information is acquired, it appears that *L. pneumophilia* is the cause of a significant number of cases of acute pneumonia, particularly in immunosuppressed patients. The complete clinical spectrum of disease caused by *L. pneumophilia* is still being defined.

13

Lyme Arthritis

In July 1975, a concerned mother telephoned the Connecticut State Health Department about an inordinate number of cases of what appeared to be juvenile rheumatoid arthritis occurring in Lyme, Conn. After several other patients were brought to the attention of investigators at Yale University Medical Center, an epidemiologic survey was undertaken. The results indicated an epidemic of a peculiar kind of oligoarticular arthritis was clustered in three adjacent southern Connecticut townships. Most of the attacks of arthritis occurred between May and September, and many of the patients remembered being bitten by a tick. Thus Lyme arthritis was born.

The disease occurs in the spring and summer months. A tick is thought to be the disease vector, although a causative organism has not yet been identified. Lyme arthritis has been reported in Connecticut, Rhode Island, Massachusetts, New York, and Wisconsin. The arthritis is preceded by a skin eruption known as *erythema chronicum migrans* (ECM) in more than half the cases. ECM begins as a small indurated red spot and eventually becomes a ring of red skin surrounding the initial lesion. The skin is hot to the touch but is usually neither tender nor pruritic.

The skin lesion *precedes* the development of oligoarticular arthritis by an average of four weeks. The knee, shoulder, elbow, temporomandibular area, ankle, wrist, and hip are the most commonly involved joints (in the order given). The arthritis lasts seven to nine days and then remits, only to recur in many of the patients at a later time without a second skin rash.

The systemic nature of the illness is illustrated by the frequent occurrence of neurologic abnormalities and cardiac conduction disturbances. Cryoglobulins are present in the serum during the active phases of both the rash and the arthritis. Other serologic tests are usually normal. The joint fluid has an inflammatory profile. Therapy is symptomatic and usually involves administration of salicylate, glucocorticoid, or both.

References: Fraser, D. W., Tsai, T. R., and Orenstein, W.: N. Engl. J. Med., *297*:1189, 1977: Center for Disease Control, International Symposium on Legionnaire's Disease: Ann. Intern. Med., *90*:491–707, 1979; Steere, A. C., Hardin, J. A., and Malawista, S. E.: Hospital Practice, *13*:143, 1978.

14

RHEUMATOLOGY

QUICK DIFFERENTIAL DIAGNOSIS OF POLYARTHRITIS

DISEASE	CLINICAL CLUE	LAB OR X-RAY
Rheumatoid arthritis	Morning stiffness. Symmetrical small joint involvement. Systemic involvement: lung and skin nodules, fevers, anemia, weakness, pleural effusions.	Positive rheumatoid factor in more than 75% of patients. Extremely low glucose in pleural effusions.
Rheumatic fever	Migratory arthritis, carditis, little soft tissue swelling, erythema marginatum, chorea, subcutaneous nodules, fever.	Antistreptolysin "O" titer. Electrocardiogram: prolonged P-R interval, premature beats.
Sarcoidosis	Ankle involvement, erythema nodosum, very little fever. Skin plaques and papules.	Paratracheal and hilar adenopathy. Restrictive pattern on pulmonary function tests. Synovial biopsy may be positive.
Gonococcal arthritis	Genital, throat, or rectal infection. Polyarticular becoming monoarticular; pustular, purpuric rash.	Urethral smear probably shows gram negative diplococci intracellularly. Joint culture positive in 40% to 75% of cases.
Reiter's syndrome	Urethritis, conjunctivitis, knee joint and back involvement, heel pain, mouth ulcers, buccal rash, rash of palms and soles.	Negative cultures. Pekin cells (giant macrophages that ingest polys) in joint fluid. High joint fluid complement.
Systemic lupus erythematosus	Rash, multisystem involvement, nondeforming arthritis. History of use of certain drugs.*	Positive ANA and LE prep, low serum complement, positive skin biopsy.
Vasculitis	Neuropathy, palpable (raised) purpura.	Positive skin biopsy. Renal involvement.
Polymyositis	Proximal muscle weakness. Similar to rheumatoid arthritis.	Elevated muscle enzymes.
Inflammatory bowel disease	Diarrhea. Sacroileitis, aortic insufficiency.	Barium enema. Upper GI series.
Viral	Mumps, hepatitis, rubella (or immunization).	SGOT, HAA, viral titers.
Osteoarthropathy	Clubbing.	Chest x ray. Periostitis of forearms.
Gout	Tophi, podagra.	Sodium urate joint crystals. Elevated serum uric acid (sometimes).
Pseudogout	Large joint involvement. History of trauma, hyperparathyroidism, degenerative joint disease, ochronosis, diabetes mellitus, hemochromatosis, Wilson's disease, hypercalcemia, and even gout.	Calcium pyrophosphate joint crystals. Chondrocalcinosis. X-rays show linear calcifications in joint space.
Serum sickness	Rash. Injection or infusion of drugs, blood products, or serum.	Decreased serum complement but often normal sedimentation rate.
Malignancy	—	X-ray of bones, chest. Examination of peripheral smear. White blood count.

*See Drug-Induced Lupus, p. 518.

14

HOW TO HANDLE JOINT FLUID

The following procedure will allow efficient and correct processing of aspirated joint fluid.

1. Aspirate the joint fluid into a *sterile heparinized* syringe (0.5 ml of heparin is drawn into the syringe and the syringe is coated; the heparin is then squirted out of the syringe).

2. The aspirated fluid is then placed into the following tubes:

Tube 1 — *A plain tube* (red top)

Fluid in this tube is used for the *gross exam* (i.e., *viscosity, color,* and *clarity*) and to determine the stability of the *mucin clot.*

Tube 2 — *An anticoagulated tube* (EDTA, heparin, or citrate; it is *not* an *oxalate* tube, as this may cause precipitation of calcium oxalate crystals)

Fluid in this tube is used for *cell counts* and *differential* (use *saline* to *dilute* the joint fluid for the cell counts, not acetic acid; acetic acid may produce a mucin clot) and for examination under *polarized light.*

Tube 3 — *An anticoagulated tube* (*not* an *oxalate* tube)

Fluid in this tube is "spun down," and the supernatant is used for chemistry determinations (e.g., glucose, LDH, rheumatoid factor, ANA, immunoglobulins, immunoelectrophoresis, complement). Simultaneous serum chemistries should also be drawn.

Tube 4 — A plain *sterile* tube

Fluid in this tube is used for *microbiological* studies. These should include gram stain, acid fast stain, fungal stain, and cultures for aerobic bacteria, anerobic bacteria, acid fast bacilli, and fungi. Cultures for the gonococcus should be done at the bedside directly into Thayer-Martin media.

EXAMINATION OF SYNOVIAL FLUID AS A DIAGNOSTIC AID IN ARTHRITIS

The precise diagnosis of the cause of arthritis can usually be made by a careful history, a clinical examination, synovial fluid analysis, and a few serologic tests. A joint effusion must be aspirated with strict sterile technique. After noting the appearance of the joint fluid, you can estimate viscosity by placing a drop of the fluid between your thumb and index finger, slowly separating the fingers, and estimating the length of the "string." Normally viscous fluid will give a "string test" of approximately 3 cm.

To check the mucin clot, mix 1 ml of joint fluid with 1 ml of 2 per cent acetic acid. Mix the two gently by agitation. A normal mucin clot is seen as a tight white ball in the test tube. To do the cell count, mix the fluid with EDTA or saline. A drop of fluid placed on a glass slide with a cover slip can be examined for cartilage debris, inclusion cells, other special features mentioned in the following chart, and crystals (through a polarized microscope). Fluid should always be sent for culture. The remaining fluid can be tested for joint complement level, glucose, protein, antinuclear antibody levels, and rheumatoid factor (see table on following page).

14

Synovial Fluid Analysis

DISEASE	APPEARANCE	VISCOSITY	MUCIN CLOT	APPROXIMATE OR AVERAGE WHITE CELL COUNT (per cu mm)	CRYSTALS	CARTILAGE DEBRIS	SERUM COMPLEMENT	JOINT COMPLEMENT	SPECIAL FEATURES
Normal	Straw, clear	Normal to high	Good (firm)	200–600	0	0	Normal	Normal	None.
Traumatic and villonodular synovitis	Cloudy, bloody	Normal	Good	2000	0	Variable	Normal	Normal	Many red cells.
Serum sickness	Yellow, slightly cloudy	Low to normal	Fair	20,000 75% PMN*	0	Variable	Low	Low to normal	1–2 weeks after serum injected. ESR may be low.
Osteoarthritis and Charcot joint	Yellow, clear	Normal	Good	1000 20% PMN	0	Fragments fibrils	Normal	Normal	None.
Rheumatic fever	Yellow, slightly cloudy	Low	Fair to good	10,000 50% PMN	0	0	Normal	Normal	Glucose >25 mg/100 ml; a few inclusion body cells.
Systemic lupus erythematosus	Yellow, slightly cloudy	Normal	Good	3000 10% PMN	0	0	Low	Low	Lupus erythematosus cells on smear; fluid antinuclear antibodies positive. A few inclusion body cells, glucose >25 mg/100 ml.
Gouty arthritis	Yellow, cloudy	Low	Poor	10,000 75% PMN	Many (urate)	0	Normal	Normal to high	Glucose >25 mg/100 ml, crystals free or intracellular (appear yellow if parallel to polarized light).
Pseudogout	Yellow, slightly cloudy	Normal to low	Good	6000 75% PMN	Few to many—calcium pyrophosphate	Variable	Normal	Normal	Crystals in cells, free, or in cartilage fragments. Weakly positive birefringence (appear blue if parallel to polarized light).
Juvenile rheumatoid arthritis	Yellow, cloudy	Normal to low	Poor to fair	10,000 75% PMN	0	0	Normal	Normal	Glucose >25 mg/100 ml.
Rheumatoid arthritis	Yellow to greenish, cloudy	Low	Poor	8000–40,000 70% PMN	Rare (cholesterol)	0	Normal to increased	Low	5–95% of PMN show inclusions. Glucose >25 mg/100 ml. Rheumatoid factor of fluid positive.
Reiter's syndrome	Yellow, turbid	Normal	Very good	20,000	0	0	Acutely low, later elevated	Normal to high	Pekin cells present (giant macrophages containing ingested PMN).
Tuberculous arthritis	Yellow, cloudy	Low	Poor to fair	15,000 40–50% PMN	0	0	–	–	Acid-fast smear positive in 25%; culture positive in 80%; biopsy positive in 90%. Glucose low, usually <35 mg/100 ml. Protein elevated; rheumatoid factor negative.
Septic arthritis	Grayish to bloody	Low	Poor	80,000 90% PMN	0	0	–	Normal to high	Rheumatoid factor negative; culture positive. Glucose <25 mg/100 ml. Inclusion body cells are present.
Post-septic arthritis	Yellow, cloudy	Low to normal	Fair	10,000–30,000 75% PMN	0	0	Low	Low	Synovial biopsy looks like rheumatoid arthritis. Glucose >25 mg/100 ml. Cultures negative. Usually follows pneumococcus or meningococcus.

*PMN = polymorphonuclear leukocyte.

MANAGEMENT OF RHEUMATOID ARTHRITIS FOR THE NONRHEUMATOLOGIST

Rheumatoid arthritis occurs in 1 to 2 per cent of the population. Management of a patient with rheumatoid arthritis requires a multi-faceted approach. The physician must educate his patient as to the nature of the disease. Reassurance that only a minority (approximately 15 per cent) of patients with rheumatoid arthritis progress to severe crippling disease is essential. Patients with high titers of rheumatoid factor, multiple rheumatoid nodules, or vasculitis or those who have had rapid progression in the past are most likely to have the most trouble with the disease.

An accurate assessment of disease activity should be made so the effects of therapy can be evaluated (see accompanying table). The therapy of rheumatoid arthritis aims at reducing pain and inflammation while maintaining as much joint function and muscle strength as possible. Three modalities are used through all periods of disease activity — rest, physiotherapy, and drugs.

Disease Activity

	MILD	MODERATE	SEVERE
Number of hours of morning stiffness	0	1.5	>5
Number of painful joints	<2	12	>34
Number of swollen joints	0	7	>23
Grip strength (mm Hg): male	>250	140	<55
female	>180	100	<45
Time to walk 50 feet (sec)	<9	13	>27
Erythrocyte sedimentation rate (mm/hr)	<11	41	>92

Rest

- Most patients with active disease will require periods of rest during the day.
- Joint rest may occasionally allow synovitis to regress more rapidly.

Physiotherapy

- Aims at relieving muscle spasm and pain, allowing each joint to go through a full range of motion, and facilitating muscle-strengthening exercises.

14

Drugs

Aspirin (the drug of choice for initiating therapy)
— Begin with 900 to 1000 mg QID.
— Appropriate dose depends on the course of the disease and the disease activity, symptoms of salicylate intolerance (tinnitus or dyspepsia), and the serum level achieved.
— Aim for a salicylate concentration of 18 to 20 mg/100 ml just prior to the next dose.
— Once a tolerated, effective dose level is found, the drug is continued at that level.
— In early rheumatoid arthritis, use salicylate exclusively for at least three months.

Newer anti-inflammatory agents (fenoprofen, ibuprofen, indomethacin, naproxen, tolmetin)
— If the patient cannot maintain or tolerate adequate salicylate blood levels, one of the newer anti-inflammatory agents may be added to the salicylate or substituted for it. Drug interactions due to displacement from albumin binding sites may alter blood levels when combined therapy is employed.

Gold therapy
— To be initiated in patients not responding to the anti-inflammatory agents.

Antimalarial drugs
— To be initiated in patients not responding to the anti-inflammatory agents.

Glucocorticoids
— Because of the chronic nature of the disease and the adverse metabolic consequences of long-term glucocorticoid therapy, these agents have a limited role in the management of rheumatoid arthritis.
— Some physicians use glucocorticoids in patients threatened with the loss of either the ability to perform necessary household tasks or their occupation while waiting for a response from the slower-acting drugs (i.e., gold, antimalarials).

Other

— Intra-articular steroid instillation may prove helpful in a problem joint.
— Consider DL-penicillamine.

Literature for Patients with Rheumatoid Arthritis

Bland, J. H.: Arthritis: Medical Treatment and Home Care (paperback edition). New York, Collier Books, 1962.

Blau, S. P., and Schultz, D.: Arthritis. Garden City, N.Y., Doubleday and Company, Inc., 1974.

Corrigan, A. B.: Living with Arthritis. New York, Grosset and Dunlap, 1971.

Crain, D. C.: The Arthritis Handbook. Jerricho, N.Y., Exposition Press, Inc., 1971.

Healey, L. A., Wilske, K. R., and Hansen, B. H.: Beyond the Copper Bracelet: What You Should Know About Arthritis (2nd Edition). Bowie, Md., The Charles Press, 1977.

Pamphlets available from the Arthritis Foundation:

Home Care Programs in Arthritis: A Manual for Patients.

Self-Help Manual for Arthritis Patients.

Reference: Decker, J. L.: Resident and Staff Physician, August 1978, p. 50.

> *Gout* — Derives from the ancient Latin *gutta*, which means "drop." The ancients thought (correctly it seems) that noxious matter dropped from the blood stream and settled in the joint, causing the swelling and pain.

MANAGEMENT OF GOUTY ARTHRITIS

Successful management of acute gouty arthritis requires a correct diagnosis. The demonstration of *needle-shaped monosodium urate crystals* in polymorphonuclear leucocytes in the fluid aspirated from an affected joint makes gout certain. Joint fluid aspiration also allows you to culture the fluid, thus helping to exclude pyogenic infection as a cause for the arthritis.

When joint fluid is not available, certain clues will allow a high index of suspicion for acute gout:

a. Abrupt onset of monoarticular or pauciarticular arthritis in a man 30 to 50 years old.

b. Positive family history of gout.

c. History of hyperuricemia.

d. Presence of hyperuricemia at the time of the attack (need not have hyperuricemia during the acute attack).

e. Rapid lowering of the serum uric acid following the use of uric acid–lowering agents.

Seventy-five per cent of patients with acute gout will respond to colchicine, as compared to only 5 per cent of patients with other ar-

14

thritic disorders. Thus, a beneficial response to colchicine is highly suggestive of acute gouty arthritis. Joints which have been frequently involved respond less promptly.

Drugs used in the treatment of gout are listed below.

Drugs to Suppress Acute Symptoms

Colchicine
- Also used as prophylaxis against recurrent attacks.
- 0.64 mg (1 tablet) orally every hour until:
  a. Relief of symptoms occurs.
  b. Diarrhea occurs
  c. A total dose of 10 to 12 mg is reached.
- One to two tablets daily after the acute attack subsides, to prevent recurrent attacks.
- May be given intravenously during an acute attack to avoid the gastrointestinal side effects.
  a. Mix 1 to 2 mg in 30 ml normal saline and administer over 30 minutes.
  b. May give a maximum of 5 mg in 24 hours.
  c. Care must be taken *to prevent extravasation of the drug,* as severe tissue necrosis may ensue.

Indomethacin
Initial dose of 50 mg, then 50 mg every six hours for two to three days, then taper quickly.

Phenylbutazone
- Initial dose of 200 mg, then 200 mg every six hours for two to three days, then taper quickly.

Fenoprofen
- Initial dose of 600 to 800 mg, then 800 mg every six hours for 24 hours, then taper.

Naproxen
- Initial dose of 750 mg, then 750 mg every 12 hours for two days, then stop.

Morphine
- In adequate doses.

Uric Acid—Lowering Agents

Probenecid
- A uricosuric agent whose sole use is to obtain and maintain a normal serum uric acid level in patients with a history of acute gout.
- Contraindicated in patients:
  a. Allergic to the drug.
  b. Having underlying renal disease.

    c. Having uric acid nephrolithiasis.

    d. Having hematologic disorders requiring administration of a xanthine oxidase inhibitor prior to chemotherapy.

    e. Having severe tophaceous gout with large pools of excess urate.

— Initial dose is 500 mg BID. The dose is titrated to keep the serum uric acid in the normal range. The total dose is usually less than 3 grams daily.

Sulfinpyrazone

— A uricosuric agent.

— Initial dose is 100 to 200 mg BID. The dose is titrated to keep the serum uric acid in the normal range. The total dose is usually 400 to 800 mg daily.

Allopurinol

— A xanthine oxidase inhibitor used to obtain and maintain a normal serum uric acid level.

— Initial dose is 300 mg administered once daily.

— The maintenance dose is usually 100 to 300 mg daily.

— Doses of 600 or 900 mg daily may be used to control drastic elevations of serum uric acid (e.g., prior to therapy of hematologic malignancies).

Reference: Klineberg, J. R.: Med. Clin. North Am., *61*:299, 1977.

SATURNINE GOUT

Saturnine gout is a uric acid arthropathy, arising as a consequence of the chronic hyperuricemia induced by lead nephropathy. Analysis of uric acid production in patients with this malady has established that production of uric acid and the uric acid pool are not significantly elevated. There appears to be a decrement in the clearance of uric acid in excess of what might be anticipated from the mild decrease in glomerular filtration rate. An interference in the tubular transport of uric acid induced by the heavy metal poisoning is thereby suggested. Patients with saturnine gout are characteristically nonazotemic initially. The chronicity of the exposure to lead-induced hyperuricemia has been invoked as the cause of the crystal-induced synovitis.

In Australia, lead nephropathy and the development of saturnine gout have been linked to the ingestion of leaded paint by children. In 1967, 37 of 43 patients admitted to the Birmingham, Alabama, Veterans Administration Hospital with acute gout were found to have gout related to lead intoxication. Patients typically had a history of long exposure to moonshine whiskey (auto battery casings are often used in the still), lacked a family history of gout, were mildly hypertensive and anemic, and had elevated urinary lead levels. Renal biopsies

14

revealed interstitial fibrosis and degenerating proximal tubular cells containing intranuclear inclusions characteristic of lead nephropathy. Consequently, physicians related the epidemic of saturnine gout to chronic moonshine ingestion.

Reference: Ball, G. V., and Sorensen, L. B.: New Engl. J. Med., *280*:1199, 1969.

MANAGEMENT OF BACTERIAL (NONGONOCOCCAL) JOINT SPACE INFECTION IN THE ADULT

Preservation of joint function and eradication of infection are the therapeutic goals in treating the patient with a septic joint. The following is offered as a guide to aid in the management of the patient with an infected joint.

I. Suspect joint infection
    1. Suspect joint infection in anyone with fever, chills, joint pain, joint tenderness and swelling, and decreased range of motion caused by joint pain. Systemic manifestations may be missing (i.e., fever, chills).
    2. Factors that predispose to joint infections:
        a. Any condition associated with *bacteremia* (chronically ill debilitated patients; patients with diabetes mellitus; alcoholics, intravenous drug abusers; granulocytopenic patients).
        b. Rheumatoid arthritis.
        c. Previous intra-articular steroid injection.
    3. Joint fluid aspiration *must* be performed in anyone suspected of having an infected joint.
    4. Search for a primary site of infection. Most joint infection results from hematogenous dissemination (e.g., soft tissue abscesses, pneumonia, urinary tract infection).
    5. X-ray the joint to exclude osteomyelitis and to provide a baseline for future comparison.
II. Antibiotics
    1. The *initial* choice of antibiotic(s) depends on:
        a. The results of the gram stain (e.g., gram positive cocci, gram negative rods).
        b. If the gram stain does not reveal an organism, and an organism is not recovered from a primary site, coverage against *both S. aureus* and the aerobic *gram negative bacilli* should be instituted in patients predisposed to bacteremia.
    2. Subsequent decisions regarding antibiotics should be made

after the organism and the sensitivities are known. The clinical response of the patient and the improvement in the joint fluid will also be factors in helping to determine subsequent decisions regarding antibiotics.

3. The organisms (excluding the Gonococcus) most likely to cause joint sepsis are:
    a. Gram positive cocci — 75 per cent (*S. aureus,* Streptococcus, pneumococcus).
    b. Gram negative bacilli — 25 per cent (usually aerobic).

4. Antibiotics should be administered parenterally for the first two to four weeks; subsequent antibiotics can be administered orally for an additional four to six weeks.

5. Intra-articular antibiotics should not be given, as antibiotic levels in the joint space are adequate when the antibiotics are given IM or IV; also, intra-articular antibiotics may incite joint inflammation, causing additional joint destruction.

III. Supportive care

1. Joint aspiration initially is performed *daily* to assess joint fluid improvement that occurs prior to the clinical response.

2. An improvement in the joint fluid is manifested by a *rise in glucose concentration, a fall in the volume, white blood count, and LDH,* and a conversion to a *sterile effusion.*

3. Aspiration is repeated as often as is necessary to *prevent rapid reaccumulation of fluid.* Excessive pressure on the synovium from fluid enhances joint destruction.

4. *Closed drainage* (i.e., repeat aspirations through a syringe) is the *preferred* method of drainage *except:*
    a. When intra-articular adhesions cause loculation of pus and prevent adequate aspiration.
    b. When the joint sepsis involves the *hip,* because closed drainage is very difficult.

5. Immobilization of the affected joint is not necessary; however, no weight bearing should be allowed until all the signs of inflammation have subsided.

6. *Passive range of motion* of the joint should begin after therapy has started and the joint fluid shows improvement.

7. *Active range of motion* exercises can be started when the signs and symptoms of inflammation have subsided.

8. Adequate analgesics in the form of *non–anti-inflammatory agents* should be used. This will allow better evaluation of the clinical response to therapy.

IV. Monitor response

1. Both the clinical response and the joint fluid analysis are used to monitor the response to therapy.

2. X-ray of the joint should be obtained every two weeks during the period of hospitalization.

14

    3. Prior to discharge the joint should be evaluated for:
      a. Swelling.
      b. Range of motion.
      c. Joint stability.
    4. After discharge, the patient should be followed for an additional three to six months, and the same joint examination should be performed each visit. X-rays of the joint are also taken at each visit.

V. Prognosis
    1. The outcome depends on three factors:
      a. The duration of infection prior to the institution of therapy. If *greater than one week,* the patient is less likely to recover with normal joint function.
      b. The virulence of the infecting organism; i.e., *S. aureus* and gram negative bacilli are more likely to result in significant morbidity than are the pneumococcus and Streptococcus.
      c. The severity of the patient's associated disease(s).

References: Ward, J. R., and Atcheson, S. G.: Med. Clin. North Am., *61*:313, 1977; Goldenberg, D. L., and Cohen, A. S.: Am. J. Med., *60*:369, 1976; Schmid, F. R.: Resident and Staff Physician, December, 1978, p. 76.

Herbert's Homily:
The only thing I know that is autoimmune is the local drunk who staggers across the street to the bar three times a day and doesn't get hit by a car.

PREVALENCE OF DIAGNOSTIC CRITERIA FOR SYSTEMIC LUPUS ERYTHEMATOSUS

Ideal diagnostic criteria are absolutely sensitive (all patients with the disease exhibit the sign) and absolutely specific (the finding is never present in any patient without the disease). Few such ideal criteria exist in clinical medicine. Usually the more specific a criterion, the less sensitive it proves to be (and vice versa). In establishing criteria for the diagnosis of systemic lupus erythematosus (SLE), 74 findings in approximately 250 patients with well-established SLE were analyzed and compared to those observed in a panel of patients with rheumatoid arthritis and a miscellany of other diseases. When the dust settled, four or more of the findings from a final list of 14 manifestations were found to be present in 90 per cent of patients with SLE (90 per cent sensitivity). Importantly, each quartet of criteria displayed a specificity of 99 per cent and 98 per cent against findings in patients with rheumatoid arthritis and miscellaneous other disorders respectively.

Given the manner in which the diagnostic criteria were established for SLE, it should not be surprising that each manifestation is not present in each case. Nonetheless, a knowledge of the individual criteria and their relative frequency helps provide a clear picture of the disease.

The American Rheumatism Association criteria for the diagnosis of SLE are given in the table on pages 516–517. The frequency of each finding at presentation and during the clinical course in 365 "pedigreed" patients with SLE is also provided. The presence of at least four of the criteria are required to establish the diagnosis. Note that these diagnostic guidelines were established prior to the extensive diagnostic experience with antinuclear and anti–double-stranded DNA antibody, serum complement levels, and cutaneous immunoglobin deposition.

Reference: Primer on the Rheumatic Diseases, 7th Edition, 1973, p. 139.

Pedigree — Apparently comes from our version of the French *pied de grue*, which means the "foot of a crane." Presumably, the three lines of lineal descent pictured in old documents resembled the imprint of a crane's foot.

14

Findings for Diagnosis of SLE

	PRESENT AT DIAGNOSIS	PRESENT AT DIAGNOSIS OR DURING CLINICAL COURSE
1. *Facial erythema* (butterfly rash): A diffuse erythema, which may be flat or raised, covering the malar eminence(s) and/or the bridge of the nose. (The periorbital regions are usually spared as a result of the protection from the sun afforded by the orbital ridge. The nasal creases are usually spared as well.)	52%	55%
2. *Discoid lupus:* Erythematous raised patches with adherent hyperkeratotic scaling and follicular plugging. Atrophic scarring may occur in older lesions. Lesions may be present anywhere on the body.	18%	19%
3. *Raynaud's phenomenon:* The characteristic two-phase reaction of cold-induced blanching followed by hyperemia on warming is noted in the patient's history or observed by a physician.	16%	20%
4. *Alopecia:* The loss of a significant amount of scalp hair is present by history or physician's observation.	58%	71%
5. *Photosensitivity:* Unusual skin reaction is present in a patient's history or seen in a physical examination. (Probably seen with decreased frequency outside the Sun Belt.)	37%	41%
6. *Oral or nasopharyngeal ulceration* (often asymptomatic and must be assessed by physical exam).	25%	36%
7. *Arthritis without deformity:* (10% of patients have polyarthralgias without arthritis). One or more peripheral joints exhibit the following in the absence of deformity: a. Pain on motion. b. Tenderness. c. Effusion or periarticular swelling. (The frequency of arthritic involvement appears to be: proximal interphalangeal (close to 100%) > metacarpal > wrists > knees (about 50%) > elbows > shoulders > ankles > distal interphalangeal joints (about 10%). (The hip joints are almost *never* involved in the primary disease).	78%	85%

	PRESENT AT DIAGNOSIS	PRESENT AT DIAGNOSIS OR DURING CLINICAL COURSE
8. *LE cells:* Two or more classic LE cells seen on one occasion, or one cell seen on two or more occasions by means of published methods.	84%	86%
9. *Chronic false positive STS:* The test is known to be positive for at least 6 months and the "false" positivity is confirmed by *T. pallidum* immobilization or Reiter's test.	27%	27%
10. *Profuse proteinuria:* Greater than 3.5 grams/day. (Some degree of proteinuria appears to be present in about half of patients, hematuria in about a third.)	17%	25%
11. *Cellular urinary casts:* May be red cell, hemoglobin, granular, tubular, or mixed.	23%	34%
12. One or both of the following: a. *Pleuritis*—either a convincing history, a rub heard by a physician, or radiographic evidence of pleural thickening and fluid. b. *Pericarditis,* documented by ECG or rub.	40%	54%
13. One or both of the following: a. *Psychosis.* b. *Convulsions.* Verified by history or physician's observation in the absence of offending drugs or uremia.	14%	16%
14. One or more of the following: a. *Hemolytic anemia* b. *Leukopenia* (WBC <4000 mm^3 on two or more occasions) c. *Thrombocytopenia* (platelet count less than 100,000 mm^3)	43%	49%

Reference: Rothfield, N.: Lupus erythematosus in Fitzpatrick, T. B., Eisen, A. Z., Wolff, K., Freeberg, I. M., and Austin, K. F. (Eds.): *Dermatology In Clinical Medicine,* New York, McGraw-Hill Book Company, 1979, p. 1281; and Rothfield, N.: Personal Communication (by permission).

14

DRUG-INDUCED LUPUS SYNDROME

The mechanism by which drugs cause a lupus syndrome is not clearly understood. Either a metabolic product or the native drug may be responsible.

Patients with drug-induced lupus rarely have serious renal disease. Rash and fever are less frequent than in the idiopathic disease; the exception is hydralazine-induced lupus, which may be identical to the idiopathic variety. On the other hand, the serositis, arthralgias, cerebritis, and liver, lung, and spleen involvement may be similar in the spontaneous and drug-evoked disorder. The drugs listed below may "induce" positive lupus erythematosus (LE) cell tests, positive antinuclear factors, and, at all times, a flagrant lupus syndrome.

Antihypertensives	*Antibiotics*
Hydralazine*	Isoniazid*
Reserpine	Sulfonamides
Methyldopa	Streptomycin
	The penicillins
Antiarrhythmics	The tetracyclines
Procainamide*	Griseofulvin
Quinidine	Aminosalicylic acid
Anticonvulsants	*Others*
Phenytoin	Oral contraceptives
Mephenytoin	Propylthiouracil
Trimethadione	Chlorpromazine
Primidone	Other phenothiazines
Ethosuximide	Methysergide
	Phenylbutazone
	Gold salts
	Clofibrate

Usually, the clinical and laboratory manifestations of drug-induced lupus disappear after the drug has been stopped. However, spontaneous flare-ups and even persistence of lupus for up to a decade have occurred despite a cessation of the offending agent. Obviously, these latter patients may have underlying systemic lupus erythematosus (SLE).

---

*The most common offenders.

ANADNAENA

On a hunch, the bright young medical student ordered antinuclear antibodies on a patient with pneumonitis and renal failure. The ANA-peripheral pattern was positive in a high titer, as was the ENA-Sm test. For final confirmation he excitedly orders a serum C_3 and an anti-DNA titer! What is going on?

There has been a recent explosion of knowledge and data about antibodies directed against a variety of "nuclear antigens" that are associated with the connective tissue diseases. The following is a brief primer.

Fluorescent Antinuclear Antibody Assay (ANA)

The ANA is an excellent screening test for the presence of connective tissue disease. Some healthy individuals older than 60 may have low titers ($\leq 1:80$) of a homogeneous pattern, but, in general, a positive assay means "disease."

Per Cent Positive ANA By Disease State

DISEASE	PER CENT POSITIVE ANA
SLE	90
Rheumatoid arthritis	25–40
Sjogren's syndrome	35–60
Scleroderma	30–67
Juvenile rheumatoid arthritis	20–25
Periarteritis nodosum	5–20
Dermatomyositis/polymyositis	5–12
Drug-induced	10–20
Myasthenia gravis	8–11
Hashimoto's thyroiditis	3–8

14

There are four ANA patterns:

Nucleolar	The "dot" pattern is seen in systemic lupus erythematosus (SLE) and scleroderma. It has no special value for prognosis.
Speckled	The speckled pattern is the least specific of the four types of ANA and is found in the gamut of collagen-vascular diseases. It is positive when antibodies are directed against ribonucleic acids, histones, ribonucleoproteins, and extractable nuclear antigens (ENA).
Homogeneous	The homogeneous pattern is not specific for any connective tissue disease. It detects antibody against desoxyribonucleoprotein, the antibody responsible for the LE cell phenomenon.
Peripheral or shaggy	This pattern is most commonly seen in active SLE. The distribution indicates antibody directed against native DNA. The peripheral pattern is often seen when lupus nephritis is present.

Antibody To Native DNA (Anti-nDNA)

The presence of circulating anti-nDNA is associated with active systemic lupus, particularly active SLE with renal disease. Together with measurements of C_3 and C_4, it may be employed to monitor disease activity and response to therapy in patients with lupus nephritis. Up to 80 per cent of patients with SLE will demonstrate anti-nDNA. Half of these patients will also have a low C_3.

Extractable Nuclear Antigens (ENA)

There are two ENAs of current clinical importance, RNP and Sm. The antibody to ribonucleoprotein (RNP) antigen is associated with a lupus-like syndrome that tends to be fairly nonvirulent and is usually not associated with renal disease. Patients with this condition have features that are common to several connective tissue disorders. It has consequently been called mixed connective tissue disease (MCTD).

Antibody to ENA-Sm (named after patient Smith) is associated almost exclusively with systemic lupus.

ENA: Anti-Sm versus Anti-RNP

ANTIBODY	PER CENT POSITIVE IN SLE	PER CENT POSITIVE IN MCTD	PER CENT POSITIVE IN RA	PER CENT POSITIVE IN CONTROLS YOUNGER THAN 60
Anti-Sm	30	8	0	0
Anti-RNP	14–26	100	0–10	0

Notes:
1. Antibodies to RNP are uncommon in severe SLE.
2. A positive anti-Sm, together with a positive anti-nDNA, is virtually diagnostic of active SLE.
3. The absence of antibody to RNP rules out the diagnosis of MCTD.
4. The presence of anti-RNP is usually associated with low or negative anti-nDNA titers and is a good prognostic sign in SLE.

References: Kurate, N., and Tan, E. M.: Arthritis Rheum., *19*:574, 1976; Hamburger, M., Hodes, S., and Barland, P.: Am. J. Med. Sci., *273*:21, 1977.

ADULT ACUTE RHEUMATIC FEVER

The diagnosis of adult acute rheumatic fever is usually difficult and requires a careful analysis of the clinical data available. The modified Jones criteria for diagnosis include:
1. Active carditis
2. Chorea
3. Erythema marginatum
4. Subcutaneous nodules
5. Migrating polyarthritis

Two major criteria coupled with any one of the plethora of minor criteria make the diagnosis highly suggestive when evidence of a preceding streptococcal infection is also present. Minor criteria such as fever, leukocytosis, arthralgia, and an elevated sedimentation rate are, of course, quite nonspecific.

14

Streptococcus — was named by Dr. A. C. T. Billroth. The roots of the word are Greek. *Streptos* means a "twisted necklace" and *kikkos,* a "seed." The name related to the long twisting chains in which the organism is found.

Carditis appears as the initial manifestation of rheumatic fever in about 20 per cent (15 per cent, 23 per cent, 40 per cent in three series) of adult patients. Chorea is now virtually unheard of as a presenting sign except in children. The subcutaneous nodules of acute rheumatic fever that appear over bony surfaces and near tendons are extremely rare. A transient dermatitis is observed in less than 5 per cent of adults and usually cannot be diagnosed as erythema marginatum.

On the other hand, evidence of a preceding streptococcal infection is almost invariable. In its absence the diagnosis of acute rheumatic fever should be seriously questioned. Nonetheless, the physician finds himself without four of his five diagnostic standbys. Polyarthritis usually remains as the sole major diagnostic criterion to suggest the diagnosis of adult acute rheumatic fever.

The features of the arthritis do, however, lend themselves to analysis. Its onset is rapid, with maximal severity reached within a day. There is gradual detumescence and decrease in pain within the next two to five days. The arthritis is both migratory and additive, with involvement of additional joints appearing prior to resolution of swelling of the joints involved earlier. Symmetric involvement is seen in only a third of cases. There may be bursal involvement and extensive periarticular tenosynovitis. The joints of the lower extremities are involved in 85 per cent of cases. Joint fluids are inflammatory in nature. Cervical spine involvement may occur more often than previously noted in rheumatic fever. Temperomandibular joint involvement is not characteristic of rheumatic fever and, if present suggests rheumatoid or osteo-arthritis. The severity of the arthritic pain may be striking and seem inappropriate to the degree of joint involvement. Arthritic signs and symptoms respond promptly and dramatically to aspirin.

Most attacks of rheumatic fever mimic previous attacks in the same patient. Since carditis can nevertheless appear as a major new manifestation with recurrent attacks, chemoprophylaxis against Streptococcus (see Antimicrobial Prophylaxis, p. 458) is recommended when the diagnosis of acute rheumatic fever is made.

References: Persellin, R. H.: Ann. Intern. Med., *89*:1002, 1978; McDonald, E. C., and Weisman, M. G.: Ann. Intern. Med., *89*:917, 1978.

Before ordering a test, decide what you will do if it is (1) positive or (2) negative, and if both answers are the same, don't do the test.

FALSE "FALSE" POSITIVES

The following are some of the frequently ordered serologic tests, the classic disease associated with a positive result, and other conditions that may give a "false" positive result.

Antinuclear antibodies

> Systemic lupus erythematosus*
> Scleroderma
> Sicca syndrome
> Rheumatoid arthritis
> Still's disease
> Periarteritis nodosa
> Polymyositis
> Dermatomyositis
> Hepatocellular disease (especially chronic active hepatitis)
> Chronic membranoproliferative glomerulonephritis
> Hashimoto's thyroiditis
> Waldenstrom's hyperglobulinemic purpura
> Myasthenia gravis
> Thymoma
> Pernicious anemia
> Ulcerative colitis
> Cytomegalovirus
> Tuberculosis, leprosy
> Lymphoma
> Drugs (see p. 518)
> Elderly normals
>   (homogeneous titer 1:40 to 1:80)

Lupus erythematosus cell

> Systemic lupus erythematosus*
> Chronic active hepatitis
> Scleroderma
> Drug hypersensitivities
> Active rheumatoid arthritis
> Tart cell (not a true LE cell)

Rheumatoid factor

> Rheumatoid arthritis*
> Systemic lupus erythematosus
> Scleroderma
> Dermatomyositis
> Polymyositis

14

---

*Classic disease.

Rheumatoid factor (continued)

    Sicca syndrome
    Pulmonary fibrosis
    Tuberculosis, leprosy
    Hepatocellular disease (especially chronic active hepatitis)
    Cytomegalovirus
    Subacute bacterial endocarditis
    Dysproteinemias
    4 per cent of normals

VDRL or STS

    Syphilis*
    Heroin addiction
    Subacute bacterial endocarditis
    Rheumatic fever
    Yaws, pinta
    Leprosy, malaria
    Mononucleosis
    Systemic lupus erythematosus
    Rheumatoid arthritis
    Smallpox vaccinations
    Some hemolytic anemias
    Some acute infections
    Hydralazine use

Fluorescent treponemal antibody-abs

    Syphilis*
    Systemic lupus erythematosus (beaded pattern)
    Mixed connective tissue disease (rare)
    Rheumatoid arthritis (rare)
    Scleroderma (rare)

*Classic disease.

OSTEONECROSIS, OR ASEPTIC NECROSIS OF BONE

Osteonecrosis is usually caused by vasculitis, vascular occlusion, or conditions associated with lipid abnormalities. It can occur in the femoral head, femoral condyles, the tibia, the proximal or distal humerus, the talus, and the navicular bone of the hand. Radiographically established osteonecrosis shows single or multiple focal areas of medullary sclerosis. Weight-bearing bones become distorted, with flattening or collapse of the cortical surface at points of stress. The differential diagnosis includes:

1. Trauma
2. Sickle cell disease

3. Polyarteritis, systemic lupus erythematosus
4. Diabetes mellitus
5. Alcoholism
6. Cushing's disease, corticosteroid therapy
7. Gaucher's disease
8. Pancreatitis
9. Caisson disease (decompression sickness)
10. Heroin abuse
11. Idiopathic:
    a. Legg-Calvé-Perthes disease (femoral head)
    b. Freiberg's disease (metatarsal head)
    c. Kohler's disease (tarsal navicular)
    d. Osgood-Schlatter disease (tibial tubercle)

GENU AMORIS

The following report is the first of what promises to be a series of "musculoskeletal misadventures for participants who are predisposed, poorly conditioned, or overenthusiastic." It is best described in the author's own words.

Intractable pain in a patient with chondromalacia patellae was found to be related to an unusual type of repetitive trauma.

Traumatic arthritis of the knee has been associated with many types of occupational and athletic injury, both acute (such as the sprains and internal derangements resulting from contact sports) and chronic (usually involving repetitive, inappropriate stress). Examples of the latter variety were common before the age of mechanization. However, in this modern era of automation and the foreshortened work week, one is not surprised to encounter new forms of articular abuse related to leisure-time activities and to the continuing search for new vistas in human experience. This case report describes such an example.

Case Report

A 31-year-old woman complained of knee pain, which had started insidiously a year previously. The pain was aggravated by weight bearing, was relieved by rest, and was accompanied intermittently by mild swelling. Because of these symptoms she had relinquished her job as a sales person and had also stopped bicycling and skiing. She had been examined by a physician seven months previously and was found to have a small effusion in one knee, which, when aspirated, revealed essentially normal joint fluid.

There were no abnormalities on general physical examination and the joints were unremarkable, with the exception of the knees, which

14

showed marked crepitus in the patellofemoral joints and pain on patellar compression. There were audible snapping and crackling sounds on performing a deep knee bend, which she was able to do with some difficulty. No effusion or instability was detected.

Laboratory studies revealed no rheumatoid factor. Sedimentation rate uric acid, protein electrophoresis, and antinuclear antibodies were normal. Radiographs of the knees, including tangential views of the patella and intercondylar views, were normal.

A diagnosis of chondromalacia patellae was made. She was advised to take salicylates and to refrain from various activities that would be stressful to the patellofemoral joints. She protested that these activities had already been virtually eliminated but promised to take even more stringent precautions against minor knee traumata.

She was seen again two months later, still complaining of incapacitating knee discomfort. Examination was unchanged except for a small ecchymosis over the lower patella on one side. In view of the unusual severity and persistence of symptoms, her daily activities were reviewed in detail, but nothing of an injurious nature was uncovered. However, at the end of the interview she confided that there was one previously unmentioned practice about which she had some concern. "You see, doctor," she said, "I always have sex on my knees." She then described a position that she and her partner had adopted about one year previously on a regular basis, after some considerable experimentation with other more conventional but vastly less gratifying techniques. This position had proved to be so satisfactory that intercourse several times daily was not unusual. Moreover, during the act, she never experienced any pain in the knees or elsewhere and thus failed to connect it in any way with her symptoms. A hard surface such as the floor, was often utilized; the patient took a kneeling position and her partner, apparently a very vigorous and athletic man, assumed certain postures that, for full comprehension, would require illustrative material beyond the scope of the report. Abandonment of this position was recommended on a trial basis, and with some reluctance the patient agreed. Two months later she reported that the knee pain had almost completely disappeared, except for minor discomfort after skating. Patellofemoral crepitus persisted but tenderness was absent.

Reference: Reprinted from Pinals, R. S.: Arthritis Rheum., *19*:637, 1976. With permission of author and publisher.

15
PREGNANCY: BEFORE, DURING AND AFTER

EFFICACY OF CONTRACEPTIVE METHODS

In the following table the efficacy of various contraceptives is assessed as the number of pregnancies during the first year of use by 100 nonsterile women.

METHOD	CORRECT AND CONSTANT USE	TYPICAL USE
Rhythm	15	25–40
Coitus interruptus	9	20–25
Oral contraceptives (combined pill)	0.34	4–10
Mini-pill (progestin)	1.5–3.0	5–10
Intrauterine device	1–3	5
Tubal ligation	0.04	–
Condom	3	10
Spermicidal agent	3	20–30
Diaphragm with spermicidal agent	3	20–25
Vasectomy	0.15	–

Reference: Adapted from Brucker, P., and Chapler, F. K.: Contraceptive counseling. In Rakel, R. F., and Conn, H. F. (Eds.): *Family Practice.* Philadelphia, W. B. Saunders Company, 1978, p. 451.

Hermaphrodite — Hermaphroditos was the handsome son of Hermes and Aphrodite. A rather self-serving water nymph fell deeply in love with him. The young man made the mistake of bathing in a pond under the nymph's control. Her prayers for union with him were apparently answered, permanently.

15

THE "PILLS"

Two types of oral contraceptive pills are currently available; combination estrogen and progestin, and a progestin alone.

Combination pills contain at least 50 μg of a synthetic estrogen and one of five synthetic progestins. The new low-dose estrogen pill contains less estrogen. Combination pills are taken for three weeks, followed by a week without pills. Their contraceptive action is mediated by pituitary-hypothalamic suppression. The consequent decrease in production of gonadotropins results in a failure of follicular development. The contraceptive failure rate is said to be less than 1 per cent.

Progestins in small quantity are contained in the second type of pill ("mini-pills"), which are taken daily. Contraceptive action results from maintaining the uterus and cervical mucus in an inhospitable state for the implantation of the fertilized ovum and migration of sperm. The failure rate of 1.5 to 3 per cent is somewhat higher than with the more conventional pills.

Synthetic estrogens	*Synthetic Progesterones*
Ethinyl estradiol	Norethindrone
Mestranol	Norgestrel
	Norethynodrel
	Norethindrone acetate
	Ethynodiol diacetate

Whether to prescribe pills, and which ones, constitutes a trade-off between the absolute efficacy (or tolerable risk of pregnancy), side effects, and the relative contraindications to the use of these agents.

CLINICAL SIDE EFFECTS

Estrogenic

> Nausea
> Edema
> Weight gain
> Headache, migraine
> Depression
> Breast tenderness
> Mucorrhea

Progestogenic

> Hypomenorrhea
> Monilial vaginitis
> (?) Depression

Androgenic

> Acne
> Hirsutism
> Weight gain
>   and
> Chloasma
> Alopecia
> Galactorrhea

15

ESTROGENIC AND PROGESTATIONAL ACTIVITY OF ORAL CONTRACEPTIVES

Estrogenic (in Order of Increasing Potency)

Zorane 1/20
Loestrin 1/20
Ovral
Zorane 1/50
Norlestrin 1 mg
Norinyl 1 + 50
Ortho-Novum 1/50
Demulen
Norinyl 1 + 80
Ortho-Novum 1/80
Ovulen
Enovid-E

Progestational (in Order of Increasing Potency)

Norethynodrel
Norethindrone
Norethindrone acetate
Ethynodiol diacetate
Norgestrel

SYSTEMIC SIDE EFFECTS (For Estrogen-Containing Pills)

1. Stroke (rate rises from 0.2 cases to 1.5 per 100,000 for women younger than 34).
2. Hypertension (2 to 5 per cent with estrogen-containing pills).
3. (?) Coronary artery disease (in women over 40 taking an estrogen-containing pill).
4. Alteration in laboratory measurements.
   a. Increase in serum lipids.
   b. Increase in red cell rigidity.
   c. Increase in renin substrate.
   d. Increase in circulating procoagulants, particularly fibrinogen and factor VIII.
   e. Increase in T_4; decrease in T_3 resin uptake, normal free T_4, increased thyroid-binding globulin).
   f. Increase in iron-binding capacity; slight increase in serum iron.
   g. Alteration in hepatic conjugation and enzymes.
   h. Increase in serum copper.
   i. Decrease in folate utilization.

j.   Decrease in 17-OH steroids and cortisol; impaired responsiveness to metyrapone.

5.   Post-pill amenorrhea.

6.   Breakthrough "bleeding" (will initially respond to more estrogen).

7.   Cyst-adenomatous disease of the liver.

8.   Increased incidence of gallbladder disease.

CONTRAINDICATIONS TO ORAL CONTRACEPTIVES

1.   Thromboembolic disease, thrombophlebitis, cerebrovascular disease, or a history of these conditions.

2.   Undiagnosed genital bleeding.

3.   Known or potentially estrogen-dependent tumor (breast, uterus).

4.   Impaired liver function; past history of cholestatic jaundice of pregnancy.

5.   Known or suspected pregnancy (fetal anomalies) — rule out pregnancy prior to prescribing.

6.   Hyperlipidemia.

7.   Gestational diabetes.

8.   Progressive hypertension.

9.   Cardiac disease.

10.   Relatively contraindicated in:

a.   Epilepsy.

b.   Hypertension.

c.   Migraine.

d.   Oligomenorrhea.

e.   Obesity.

f.   Persons with a family history of cerebrovascular and cardiac disease.

g.   Persons who are heavy smokers.

h.   Persons over 40.

i.   Lupus.

j.   Porphyria.

Reference: Brucker, P., and Chapler, F. K.: Contraceptive counseling. In Rakel, R. E., and Conn, H. F. (Eds.): *Family Practice.* Philadelphia, W. B. Saunders Company, 1978.

15

...AND THE INTRAUTERINE DEVICE

1. Failure rate 1 to 3 per cent (same as for "mini-pill").
2. Approximately 25 per cent of women require removal secondary to menorrhagia or cramping or have a spontaneous expulsion in the first year.
3. Increased incidence of uterine infection.
4. If pregnancy occurs, increased incidence of septic abortion and tubal pregnancy.
5. Uterine perforation (1/1500 insertions).
6. Contraindications to use include:
    a. Pregnancy — rule out pregnancy prior to insertion.
    b. Presence or suspicion of gynecologic malignancy.
    c. Pelvic inflammatory disease.
    d. Cervicitis.
    e. Previous ectopic pregnancy.

POST-PILL AMENORRRHEA

Delayed reappearance of the menses after the discontinuance of combined estrogen-progestin contraceptive pills is a common occurrence. Some 98 per cent of patients will have the return of normal menstral function within one year. When endometrial atrophy is the cause, the reappearance of menses usually occurs within three months. The return of function is somewhat slower when hypothalamic-pituitary suppression is the etiology. Nonetheless, menses usually appear within six months.

In general, women experiencing problems with their menses prior to taking the pill have a higher incidence of difficulty after its discontinuance. The possibility that an underlying disorder such as marginal pituitary insufficiency has been masked during the period of contraception is an important consideration.

An evaluation of patients with post-pill amenorrhea is recommended in all patients in whom normal menses have not returned in six months. The evaluation starts with a consideration of possible pregnancy and menopause. The approach to this problem is described in Cessation of Menses, page 189.

DRUGS IN PREGNANCY

We possess little information on the effects of most drugs on the human fetus. Since it is difficult to safely perform controlled studies on pregnant humans, our data are frequently second-hand — we depend on animal studies and guilt by association. This research is frequently unclear because of polydrug use, nutritional factors, inaccuracy of information, differences in doses used, and other similar variants.

It is difficult to assess the *degree* of risk of any therapeutic modality. The fetal effects of a medicine must always be balanced by the clinical indications for a medicine's use and the implications of not using it. *It is always best to avoid medication whenever possible.*

The following list discusses some current findings about drug use in pregnancy.

Antihistamines: appear to be safe.

Anti-infectives:

Amantadine —	cardiovascular lesions (one case report).
Aminoglycosides —	possible kidney or ear toxicity; fetal blood levels may exceed MIC for many organisms.
Ampicillin —	no anomalies noted; depresses maternal estriols, may reach therapeutic concentration in the fetus.
Cephalosporins —	does not reach therapeutic concentrations in the fetus; no anomalies reported.
Chloramphenicol —	no anomalies noted; gray baby syndrome if given near term.
Chloroquine —	case reports of deafness, eye problems, thrombocytopenia.
Clindamycin —	no anomalies reported; may reach MIC in fetus.
Dicloxacillin —	no anomalies reported.
Erythromycin —	no anomalies reported; may concentrate in fetal liver.
Ethambutol —	no fetal anomalies assocated with use.
Isoniazid —	conflicting reports of anomalies.
Lincomycin —	no associated anomalies found even after seven-year follow-up.
Mandelic Acid —	depresses maternal estriol excretion.
Methenamine —	depresses maternal estriol excretion.
Neomycin —	depresses maternal estriol excretion.
Nitrofurantoin —	no anomalies reported.
Methicillin —	no anomalies reported.
Penicillin —	no anomalies reported.
Quinine —	abortion; eye, ear, heart, kidney, and limb anomalies.
Rifampin —	no anomalies noted.
Sulfonamides —	if used near the time of delivery, may displace bilirubin from the binding sites, resulting in increased tendency to kernicterus.

15

Tetracyclines —

tooth discoloration, enamel hypoplasia, depressed skeletal growth, eye cataracts.

Antineoplastics:

Aminopterin
Azathioprine
Busulphan
Chlorambucil
Fluorouracil
Mercaptopurine
Methotrexate
Nitrogen mustard
Vinblastine

— cases of normal infants are reported; many other reports of abortion, ovarian and thyroid hypoplasia, drug intoxication, cleft lip and palate, eye or ear defects, CNS problems, bone abnormalities, growth retardation, and immunologic deficiency. The denominator is not known.

Autonomic drugs:

Ergonovine —

Poland anomaly (muscle, bone and digit abnormalities).

Blood formation and coagulation:

Coumarins

— predisposition to hemorrhage by depression of vitamin K–dependent clotting factors, bone malformations, nasal bone hypoplasia, low set ears, and palate defects.

Heparin —

does not cross the placenta.

Iron Dextran —

may cross the placenta; no anomalies reported.

Cardiovascular drugs:

Diazoxide —

associated with four cases of alopecia.

Digoxin —

no anomalies noted, equal concentrations in mother and child.

Propranolol —

possible growth retardation, hypoglycemia, bradycardia, small placenta, heart block.

Reserpine —

newborn may show lethargy, hypothermia, or nasal congestion; no reports of anomalies.

Central nervous system drugs:

Analgesics:

Alcohol —	Fetal alcohol syndrome: low birth weight and length, joint and cardiac anomalies, learning disabilities and retardation, CNS depression if near time of delivery.
Anesthesia —	higher spontaneous abortion rate in women anesthetists and wives of anesthetists; anomalies three times more common in nurse anesthetists.
Pentazocine —	case reports of withdrawal signs and symptoms after chronic maternal use.
Propoxyphene —	no anomalies reported; cases of newborn withdrawal after chronic maternal use now reported.
Salicylates —	some associated anomalies; depresses maternal urinary estriols; may delay onset of labor and increase length of labor; newborn blood coagulation or toxicity problems; bilirubin displacement.
Acetaminophen —	possible kidney toxicity or bilirubin displacement.

Anticonvulsants:

Phenytoin —	multiple physical anomalies, growth and mental deficiencies, coagulation defects.
Phenobarbital —	(guilty by association?) is associated with multiple anomalies and possible withdrawal syndrome in the neonate; may enhance enzyme activity to decrease the amount of hyperbilirubinemia.
Trimethadione —	primarily heart and facial clefts; also developmental delays.

Psychotherapeutics:

Amitriptyline —	conflicting reports; reported anomalies are primarily skeletal.
Imipramine —	some report normal offspring; others report limb defects and facial clefts.

15

Diazepam — conflicting reports of increased incidence of cleft palate in some studies; use near term may result in infant with apnea, hypothermia, hypotonia, poor feeding.

Chlordiazepoxide — newborn withdrawal reported; conflicting reports of increased defects among infants exposed to this drug in early pregnancy; may also produce hypotonia, hypothermia if used near term.

Meprobamate — reports of anomalies if used in early pregnancy; other studies report no harm.

Haloperidol — use in early pregnancy associated with some limb anomalies.

Thalidomide — a classic teratogen: limb, eye, ear, heart, GI, GU anomalies; also stillbirth and neonatal deaths.

Phenothiazines — one case report of limb anomalies; may impair temperature regulation, induce fetal enzymes, inhibit lymphocyte rosette formation.

Lithium — reports of ear, heart, and CNS anomalies; lithium intoxication may be present at birth (floppy, cyanotic, hypothermic).

Barbiturates — see Anticonvulsants.

Bromides — case reports of short stature, small head, or lethargy and hypotonia at birth.

Ethchlorvynol — newborn lethargy, hypotonia, irritability, and jitteriness.

Diuretics:

Thiazides —

associated (rarely) with thrombocytopenia and bone marrow depression; may inhibit excretion of uric acid, slight depression of maternal estriol values.

Furosemide —

may depress uric acid elimination.

Hormones and synthetic substitutes:

Fertility:

Clomiphene citrate —

multiple pregnancy; reports of anencephaly, spina bifida, or multiple other anomalies.

Contraceptives:

Estrogen/progestin combinations —

conflicting reports; possible higher incidence of chromosomal anomalies in the spontaneous abortions of women who became pregnant 6 to 12 months after stopping the pill; many reports of normal infants; no masculinization of female fetus reported; possible association with higher bilirubin levels in newborn.

Progestin —

associated with more limb defects; also increased VACTERL (vertebral, anal, cardiac, tracheoesophageal, renal, and limb) anomalies after early pregnancy exposure.

Progesterone or androgen-like —

possible masculinization of female fetus.

15

Estrogen compounds —	altered sexual behavior; feminization of male fetus?
DES (diethylstilbestrol) —	vaginal adenosis in females exposed *in utero* before twelfth week of pregnancy; vaginal cellular changes reported in 90 per cent; clear cell adenocarcinoma of cervix and vagina associated.

Corticosteroids:

Cortisone —	no firm evidence of human anomalies (contrary to mouse data).
Prednisone —	case report of congenital cataracts.
Betamethasone —	being used experimentally to enhance lung maturation in the fetus; may depress maternal estriol determination.
Dexamethasone —	being used experimentally to enhance lung maturation in the fetus.

Hypoglycemic agents:

Insulin —	no placental transfer; benefits fetus through maternal blood sugar control if diabetic.
Tolbutamide, chlorpropamide, phenformin —	some association with anomalies; may result in prolonged newborn hypoglycemia, poor control of hypoglycemia in the mother, displacement of bilirubin in the newborn.

Thyroid agents:

Iodides —	may cause goiter (with or without tracheal obstruction), hypothyroidism, mental retardation.
Propylthiouracil, methimazole —	congenital goiter seen.
Desiccated thyroid —	no significant placental transfer.

Serums, toxoids, and vaccines:

Generally, vaccinations should be avoided during pregnancy. Infection by the virus can be subtle at birth. Viral particles have been isolated from the placenta and fetus in many cases. Reports of malformations are sporadic. Measles is associated with an increased incidence of neural tube tumors and malignancies; pertussis is associated with abortion. Rabies vaccine is associated with physical and mental retardation. Rubella is possibly teratogenic. Avoid vaccination two to three months before conception: Smallpox vaccine may produce abortion if given in the first trimester.

Miscellaneous:

Podophyllin —	reports of anomalies after use in pregnancy; case report of fetal death after maternal treatment at 34 weeks' gestation.
Phytonadione —	possible neonatal jaundice and hemolysis; increased bilirubin; may be prophylactic against coagulation defect of phenytoin.
Vitamin A and D —	large doses associated with malformations and mental retardation.
Methyl mercury —	Minamata disease, palsies, deformities, mental retardation, impaired motor ability.
Agricultural chemicals —	possible malformations reported.
Food additives —	Chlorobiphenyls: cola-colored baby syndrome.
Iron, vitamins, antacids —	associated with an increased incidence of malformations if used during the first 56 days of pregnancy.
G-6-PD deficiency —	possible hemolysis for fetus is associated with the following drugs: acetanilid, ASA, antimalarials, phenacetin, sulfonamides, nitrofurantoin, naldixic acid, mestranol, phenylhydrazine, fava beans (see drugs and G-6-PD deficiency, p. 397).

Abused drugs:

Amphetamines —	possible neonatal withdrawal after maternal use; associated with cardiac and GI anomalies.
Nicotine —	intrauterine growth retardation (IUGR), increased perinatal mortality.
Alcohol —	Fetal alcohol syndrome (see analgesics).
Cocaine —	no documented effects.
Marihuana —	some case reports of abnormalities or possible chromosomal disruption.
Heroin —	intrauterine addiction, growth retardation, newborn withdrawal syndrome, less respiratory distress syndrome (RDS).

15

Methadone —	intrauterine addiction and newborn withdrawal.
LSD —	increased spontaneous abortion (?), possible chromosomal anomalies.

References: Clin. Perinatol. 1974, 1975, and 1976; Nishimura; H. and Tanimura, T.: Clinical Aspects of the Teratogenicity of Drugs. New York, Elsevier North Holland, Inc., 1976; Tuchmann-Duplessis, H.: Drug Effects on the Fetus. Littleton, Mass., Publishing Sciences Group, Inc., 1975; Clin. Obstet. Gynecol., *18*:141–163, 1975; Morselli, P. L., et al. (Eds): Basic and Therapeutic Aspects of Perinatal Pharmacology. New York, Raven Press, 1975.

RASHES IN PREGNANCY

Most physicians are aware of the common dermatologic changes that occur with pregnancy, such as pigmentation, stretch marks, and hair and vascular changes. For the most part these changes are painless and of little consequence, save for cosmetic appearance. There are, however, skin diseases associated with pregnancy that are uncomfortable, disabling, or even fatal. Fortunately, these conditions are rare.

Classification of Skin Changes and Diseases Associated with Pregnancy

Group I. **Skin changes of probable hormonal cause**

1. Pigmentation
   a. Hyperpigmentation of areolae, axillae, abdomen (linea

nigra), perineal area

    b. Chloasma gravidarum (melasma, mask of pregnancy)

2. Striae gravidarum

3. Hair growth: post-partum telogen effluvium (temporary hair loss)

4. Vascular

    a. Vascular spiders (nevi aranei)

    b. Palmar erythema

    c. Granuloma gravidarum (pedunculated, red, friable oral lesion)

Group II. **Skin diseases unique to pregnancy** (See chart on following page)

1. Herpes gestationis

2. Prurigo gestationis

3. Papular dermatitis of pregnancy

4. Pruritus gravidarum

5. Idiopathic jaundice of pregnancy

Group III. **Skin diseases frequently associated with pregnancy**

1. Impetigo herpetiformis

15

DISEASE PROCESS	INCIDENCE	ONSET	LOCATION OF LESIONS	TYPE OF LESION	SYMPTOMS	ASSOCIATED LABORATORY ABNORMALITIES	THERAPY	COURSE OF DISEASE	MATERNAL/ FETAL MORBIDITY-MORTALITY	DIFFERENTIAL DIAGNOSIS
Herpes gestationis	Rare 1:3000	Second half of pregnancy and post-partum	Extremities, abdomen, buttocks, mucous membranes (20%) (tendency to symmetry)	Erythematous papules, vesicules, bullae	Pruritus, few mild systemic manifestations (fever, chills)	Eosinophilia, positive immunofluorescence, elevated chorionic gonadotropin	Systemic corticosteriods	Progressive throughout pregnancy, resolution at parturition, frequent recurrences with succeeding pregnancies	Maternal—none Fetal—reports variable	Dermatitis herpetiformis, pemphigoid, erythema multiforme, drug reactions
Papular dermatitis of pregnancy	Rare 1:2000	Anytime during gestation	Generalized eruptions	Erythematous papules (3–5 mm)	Pruritus, no associated systemic symptoms	Elevated urinary chorionic gonadotropin levels, decreased estrogen and cortisol level	Systemic corticosteriods	Progressive throughout pregnancy, resolution at parturition, frequent recurrences with succeeding pregnancies	Maternal—none Fetal—increased mortality rate	Dermatitis herpetiformis, herpes gestationis, infestations, drug reactions
Prurigo gestationis	2% of all pregnancies	Second half of gestation	Extensor surfaces of extremities, trunk (tendency to symmetry)	Small papules (1–2 mm)	Pruritus, no associated systemic symptoms	None	Antipruritics	Progressive throughout pregnancy, resolution at parturition, frequent recurrences with succeeding pregnancies	Maternal—none Fetal—none	Pruritus gravidarum, papular dermatitis of pregnancy infestations, drug reactions
Pruritus gravidarum and idiopathic jaundice of pregnancy	17% of all pregnancies (pruritus)	Last trimester	Localized to abdomen or generalized	No primary lesion	Pruritus, no associated systemic symptoms	Elevated bilirubin (in idiopathic jaundice of pregnancy)	Antipruritics	Resolution at parturition, frequent recurrences with succeeding pregnancies	Maternal—none Fetal—increased prematurity rate	Infestations, drug reactions
Impetigo herpetiformis	Rare	Second half of gestation (usually)	Groin, inner thighs, extremities, mucous membranes (occasionally)	Small pustules (may coalesce)	Pain, severe systemic symptoms common (high fever, chills, vomiting, diarrhea, arthritis, splenomegaly, lymphadenopathy, septicemia)	Hypercalcemia, hyperphosphatemia	Systemic corticosteroids	Progressive throughout pregnancy, resolution at parturition, recurrences rare	Maternal—increased mortality rate Fetal—increased number of stillbirths	Dermatitis herpetiformis, pustular psoriasis, erythema multiforme, pemphigus

Reference: Wade, T. R., Wade, L. L., and Jones, H. E.: Obstet. Gynecol., *52*:233, 1978.
Table reproduced with permission of author and Obstetrics and Gynecology.

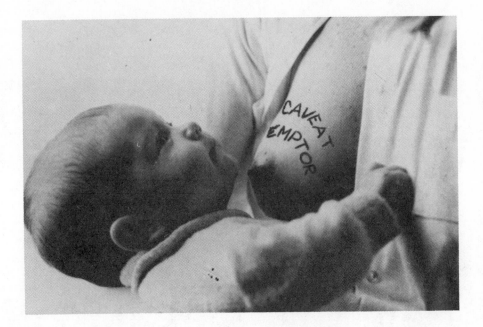

FIG. 15–1

NURSING CHILDREN BEWARE!

More women are now nursing their children. There is an abundance of drugs to prescribe for the breast-feeding mother but a paucity of information concerning which drugs may interfere with milk production or which may reach the infant via the breast milk. Though the data are scanty, the table on pages 546–547 offers several considerations about drugs to avoid or use with caution.

The drugs most likely to enter breast milk are those that are lipid soluble, have a molecular weight of less than 600, are not ionized at the plasma pH of 7.4, and are not tightly bound to plasma proteins.

The drugs excreted in breast milk may not necessarily be toxic to the infant if the amount is small or if the drug is bound to calcium. Some drugs are not toxic to the infant but have an adverse effect on the mother's milk production.

Reference: Fig. 15–1 reproduced courtesy of Kathryn Abbe, photographer, and with permission of publisher from Eiger, M. S., and Olds, S. W.: The Complete Book of Breastfeeding. New York, Workman Publishing Co., 1976, p. 121.

15

DRUG	EVALUATION	COMMENT
Anticoagulants		
Heparin	Safe	17,000 M.W.
Dicumarol	Probably safe	125 cases reported without abnormality
Warfarin	Probably safe	Most is bound to plasma proteins, ionized
Phenindione	Not safe	Affects infant prothrombin time.
Antihypertensives and diuretics		
Reserpine	Contraindicated	Infant lethargy, nasal stuffiness, and diarrhea
Propranolol	Safe	
Guanethidine	Safe	
Methyldopa	Unknown	
Chlorothiazide	Caution	One case of infant thrombocytopenia
Other diuretics	Only if necessary	May decrease milk production
Antimicrobials		
Chloramphenicol	Contraindicated	Bone marrow depression
Metronidazole	Contraindicated	Blood dyscrasias, neurologic disorders
Tetracycline	Only if necessary	Although bound to calcium, may cause discolored teeth and enamel hypoplasia
Nalidixic acid	Caution	Hemolytic anemia in infants with G-6-PD deficiency
Sulfonamides	Caution	G-6-PD–dependent hemolytic anemia potentiates kernicterus
Chloroquine	Probably safe	
Quinine	Caution	Thrombocytopenia reported
Pyrimethamine	Caution	Human milk levels documented for this toxic drug
Isoniazid	Caution	Milk levels equal to mother's plasma level. Monitor infant's hepatic function.
Penicillins	Safe	
Drugs affecting the CNS		
Alcohol	Safe	Avoid prolonged ingestion of large amounts
Chloral hydrate	Safe	
Meprobamate	Contraindicated	*Official FDA warning!* Milk levels 200–400% of mother's plasma level
Diazepam	Caution	Accumulated in infant; may cause drowsiness
Lithium	Caution	50% of plasma level is in milk
Thorazine	Unknown	
Compazine	Unknown	
Stelazine	Unknown	
Imipramine	Unknown	
Amitriptyline	Unknown	
Phenobarbital	Probably safe	May induce hepatic microsomal enzymes.
Phenytoin	Caution	May induce hydroxylating enzymes
Primidone	Caution	May cause undue somnolence

Other drugs

Drug	Rating	Comments
Aspirin	Safe	Large doses may alter platelet function
Propoxyphene	Safe	
Acetaminophen	Unknown	
Methadone	Safe	
Heroin	Contraindicated	Drug excreted in breast milk
Codeine	Probably safe	May impair milk production; none detected in breast milk
Morphine	Probably safe	May impair milk production; none detected in breast milk
Marihuana	Safe	
Antihistamines	Safe	May impair milk production
Atropine	Caution	Does impair milk production; has anticholinergic effects on infant
Ergot alkaloids	Contraindicated	Suppress lactation, cause ergotism in infants
Nicotine	Caution	Decrease to less than 15 cigarettes per day because of nicotine intoxication
Iodine	Caution	May inhibit thyroid function
Propylthiouracil	Contraindicated	300–1200% higher in milk than in mother's plasma
Theophylline	Probably safe	Monitor for side effects

Laxatives

Drug	Rating	Comments
Cascara	Contraindicated	Diarrhea
Danthron	Contraindicated	Diarrhea
Senna	Safe	
Milk of magnesia	Safe	
Softeners	Safe	
Bulk formers	Safe	
Phenolphthalein	Unknown	

Hormones

Drug	Rating	Comments
Insulin	Safe	Destroyed in GI tract
Epinephrine	Safe	Destroyed in GI tract
Corticotropin	Safe	Destroyed in GI tract
Thyroxine	Safe	Excreted in insignificant amounts
Oral contraceptives	Unknown	Long-term effects unknown; controversial
Prednisone	Unknown	Long-term effects unknown

Radioactive drugs

Drug	Rating	Comments
Active therapy	Contraindicated	Don't breast feed
Tracer doses	Caution	Don't breast feed for 72 hours
Radioactive albumin	Caution	Don't breast feed for 10 days

Reference: Hervada, A. R., Feit, E., and Sagraves, R.: Perinatal Care, 2:19, 1978.

15

PANDORA'S JUG

It probably was Pandora that put us all in business. Zeus was outraged at the theft of fire and its presentation to man by Prometheus. Accordingly, he had a virgin of dazzling beauty fashioned from clay and water. Hermes, the trickster, helped make her perfidious and deceitful. Prometheus' brother, despite a warning about accepting any gift from the outraged Zeus, was enchanted by Pandora's beauty and welcomed her. Pandora brought a great vase with her which now is incorrectly called Pandora's box. On raising its lid, all the terrible afflictions that filled the vase escaped and were spread over the earth. Only hope remained. Thus, at least according to the Greeks, misery made its first appearance with the arrival of the first woman on earth.

DRUGS, ORGANIC DISEASE, AND SEXUAL DYSFUNCTION

Sexual dysfunction can occur as a complication of the use of a variety of drugs. The male may develop impotence (erectile dysfunction), retrograde ejaculation, or failure to ejaculate. The female may develop delay or failure in reaching orgasm. Psychological factors are the most common cause of male impotence, but organic disease or drug complications may be responsible. If there is consistent failure to obtain or maintain an erection during sexual activity with different partners, with masturbation, during sleep, or upon awakening, then one of the organic factors listed below is likely to be responsible:

1. Diabetic neuropathy (there is usually other evidence of peripheral neuropathy).
2. Vascular occlusive disease — Leriche's syndrome.
3. Generalized poor health or debility — chronic cardiac, pulmonary, or renal disease.
4. Surgical complications — post-prostatectomy, aortic bypass, sympathectomy.
5. Neurologic diseases — spinal cord tumors, multiple sclerosis, peripheral neuropathies.
6. Endocrine abnormalities — adrenal, thyroid hypo- or hyperfunction.
7. Urologic conditions — Peyronie's disease, priapism (especially Sickle Cell Anemia).
8. Drug abuse — acute and chronic abuse of alcohol, heroin, methadone, amphetamines, or barbiturates.

9. Aging.
10. Complications of drug therapy (see below).

Antihypertensive drugs commonly cause impotence, but they may also cause ejaculatory dysfunction or, occasionally, loss of libido. Guanethidine, methyldopa, and reserpine are the most widely appreciated agents. The incidence of sexual dysfunction with clonidine appears to be similar to the incidence with methyldopa. Dysfunction may occur in 20 to 30 per cent of patients using either drug. Impotence can occur with propranolol, although the incidence is probably low (5 to 10 per cent). When impotence occurs with one drug, it may be possible to switch to another drug (which may cause impotence in other patients) and recover sexual function.

The therapeutic agents that have been implicated in producing sexual dysfunction are listed below:

1. Antihypertensives — guanethidine, reserpine, methyldopa, clonidine; less commonly, prazosin, propranolol.
2. Diuretics — spironolactone, chlorthalidone, thiazides.
3. Anticholinergic drugs.
4. Psycho-active drugs: antidepressants (tricyclics, MAO inhibitors), phenothiazines, lithium, sedatives (chlordiazepoxide, diazepam).
5. Estrogens.
6. Vincristine.

References: Levine, S. B.: Ann. Intern. Med. *85*:342, 1976; The Medical Letter, *19*:81, 1977.

CRITERIA FOR GONADAL SHIELDING IN DIAGNOSTIC RADIOLOGY

Specific-area gonadal shielding should be used when: (1) the patient has reproductive potential, (2) the gonads will lie within the primary x-ray field or in close proximity (5 cm despite proper beam positioning), and (3) the clinical objectives of the examination will not be compromised.

Reference: Specific Area Gonad Shielding. Federal Register, *41*:30327–30329, July 23, 1976.

15

REPRODUCTION, SEXUALITY, AND CANCER THERAPY

Questions regarding fertility, sexual function, and childbearing are frequently asked by patients who have been treated for cancer or by their partners. Because of improved radiation and chemotherapeutic programs, long-term survival is now possible in many malignant diseases. Thus, an increasing number of patients reach and survive their years of reproductive potential. Pretreatment discussion and continued counseling regarding the effects of these therapies on fertility, the risks of fetal malformation, and future childbearing capabilities are extremely important. The majority of material to be discussed herein relates to the aftermath of the therapy of Hodgkin's disease. As an increasing number of patients cured of childhood acute lymphocytic leukemia attain adulthood, additional coherent data will become available. Some general considerations will be noted.

Effects of Radiation and Chemotherapy on Male Fertility

Both radiation therapy and chemotherapy are known to produce decreased fertility and, in most males, a prolonged period of sterility. The effects on the gonads are related to the age of the patient and the dose received by the testes. Despite the gonadal shielding used during the "inverted Y" radiotherapy for Hodgkin's disease, the low-dose scatter radiation received by the testes is sufficient to cause sterility. Depending on radiotherapeutic technique and the equipment employed, the dose to which the testes are exposed has been found to vary from about 100 rads to up to 300 rads over the five to six weeks of therapy. Fertility is more severely affected by this fractionated dose than if the same level of radiation were delivered in a single or a few doses.

Oligospermia, azoospermia, and decreased sperm viability and motility are also seen in men receiving single-agent and multiple-drug chemotherapy, especially when alkylating agents are used. Testicular biopsies show a depletion of germinal cells, and the tubules are lined with only Sertoli cells. Peritubular fibrosis may also be evident. Rare viable motile sperm have been found on semen analysis one year after completing multidrug combination chemotherapy (MOPP); however, the sterility induced by such multidrug therapy appears to last a minimum of three to four years. Therapy of this type may result in gynecomastia in pubescent males.

Prior to the initiation of these therapies it is wise to advise men to utilize the services of a "sperm bank." The sperm are kept frozen under liquid nitrogen. Although the fertility of stored sperm cannot be guaranteed, successful induction of pregnancy has been reported with sperm kept frozen for up to 10 years. There does not appear to be an increased risk of birth defect when stored sperm are employed. The cost for sperm storage generally includes an initial processing fee of approximately $150 for three ejaculates. The annual storage charge is currently about $25. For more information on sperm banking, we would suggest contacting Idant Corporation in New York City, (212)-935-1430.

Effects of Radiation Therapy and Chemotherapy on Female Fertility

The damaging effects of irradiation used in the treatment of Hodgkin's disease ("inverted Y") to the female gonads has been somewhat modified by oophoropexy at the time of staging laparotomy. Pregnancy following total nodal irradiation has been reported as early as two years after the cessation of treatment. When transplanted laterally, the ovaries appear to be less affected by the radiation than when they are transplanted to the midline. However, despite improved shielding techniques and ovarian placement procedures, the ovaries receive internally scattered irradiation (usually less than 100 rads), which may cause permanent sterility. In women of childbearing age, approximately a third become prematurely menopausal, a third become amenorrheic or experience change in their menses, and a third continue to menstruate regularly following radiation therapy. The effect of radiation therapy on the ovary also appears to be related to the age of the woman. The ovaries of younger women appear to tolerate higher doses of irradiation before permanent sterility occurs.

The effects of combination chemotherapy (such as with MOPP) on the ovaries are not as well known as the effects on the testes and are not as easily assessed. As with radiation therapy, approximately two thirds of the patients either become menopausal, amenorrheic or experience changes in their menstrual bleeding as a result of ovarian failure or progressive ovarian insufficiency. No more than a third and perhaps as few as 10% of patients continue to menstruate normally. It appears that the "older" ovary is more affected by smaller amounts of chemotherapy. Recovery may occur after a period of years. A few women have become pregnant while receiving multi-agent chemotherapy.

Although successful pregnancies have been reported following both radiation and chemotherapy, one must remember that the real denominator is not known. There are no statistics on the number of women who have unsuccessfully attempted conception after being treated with either or both of these modalities.

Teratogenicity, Survival, and Birth Control Counseling

Follow-up examinations of children born to survivors of Hiroshima and Nagasaki and similar studies of the progeny of patients treated for malignancy with either radiation or chemotherapy indicate that the incidence of fetal abnormality or subsequent leukemia and cancer may not be significantly increased. Since recessive genetic changes are not always apparent in the first generation, we must await future generations for more accurate data. Although it appears that chemotherapeutic agents may be administered with relative safety during the

15

third trimester of pregnancy, these agents and radiation therapy should be avoided, when possible, particularly during the first trimester.

We suggest birth control counseling at the time of diagnosis. (See Efficacy of Birth Control Methods, p. 529). Pregnancy prevention should continue at least through the period of highest risk for relapse so that a better estimate of the permanency of remission may be obtained. When complete remission is attained, we usually advise the continuation of birth control, which will provide a period during which the permanency of the remission may be assessed.

The ultimate arbiter in these matters is, of course, the patient. Many are anxious to have or adopt children. The family and their children-to-be deserve your best estimate of the patient's chance of survival. These data may then be factored into the decision regarding natural or acquired parenthood.

The evaluation of sperm count and motility is straightforward. At times, a full evaluation of ovarian function may be required, which when the most rigorous documentation is necessary mandates ovarian biopsy. Keep in mind that if the thyroid is in the radiation field, there is a significant incidence of post-irradiation hypothyroidism even with adequate shielding of the gland.

Effect on Libido and Sexuality

One must remember that it is not uncommon for "normal, healthy" men and women to experience periods of sexual dysfunction, often related to either physical or emotional stress. Illness, in general, affects an individual's sexuality and sexual responsiveness. The fears and uncertainties accompanying the diagnosis of cancer, financial worries, altered body image, and the feeling of physical *un*well-being may understandably change the patients's or the partner's usual sexual patterns.

In males, hormone replacement with testosterone is not helpful in alleviating the impotence caused or augmented by drugs (e.g., vincristine) or in aiding sperm production. In young females experiencing early menopause, estrogen replacement may decrease hot flashes and improve libido, sexual function and self-image.

The patient and his or her partner should be informed about these possible changes in sexual feelings and functioning in an effort to obviate additional undue stresses that may appear. The patience and compassion of all parties are, of course, part of the curative therapy.

References: Chapman, R. M., Sutcliffe, S. B., Rees, L. H., et al. Lancet,: 285, 1979; D. Angio, G. J.: Cancer, *42*:1015, 1978; LeFloch, O., Donaldson, S. S., and Kaplan, H. S.: Cancer, *38*:2263, 1976; Speiser, B., Rubin, P., and Casarett, G.: Cancer, *32*:692, 1973. Chapman, R. M., Sutcliffe, S. B., and Malpas, J. S.: J.A.M.A., *242*:1877, 1979.

Thanks to Diane Cass, R.N., N.C. for this contribution.

16
POTPOURRI

BOOKMAKING INDICES

Now that you've read the book it's time to cash in on what you've learned!

The probability that a particular anemic patient will have an iron, folate, or B_{12} deficiency was calculated for 1000 ambulatory and 206 hospitalized anemic patients in Rochester, N.Y. The betting line is based on the MCH and MCV obtained from the Coulter counter and the serum iron, transferrin saturation, B_{12}, and folate determinations. Set your bets using the "spread" suggested by this form sheet and you can pick up some spare change from your colleagues. You can then reimburse your patients for the additional tests you ordered to prove yourself right. (See MCVMCHMCHC, p. 376, for more information.)

Setting it up:

Anemia: males < 13 grams/dl
females < 12 grams/dl

For iron deficiency:

Low transferrin: < 16 per cent saturation

Index finding	Past performance	Hospitalized	Ambulatory
MCH < 27 pg	Transferrin saturation is low	52%	67%
MCH > 27 pg	Transferrin saturation is low	9%	21%
MCH > 30 pg	Transferrin saturation is low	4%	14%

Tips:

1. The incidence of true iron deficiency is highest in the ambulatory patients with the low MCH. There's more anemia of chronic disease (in which the MCH may be low but the transferrin saturation may not be) in a hospitalized, as compared to an ambulatory, patient population.

2. Shade your odds against iron deficiency with a large Italian or Greek patient group. (See Discriminate Function, p. 377, for an extra edge.)

3. Females in their reproductive years are always iron-deficient unless the price is *really* right. (See Monthly Blood Loss, p. 382.)

For B₁₂ and folate deficiency

For long-shot bettors:

Index finding	Past performance	
MCV < 95 cu μ	Low B₁₂ or folate	0.1%
MCV > 95 cu μ	Low B₁₂ or folate	18.0%

For really easy money (a lock):

Index finding	Chances of finding
MCHC > 38	Hereditary spherocytosis or cold agglutinin present

Tips:

1. Don't bet against the patient with the MCV < 95 having a low B₁₂ or folate. Although it's a 1000:1 shot against, you'll owe the patient about $50 for the tests. Even if you lay 100:1 against, you still risk $5000 to break even and you might get busted.

2. The MCHC is a money-maker! You can check it out at low cost with a smear. The MCHC is elevated in hereditary spherocytosis and may be spuriously elevated by the presence of a cold agglutinin. The latter results from a true hemoglobin determination (cells are lysed) and a spuriously high MCV, low red count, and low calculated hematocrit caused by red cell clumping.

Reference: Mostly derived from serious data presented by Griner, P. F., and Oranburg, P. R.: Am. J. Clin. Pathol., *70*:748, 1978.

3,4—IT'S A NATURAL!

You can make your points in Hematology by remembering 3,4. These include:

34	Milligrams of bilirubin produced per gram Hb
3.4	Milligrams of iron per gram Hb
3.42	Nuclear lobes/neutrophil: the upper limit of normal when averaging 100 or more neutrophils
1.34	Cubic centimeters of oxygen carried by each gram of hemoglobin (if you don't mind stretching the rule of 34's a little)

Reference: Sills, R.: Personal communication, 1977.

CIGARETTE SMOKING AND DEATH

Mortality ratios from a variety of diseases are consistently higher for cigarette smokers than for nonsmokers. Overall, the chances of a cigarette smoker dying from the gamut of disorders listed here are increased by 70 per cent (mortality ratio 1.7). Life expectancy is shortened at any age but appears most truncated in *both* men and women between the ages of 45 and 54. Specific mortality ratios depend on the total years of smoking, volume, patterns of inhalation, and age of initiation of smoking. Coronary artery disease, lung cancer, and chronic obstructive lung disease are the chief culprits in the increased mortality.

Overall, the mortality rate for pipe and cigar smokers is higher than that for nonsmokers but less than for cigarette smokers. Reformed cigarette smokers display declining mortality ratios as their years of abstinence increase.

The mortality ratio of active cigarette smokers, by cause of death, for *eight prospective epidemiologic studies* is given in the table on the following page.

16

	A	B Age in years 45–64	B Age in years 65–79	STUDY C	STUDY D	STUDY E	STUDY F	G Sex M	G Sex F	H
All cancers		2.14	1.76	2.21	1.62		1.97			
Lung and bronchus	14.0	7.84	11.59	12.14	3.64	14.2	10.73	7.0	4.5	15.9
Larynx	13.0	6.09	8.99	9.95	13.59		13.10			
Buccal cavity		(9.90)	(2.93)	4.09	7.04	3.9	2.80			1.0
Pharynx				12.54	2.81					
Esophagus	4.7	4.17	1.74	6.17	2.57	3.3	6.60			0.7
Bladder and other	2.1	2.20	2.96	2.15	0.98	1.3	2.40	1.8	1.6	6.0
Pancreas	1.6	2.69	2.17	1.84	1.83	2.1		3.1	2.5	
Kidney		1.42	1.57	1.45	1.11	1.4	1.50			
Stomach		1.42	1.26	1.60	1.51	1.9	2.30	0.9	2.3	0.8
Intestines				1.27	1.27	1.4	0.50			0.9
Rectum	2.7	(1.01)	(1.17)	0.98	0.91	0.6	0.80			1.0
All cardiovascular				1.75			1.57			
Coronary heart disease	1.6	1.90	1.31	1.74	1.96	1.6	1.70	1.7	1.3	2.0
Cerebrovascular lesions	1.3	2.03	1.36	1.52	1.14	0.9	1.30	1.0	1.1	1.8
Aortic aneurysm (non-syphilitic)	6.6	1.38	1.06	5.24		1.8		1.6		
Hypertension		2.62	4.92	1.67		1.6	1.20	1.3	1.4	
General arteriosclerosis	1.4	1.40	1.42	1.86	2.51	3.3	2.00	2.0	2.0	1.0
All respiratory diseases (nonneoplastic)				10.08			2.85			
Emphysema and/or bronchitis	24.7	6.55	11.41	14.17			2.30	1.6	2.2	4.3
Emphysema without bronchitis				4.49		7.7				
Bronchitis				2.12		11.3				
Respiratory tuberculosis	5.0				1.27					
Asthma				3.47						
Influenza and pneumonia	1.4	1.86	1.72	1.87		1.4	2.60			2.4
Certain other conditions										
Stomach ulcer	(2.5)	4.06	4.13	4.13	(2.06)					
Duodenal ulcer		2.86	1.50	2.98		6.9	2.16			0.5
Cirrhosis	3.0	2.06	1.97	3.33	1.35	2.3	1.93	2.4	0.8	4.0
Parkinsonism	0.4			0.26						
All causes	1.64	1.88	1.43	1.84	1.22	1.52	1.70	1.4	1.2	1.78

Reference: Surgeon General's Report on Smoking and Health, 1979; Morbidity and Mortality Weekly Report 28, January 12, 1979.

OTHER ADVERSE EFFECTS OF SMOKING

Smoking is a well-recognized etiologic agent in certain cancers, chronic obstructive lung disease, and cardiovascular disease. Smokers may also have altered response to some drugs, different "normal" values in certain diagnostic tests, and altered absorption and metabolism of important macro- and micronutrients.

The major effect of smoking on drug pharmacology is the ability of various tobacco constituents to enhance drug metabolism by microsomal enzyme system induction. For example, theophylline has a half-life of about four hours in smokers compared to about seven hours in nonsmokers. Smokers will, on the average, need 1½ to two times as much of the drug as nonsmokers to achieve the same therapeutic effects. Similar effects have been reported with tranquilizers, analgesics, and antidepressants. A corollary is that smokers who cease smoking may have decreasing drug requirements. Thus, the potential for drug toxicity on doses that were previously therapeutic while they were smoking increases.

Smokers have been reported to have higher "normal" blood levels of white blood cells, hemoglobin (see Smoker's Polycythemia, p. 409), and carcinoembryonic antigen. Smoking has been reported to reduce the clotting time by potentiating platelet aggregation.

Smokers have alterations in both carbohydrate and protein metabolism. Plasma levels of vitamin C, vitamin B_{12}, vitamin B_6, and several minerals are decreased in smokers unless they are given additional supplementation. These adverse interactions between macro- and micronutrients and tobacco are especially significant in pregnant patients. Babies born to smoking mothers are smaller and have a greater risk of perinatal mortality.

Reference: FDA Drug Bulletin, *9*:4, 1979.

PROPHYLAXIS AGAINST MALPRACTICE

Malpractice litigation is one of the most unpleasant situations that a physician can face in medical practice. The following recommendations to help avoid unjustified suits are a summary of a special session on malpractice held during the 1978 annual meeting of the New York State Medical Society. Remember that good medicine is the best defense against malpractice. Peer review and continuing medical education to maintain the quality of your practice are mandatory.

Patient

1. Establish and maintain a friendly cooperative atmosphere.
2. Answer questions freely and honestly.

16

3. Know your limitations and don't attempt to handle problems beyond your ability.

4. Know the drugs you prescribe in detail. Explain potential interactions and side effects to the patient.

5. Don't needlessly protract treatment, especially if it isn't working.

6. Don't sue for collection of delinquent accounts if a patient has had unsatisfactory medical results.

Medical Records

1. Keep meticulous records and document everything.

2. Never alter a record or a chart at anytime for any reason.

3. Don't countersign a chart if you haven't personally seen the patient.

4. Avoid levity in chart entries.

5. Don't describe another doctor's findings unless you have also confirmed them.

Hospital

1. Make sure your orders are being carried out.

2. Don't undertake a treatment program that the hospital isn't equipped to handle.

3. Order that patients who are sedated heavily or agitated be restrained, kept in bed with side rails up, or assisted when they are allowed out of bed.

4. Make sure you know the results of the tests you order and document them in the chart.

Interaction with Other Health Workers

1. Communicate with the referring physician or the physician to whom you are referring the patient.

2. Don't discuss patients or comment on the quality of another doctor's work in public places (e.g., elevators) or social settings.

Do not be deterred by fear of malpractice litigation. Practice the best medicine you can in a compassionate manner.

"Lawyers are the only persons in whom ignorance of the law is not punished."

Jeremy Bentham

If good intentions are combined with stupidity, it is impossible to outthink them.

INFORMATION FOR SENIOR CITIZENS

In addition to the aid that may usually be obtained from civic or fraternal organizations, unions (for members), and the Veterans Administration (for veterans), a number of national organizations are available for help and information. Included are:

American Association of Retired Persons/National Retired Teachers Association (AARP/NRTA), 1909 K Street NW, Washington, D.C. 20049

National Council of Senior Citizens (NCSC), 1511 K Street NW, Washington, D.C. 20005

National Association of Retired Federal Employees (NARFE), 1533 New Hampshire Avenue NW, Washington, D.C. 20036

Gray Panthers, c/o Tabernacle Church, 38th & Chestnut Streets, Philadelphia, Pa. 19104

Task Force on Older Women of the National Organization for Women (NOW), 3800 Harrison Street, Oakland, Cal. 94611

For ages 50 to 64:

Action for Independent Maturity (AIM), 1909 K Street, NW, Washington, D.C. 20049

There are also organizations of professionals who work with and on behalf of the elderly: National Council on the Aging (NCOA), 1828 L Street NW, Washington, D.C. 20036; The Gerontological Society, One Dupont Circle, Washington, D.C. 20036; American Geriatric Society, 10 Columbus Circle, New York, N.Y. 10019

SERENDIPITY

Serendipity is the faculty of finding agreeable things by accident. The word was originally coined by Horace Walpole, an eighteenth century man of letters on inspiration from the Persian fairy tale *The Three Princes of Serendib,* whose heroes made fortuitous discoveries by chance. Serendib is actually the old Arabic word for Ceylon (now Sri Lanka) and it represents a corruption of the sanskrit compound word for the island dwelling place of lions. Thus, the ancient sailors of the Indian Ocean and the Persian fairies contributed to the lexicon of modern medicine.

STRESS

Medicine is a demanding mistress. Physicians work about 15 hours a week longer than the average professional, spend 3.5 more weeks per year on the job, and have inordinately high rates of suicide, drug addiction, and marital problems. A certain amount of stress comes with the territory; however, some of it is generated by poor mental health habits and can be eliminated. The tips listed below might help you eliminate some of the unnecessary stress in your life.

16

1. There is not enough time for everything. Set life goals and assign priorities to your time based on these goals. That way you won't be frustrated by using your time and energy in activities that do little to further your progress toward these life goals.

2. Schedule your time based on your goals and priorities. Disorganization leads to inefficiency, unfulfilled tasks, acute and chronic guilt, and anxiety.

3. Keep yourself healthy. Exercise regularly, eat a balanced diet, sleep, and avoid all of those things you tell your patients to avoid.

4. Learn to relax. Set aside a little time each day for a relaxation break to give your mind a rest.

5. Do not neglect your family. The combination of an unhappy, unsatisfactory family situation and the stresses and demands of medical practice can be devastating.

6. Learn how to play. Don't be a workaholic.

7. Develop a cadre of friends with whom you can be an ordinary human being.

8. Don't become so concerned over goals and outcome that you lose the pleasure inherent in the process. It is just as important to smell the roses as it is to grow them.

9. Seek professional help before it's too late.

Reference: Woolfolk, R. L., and Richardson, F. C.: Physicians and stress — how to cure yourself. Current Prescribing, March 1979, p. 75.

DON'T EVER SAY. . .

You know! (protect us from the ubiquitous you know!)
Essentially (it is, or it isn't!)
At that time (in case presentations)
In my clinical experience . . . (stand back!)
Workup (you do patient evaluations; let the others do "workups")
Therapeutic *regime* (regimen is bad enough)
O.K.

Experience is the name everyone gives to his mistakes.

FREEBIES

There are many valuable educational materials you can get free of charge. These are some of our favorites, given in no particular order. Thanks to these and other institutions for making these resources available.

Physicians' Desk Reference

You really would find it difficult to practice medicine without this book. The PDR provides you with a comprehensive list of all commercially available drugs — approximately 2500 currently. Drug descriptions, indications, action, adverse side effects, dosage, and dosage forms are provided. You may receive a complimentary copy of this book, which is revised yearly, by writing to:

PDR
Physicians' Desk Reference
Box 58
Oradell, N.J. 07649

Morbidity and Mortality Weekly Report (MMWR)

This weekly bulletin produced by the Center for Disease Control provides you with up-to-date information on current infectious problems in the United States and the rest of the world. In addition, other news of epidemiologic interest appears in this eight-page booklet. You can get on the mailing list by writing to:

U.S. Dept. of Health, Education and Welfare
Public Health Service, Center for Disease Control
Atlanta, Ga. 30333

Mayo Clinic Proceedings

This informative journal is published monthly by the Mayo Foundation as part of its program of medical education and is sent regularly without charge, upon request, to any physician or person who has a doctorate in a field allied to medicine. It is also available to medical students in the United States who are in their last two years of school. Students asking to receive the Proceedings should state their year of graduation. Requests for Proceedings should be sent to:

Mayo Clinic Proceedings
Room 1042, Plummer Building
Mayo Clinic
Rochester, Minn. 55901

When requesting the journal, be sure to enclose your full name and complete address and indicate specialty or type of practice.

16

Hospital Practice

This informative monthly journal contains current medical news and lucidly written review articles, accompanied by superb illustrations and tables. You will never want to throw yours away. You can get on the mailing list by writing to:

Hospital Practice
Hospital Practice Publishing Co., Inc.
575 Lexington Ave.
New York, N.Y. 10022

Ca — A Cancer Journal for Clinicians

This journal is published bimonthly by the Professional Education Committee of the American Cancer Society with Arthur I. Holleb, M.D., as editor-in-chief. Excellent articles oriented toward the practicing clinician are included. It is invaluable as a source of cancer statistics. Appropriate stress is placed on epidemiology, carcinogenesis, and cancer prevention. You can get it by writing to:

Ca — A Cancer Journal for Clinicians
777 Third Ave.
New York, N.Y. 10017

Resident and Staff Physician

The editor-in-chief is Alfred Bollet, M.D. The photoquizzes have graced many a bulletin board and examination page. The articles are often just what you're looking for. Of late, the content has become increasingly analytic and involves some of the more controversial and practical matters in medicine. House officers, "full-time" physicians, and physicians at medical schools can get it by writing to:

Resident and Staff Physician
80 Shore Road
Port Washington, N.Y. 11050

Medical Aspects of Human Sexuality

A real change of pace. Everything you were afraid to ask but really should know. Courtesy subscriptions are available for house staff in teaching hospitals and physicians in the various primary care disciplines by contacting:

Hospital Publications, Inc.
360 Lexington Ave.
New York, N.Y. 10017

Ciba Clinical Symposium

Superb illustrations and increasingly good to excellent text. Not always directed at the internist, but a "must" when it is. You can get on the mailing list by writing to:

Medical Education Division
CIBA Pharmaceutical Company
Summit, N.J. 07901

What's New in Cancer Care

A critical up-to-date summary of the state of the art in subjects in cancer care. The newsletter is prepared by the West Coast Cancer Foundation for the practicing physician, with Stephen K. Carter, M.D., as editor. References are extensive. To get on the mailing list, write to:

West Coast Cancer Foundation
What's New in Cancer Care
50 Francisco Street, Suite 200
San Francisco, Calif. 94133

Clinical Diagnosis Quiz in Oncology

Published eight times annually. Each issue is a quiz with complete and illuminating answers provided. Evaluation, decision-making, and therapy in both solid tumor and hematologic oncology are covered. Included are issues devoted to specific diseases, pharmacology, supportive care, and medical aspects of oncology. Always current, it is excellent for classroom use. Key references are provided. Robert Comis, M.D., is the editor. It is *de rigueur* for board review in hematology and oncology. You can get it by writing to:

Creative Medical Publications, Inc.
Cancer Treatment Edition
1 Adler Drive
East Syracuse, N.Y. 13057

Roche Handbook of Differential Diagnosis

Presents the differential diagnosis based on key signs or symptoms. The concise style permits a "quick study." Write to:

Roche Laboratories
Nutley, N.J. 07110

"May there never develop in me the notion that my education is complete, but give me the strength and leisure and zeal continually to enlarge my knowledge."

16

Maimonides

NAME INDEX

SUBJECT INDEX